Aloe Vera
The New Millennium

Aloe Vera
The New Millennium

The Future of Wellness
in the 21st Century

*by Bill C. Coats, R.Ph.,
C.C.N. with Robert Ahola*

iUniverse, Inc.

New York Lincoln Shanghai

Aloe Vera The New Millennium
The Future of Wellness in the 21st Century

iUniverse, Inc.

For information address:
iUniverse, Inc.
2021 Pine Lake Road, Suite 100
Lincoln, NE 68512
www.iuniverse.com

ISBN: 0-595-27945-7

Printed in the United States of America

Dedicated to the memory of Dr. Robert H. Davis—a pioneer of science, a compassionate health professional, and a fallen comrade.

Acknowledgments

With everlasting gratitude to all the pioneering health professionals who have put all biases aside and embraced the potentials of this plant and let your voices be heard in very important ways. Although you now number in legion, our individual appreciation for all you have done goes beyond personal measure. Thank you so much.

Authors' Note

The contents of this book are not intended in any way to reflect the approval of any state, local, or federal regulatory body. However, what is written here is documented and referenced. It represents the accumulated findings of medical professionals and summaries of tests in legion by scientific research groups, cosmetologists, independent laboratories, and through interviews with individuals who have experienced remarkable healings with Aloe Vera or products extracted from it.

Contents

1). **The New Face of World Health.** It has been predicted by Paul Zane Pilzer and other prophets of the new millennium that wellness will be the next $1 trillion industry. More than a prediction, it is a movement that is already well under way. This introductory chapter will cover three main topics: a) the current crisis in health care, medicine and "the sickness industry;" b) the new public awareness of the wellness industry in all its forms; c) the emergence of natural alternatives with an emphasis on Aloe Vera and its expanded role in that field.

....1

2). **Aloe Vera. Q & A..** This chapter makes it easy and fun to learn about this amazing plant. Featured in this chapter are *20 Questions: What Most People Ask About Aloe.* Easy answers to Aloe's secrets written in a way that anyone can understand.

....14

3). **Aloe Super Stars.** It is widely known but little discussed that stabilized Aloe Vera products have long been held in high regard in the world of professional, Olympic, and collegiate athletics. In fact, our own Aloe Vera formulations have been used to treat athletes in the NFL, NHL, the National and American Leagues of professional baseball, the Olympics, and a number of NCAA colleges and universities. At last, we offer Aloe Vera's brief but colorful journey through the world of competition athletics, and the impact it has made with thousands of athletes and dozens of sports organizations in the last three decades.

....35

4). **Major Milestones.** "The Magnificent 7" events in the history of the healing plant. From toxicology to autoimmune diseases, this chapter will mark the turning points in the research, development laboratory breakthroughs in the progress of Aloe Vera and their impact on the rest of the industry. In it, you will find some groundbreaking discoveries and some remarkable projections for the new hybrid "super-aloe" and its uses.

....55

5). Autoimmune Diseases Meet the "Aloe Vera Orchestra." In this chapter we offer some seemingly radical notions on why only Aloe Vera seems to work on some of the most challenging diseases known to modern science. In it, you will be introduced to what is known as "The Conductor-Orchestra" explanation for Aloe Vera's remarkable ability to synergize the healing process, and "The Thermos Theory," our own somewhat simplified version of what makes it perhaps the most inscrutable healant known to science. We'll also look at its success with what many believe to be the most difficult of all syndromes to treat—autoimmune diseases. From diabetes mellitus to lupus erythematosus, we will cite some dramatic case histories and how Aloe Vera has treated them with notable success.

....99

6). Memories and Miracles. Replete with anecdotes, this chapter might be a sidebar to the clinician but a Godsend to the average reader. That's because it brings us, at last, in touch with the human element where the poetry of healing truly begins. Touching upon everything from lung tumors to parrots with frostbite, it will bring Aloe Vera into a context of usage that everyone can understand—often as a last best hope for the individual's struggle to regain command of his health his life and his future.

....126

7). AIDS, Cancer and the Aloe Answer. This chapter gets to the heart of some of the most profound and controversial advances in Aloe Vera research and therapy in the last 10 years. Some of them bring new hope. Others revisit old debates. All are essential to understanding the expanded role the healing plant now faces in the changing arena of world health. Whatever you find on these pages will stir you to question and to rethink some long held positions about dread diseases and just how we go about treating them. At best it is in itself a Handbook for Hope. At its worst it is food for much consideration, research and examination. In either case, the reader will emerge from this chapter better informed and more willing to consider intelligent alternative therapies for these two pandemics.

....152

8). More than Skin Deep. This chapter will engage us in the myths and realities of Aloe Vera's role in the personal care industry. By the same token, it has continued to make such dramatic contributions in areas such as plastic surgery, esthetics and cosmetology that it has come to be viewed as indispensable by many authorities in skin care technology. But understanding both the impact and exploitation of Aloe is a matter of education. So we dedicate the following pages to establish-

ing a set of guidelines for use of Aloe Vera in personal care, and to set the record straight about what works and what doesn't.
....185

9). Animal Planet. Sometimes it is difficult for us to grasp that part of our role in the stewardship of this planet entails the care, feeding and healing of our creature companions. In this chapter we give you a look at many of the new innovations that are being employed to treat our creature companions with greater compassion, insight and understanding. From special Aloe Vera treatments for dogs and cats, we also take a good long look at some treatments for horses, cattle and some of our barnyard friends.
....225

10). Aloe's Perfect World. What the future of wellness has to offer, and what Aloe is already doing to change it for the better. Here we examine the best of all possible worlds and why Aloe, in all its variations, will play an important role in it.
....273

Notes 279

References 281

Index 295

Introduction

The Age of Aloe

This book is being written with one premise in mind: New works on break-through subjects should not tread long on old ground.

In the last ten years, Aloe Vera as a health industry phenomenon has become well known for all the right reasons and some very wrong ones. Among research scientists and health professionals it has finally come into high regard for its remarkable powers and its broad spectrum of uses. Research studies in legion show this.

To the public at large, it is still something of a pop ingredient in scores of mass-market cosmetics, shampoos, shaving creams, lotions and drinks. At this point, it has been "vernacularized" into a kind of awareness pudding. It has now become a part of the idiom of homilies that no longer make an impact on the public's decision to buy.

People have some vague understanding that it is somewhat effective as a topi-cal agent—good for the skin, hair, and possibly as a superficial topical healant (for sunburn and skin rashes). As such, it is merely a name on the marquee. Awareness of it is often jaded if not dismissive—in a category with Vitamin E, eucalyptus, Vitamin C and menthol.

Understandably, such superficial references tend to trivialize this remarkable plant in a way that undermines its pharmaceutical clout. This has much to do with the expediency of mass-marketing product development, and the tendency of major product companies to push the "next big thing."

But truth is as relentless as it is inevitable. And the complex challenges of world health in this new millennium demand that even more serious attention be paid to a healant that, by now, has proved its worth time and again.

Since we have volumes of data to support our case on behalf of the healing plant, this will not be the hard part. The challenge rests with being able to simplify it in ways that everyone can understand.

In our previous books about Aloe, the thrust of our communication has been toward the health professional, the wellness specialist, clinicians, research scientists and skeptics. And though, in our earlier works, my associates and I have always been mindful of keeping our messages as simple and direct as possible, the language of biotechnology inevitably creeps into the conversation and takes us down paths where the language of science often overrides the need for simplicity.

We write this book with a more generous intent. Although, for the sake of credibility, the voice of the scientist and health professional will be expressed on these pages, we wanted to create a body of work that the average interested lay person could read, relate to, enjoy and put to use. We do that for a number of practical reasons.

First, the new millennium, the roaring 2000s, will present challenges and even threats to world health that we could have only imagined a couple of decades ago.

Second, those of us who are willing to look upon the future for the opportunity it is will realize that we stand upon the threshold of total wellness, extended longevity and quality of life that has never been available to the generations that have gone before us.

Third, we are facing what might be defined as a revolution in health awareness, one that has never been available to anyone before now. So much life altering information is being offered to us, much of it on a daily basis, that we would be doing ourselves and our loved ones a disservice were we not to pay heed to it and act accordingly.

This book is dedicated not only to enabling the health conscious reader to have a better understanding of Aloe Vera and its integral role in the health revolution that is now taking place, it is also being written with the hope and the prayer that will reach our readers with a whole new awareness—that will open their eyes to the glorious panorama for the future of wellness that is now being constructed around them.

Chapter 1

The New Face of World Health

Currently, the potentials for a revolution in world health consciousness have achieved critical mass. What lies ahead will be a set of dynamic opposites on a global scale. In many ways, especially due to our callous indifference to the environment and the pandemics of disease that arise from it, the decades ahead will be ones of crisis and peril. For the health-conscious individual who applies a cultivated awareness, time future will offer the best of all possible worlds. And Aloe Vera, as it has always done, will have a very positive role to play in it.

Global health issues in the 21st century read very much like the first lines of Charles Dickens' *A Tale of Two Cities.* Indeed, when it comes to our personal balance horizons, we live both in "the best of times" and "the worst of times."

We sit on the threshold of new discoveries that are certain to transform the concept of wellness as we have come to know it. Such biotech buzzwords as *genomics, stem-cell research, microbotics, organotherapy* and *cloning,* though they involve aspects of our quest for wellness that are largely experimental, are slowly but inevitably coming into common usage. And if they're not already embraced as familiar terms by the public at large, they are at least a part of the awareness of every health-conscious individual in what is recognized as the modern civilized world. Without exception, these are subjects that will be the focus of biotechnology in the decades to come. In truth, they promise liberation if not a complete revolution in the search for perfect health and longevity as we know them.

At the same time, the inhabitants of our planet—both humankind and its creature companions—have been assailed by microbial mutations that are so powerful and so pervasive as to have branded this as the "Age of the Supervirus." A bit oversimplified, no doubt. But is it overstated? Some medical experts think not.

1

From relentless outbreaks of the *Ebola* virus on the continent of Africa to pernicious strains of flesh-eating *Staph Aureus* even in the U.S. and Canada, we have seen modern science fall helpless time and again against what seems to be an advance guard of microbes now laying waste entire populations in the Third World and even threatening our own. *HIV* (Human Immunodeficiency Virus) has claimed nearly 38,000,000 victims in the world today. Nearly 17 million of those are women. In such nations as Uganda, Tanzania, Nigeria, Thailand, Indonesia and Brazil, *AIDS* has reached epidemic proportions. And, as of this writing, Spain now has the highest per capita incidence of HIV of any nation.

Even in the "developed world," new strains of old pandemics such as *tuberculosis* and *smallpox* have re-emerged as both persistent and resistant to all modern forms of treatment.

Aberrations in our food chain, many of them caused by the expedient economics of factory farming, have brought us to experience animal pandemics of such diseases as hoof and mouth, "mad cow" disease, and massive outbreaks of *salmonella* and *E-coli* from tainted beef, pork, and poultry.

So commonplace have these occurrences become that—even when the outbreaks are severe—they no longer attract appropriate media attention beyond the predictable sensations of the moment. That's because they're no longer news items that draw much attention. Instead, they're merely viewed as the collateral damage that comes with living on a busy planet. Meanwhile, the underlying causes—the expedient morality of factory farming and the inclinations among health ministries in various countries to trot out "the usual suspects"—continues to be addressed on an *ad hoc* basis, with no proportionate concern for the long term implications.

Beneath the surface, we seem to have hit critical mass in the disparity of health measures that face our 21st century world. And the new global class struggle may not be one of politics, race or religion at all. It might well become an issue of who can and cannot afford to be healthy. This is not a struggle that is adversarial. Often, it is not even conscious. Still it exists.

With the advent of new discoveries in diet, exercise and nutritional supplementation, extended longevity for the health-conscious American citizen is virtually assured. As of the year, 2000, the average American male was told he could enjoy a life expectancy of 77 years, the average female, one of 80. What's more, with the introduction of nutrients such as Human Growth Hormones (HGHs), essential fatty acids, and live enzyme preventive therapy, we may be beginning to see the end of old age as we have come to know it. Many projections for the next generation of geriatrics (the Baby Boomers) promise what can only be described as the longevity of thriving—people flourishing in good health even into their centenarian years.

Like so many new breakthroughs, that horizon of redemption is immediately open only to those who are willing to embrace the power of human initiative. That points directly to those who are either financially well-to-do or intent enough upon their health to pursue a path of alternative therapy and education.

"Education" is a key word here, because it is only through the tireless pursuit of health awareness that the average American can break out of the box in what are arguably the most important areas of their lives—their wellness, their fitness, their personal longevity, and their quality of life.

"The Box" in this case is a euphemism for conventional medicine, and it is already clear that a majority of adults in the United States have become aware of its limitations. So have many health professionals, including allopaths (M.D.s) and traditional scientists. And in keeping with our fascination for the paradox of world health, we point to some of declarations of opposition:

• Currently, the American public spends close to $1.4 trillion on health care, medicine, and the "technology of sickness." It is a cost that some market indicators say will rise to nearly $3 trillion in the next ten years.

• It has been predicted, if current trends continue, that by the year 2010, the average American worker will be spending nearly 50% of his or her annual income on health care, medicine, and health insurance.

• Much of that care will be inadequate, toxic, or too expensive to offer any consistent solutions for the people who need them most.

• As of the year 2005, Medicare may be the next casualty of a health care system run amok. A recent article by David Gergen in *U.S. News & World Report* indicated that patients with Medicare benefits are being either shunned or flatly rejected by an increasing number of doctors, hospitals and medical clinics. That's because the costs of Medicare "benefits" have risen, although payments to HMOs and health professionals have not. In fact, the average office visit to a doctor costs that physician in excess of $100, while Medicare's maximum allowable is only $60. So, many doctors are losing about $40 per visit from this nation's seniors. Small wonder that many clinics and HMOs are no longer accepting any patients who fall in the 60 plus age-range category. They simply can't afford the Medicare baggage they'll be bringing with them.

• Many practicing physicians are aware of this and other challenges of repression that are innate to the current health care system. In truth, a number of physicians (nearly 15% by some estimates) are either seeking early retirement from their careers or simply moving into another line of work. The principal reason? Due to restrictions incurred by HMOs and Medicare, many physicians feel that they're not being allowed to apply their skills in the Hippocratic tradition—with the best interests of the patients as the ultimate consideration. Instead, they're often forced to modify their diagnoses and treatments to preclude the possibility malpractice claims. Or else, they're hobbled by insurance restrictions against providing their patients with the best possible treatment for their conditions. So, in today's climate of critical mass, many physicians now feel that the economics of health care are actually keeping them from doing their jobs.

• To add further fission to the impending Medicare meltdown, prescription drugs for the aged have been severely cut down and may not even pass congressional accord. So it is anticipated that the average senior citizen will probably have to foot the bill for at least half of the cost of their prescriptions every year.

• Unfortunately, at this point it comes as a surprise to no one that, even if those in need get their prescriptions filled, we're all more than likely paying too much for them—by billions of dollars. Recent studies reported in publications such as *The Washington Post* indicate that "dumb prescriptions" are being written for the latest vogue pharmaceutical products for such conditions as pain, inflammation, and other controllable syndromes that run into exorbitant and unnecessary costs. These designer drugs being hyped by drug detail men who ply physicians with an estimated $11 billion per year in perks to push them. Doctors, human and susceptible, fall under the spell and prescribe them when comparable generic brands or even OTC brands would do for a fraction of the cost. The price to the paying public climbs into the tens of billions of dollars. And that is pain of a different kind.

• According to recent studies by the FDA, people have become increasingly reluctant to use prescription drugs at all. Often due to some rather ambiguous marketing practices by some pharmaceutical companies that downplay the relative toxicity of many drugs, nearly 30% of all patients have reported side effects from their continued use that have ranged from unpleasant to violently traumatic. And "side-effect" deaths from prescription drugs or improper administration of drugs are dramatically on the rise.

• Physicians and health professionals are also starting to catch onto the dangerous game of "side-effects ping pong'" and the heavy toll it takes on patients. No doubt it's one of the many reasons that, since the year 2000, 21% (over 1/5th) of all M.D.s admit to having resorted to what might be referred to as alternative or "wellness" therapies to treat their patients.

• In that regard, their own patients are well ahead of them. According to a study reported in *U.S.A. Today* in 1998, 58% of all American's had resorted to some form alternative therapy to treat their health challenges. As of this writing, that number has increased considerably.

• Not surprisingly, the United States of America is the healthiest, best fed nation in the world—and the fattest. As recently as the 2001, over 61% of all Americans were said to be overweight, 27% of those clinically obese.

• Obesity and excessive weight gain are now acknowledged as primary causes of such conditions as diabetes, chronic fatigue syndrome, heart disease and various kinds of systemic cancer.

• Once again, mass market food consumption, like drug consumption, is often the final effect of megabuck media expenditure by food-tobacco and beverage companies. And the average, uninformed American is inundated with advertising that convinces them that somehow high fat, high sodium, excessive sugar junk food diets are what they need to truly find true pleasure in what they eat. This is an easy sell, because it is an instinct innate to the survival matrix of the creature *homo sapiens* that we are attracted to high fat foods that will stay with us over the long and difficult seasons of winter. Since prolonged exposure to the elements has not been a major consideration in the civilized world for centuries, our bodies carry with them a technology of desire that is both outdated and dangerous.

One element of our health-conscious society is aware of this. The other is not. (The other is often grossly misled by mass-market food companies into buying junk disguised as nutrition. Victimized by expedient and misleading advertising, they are directed toward "low fat," and dietetic foods that are so high in sugar, salt, and partially hydrogenated oils that they are virtually poisoning themselves while pursuing the illusion of healthy living.) So the silent class struggle continues. But it continues with great sympathy for the uninformed, and with the understanding that many processed foods, just as cigarettes and alcohol, should carry their own warning labels.

• After reviewing previous statistics about health and overweight, we have to conclude that about 39% of the U.S. population might be classified as being at high levels of health awareness. This group has been redefined by economist Paul Zane Pilzer and others as a *healthocracy.*

• A New American "healthocracy" is forming the vanguard of what might well be defined as a new class structure in modern society—those who are on the wellness path and those who are not; in other words, the "haves and have-nots" of wellness awareness. Very often, this vanguard comes from leaders in film, television, entertainment, professional sports, politics and even the higher echelons of business management. This health-first model quickly spreads to anyone who is image conscious and strongly reliant upon appearance and personal energy as aspects of their career success potential.

• This healthocracy is not an exclusive club. It is open to anyone willing to make the choice and take the initiative to join it. There are no restrictions and no requirements per se, except those of personal discipline, a desire to learn about one's true health potentials. With them, invariably comes a willingness to spend a little extra on preventive "wellness" maintenance, rather than reactive "sickness" treatments and therapy. That is a part of the package, and unfortunately one many people are not willing to open.

• Part of the problem lies in the fact that, prior to the year 2000, most health insurance carriers were not willing to pay for "preventive therapy" of any kind. So people were not only not encouraged to pursue the path of prevention, they were financially discouraged from doing so.

• The average American worker with a family of four pays over $5000 a year for health insurance coverage. And, until recently, virtually none of it has gone for preventive health care. Now, however, many health carriers are covering premium allowances for regular annual physicals. They're also viewing their obese policy-holders as far greater health risks and charging them appropriately higher premiums.

• The new American healthocracy began to bring its influence to bear in the late 1990s when some leading health professionals, along with film celebrities, sports figures and key legislators helped spearhead the Hatch/Harkin "Freedom of Health Information Act" of 1996. This act, passed over opposition from the FDA and many pharmaceutical companies, is multi-faceted. But its most pressing line-item rests with its allowance of public access to natural food-based supplementation and GRAS qualified products, as well as published information about them. (GRAS products are "foods" that are *Generally Regarded As Safe* by the USDA and therefore fit for human consumption without excessive FDA restriction or government oversight. It is only when those foods are reformulated or concentrated and set forth in pharmaceutical formulations that the rules change.)

• Even though passed, this act and its appropriate line items have been a bone of contention with the pharmaceutical companies, and is being fought by them on a regular basis. The Freedom of Health Information Act, although under constant attack, is now a reliable constant of American life. Millions of people in the U.S. are the beneficiaries of it. And healthy foods and food-based supplementation are both, for the time being at least, safe.

• The wellness potentials that accompany or intake of vitamins, minerals, enzymes, hormones, and food-based herbal formulas are not enjoying the same sunny reception in other parts of the world. In fact, the individual's right to use them is in grave danger in what presents itself as a bastion of economic progress—The European Economic Union.

• In the nation of Germany, new health ministry initiatives introduced as legislation before the Bundestag intends to restrict all nutrient supplementation in any form to MDRs (minimum daily requirements) that were set as universal standards prior to World War II. According to the new bill set forth, any supplementation, food, herb, or plant formulation that exceeds those minimums will be proscribed by government health ministry to face one of two choices: Either lower your nutrient content to accepted minimums or be sold by prescription. What's more, any health and nutrition companies failing to comply with these strict guidelines may be banned from doing business in Germany.

Because of its strong ties to other EEU nations, Germany's legislative initiative has gained momentum in of France and Belgium as well. And thus far only the United Kingdom has risen up to reject any initiatives that even suggest government control over an individual's freedom of choice in such deeply personal areas as health and wellness.

Still, the specter looms, and we must all remain vigilant, because the future of our wellness depends upon it. By the way, the "we" in this case belongs to members of the self-chosen, deeply driven healthocracy who are now reading this book.

The "Perfect World" of Future Health.

One of the dangers of writing about future potentials of health, science and technology is law of geometric progressions. So our predictions are virtually outdated before they even reach paper. Still, it is our present understanding that gives wings to the future, and helps to form the pallet of our present hopes and dreams. And what we perceive in the present paints a positive canvas indeed.

All research in science and health points to a number of discoveries that may well revolutionize the treatment of the diseases of the future for all time.

• In the still experimental field of *microbotics*, chip implants called *nanocytes* or *nanobots*, invisible to the human eye, may be inserted into the human system to help heal pain, allergies and chronic syndromes. They can also be formulated to stop the onslaught of dread diseases and perhaps even heal deadly pandemics. Furthermore, these nanocytes, properly encoded, might well provide the perfect vessels for perennial immune system stimulation and provide the "magic bullet" that will slow the aging process to a crawl.

• Initial findings in *stem cell research*—reproductive tissue from the human embryo—have led us to believe that there now exists a new therapeutic paradigm that will change the way we treat disease forever. This new kind of genomic science will eventually enable patients to grow new tissue to fight diseases such as cancer and heart disease and may even be able to regenerate entire human organs such as the liver, kidney, and lung. These foster the further development not only of genomics but also of cloning itself. And when you consider the implications of being able to replace entire glands and organs with ones cloned from the same tissue, the positive aspects of cloning far outweigh the eerie perceptions of replicating complete human beings. Nevertheless, stem cell research follows microbotics closely in terms of both its proponents and its potential for controversy.

In both cases, the moral and political implications of such revolutionary therapies are certain to slow their successful development for years if not decades. Meanwhile, we must live in the present, and deal with the challenges that come to us now in this year, in this decade. Given the progress that has been made in the past ten years in the areas of natural, non-invasive therapies and healthy "wellness" alternatives, we have whole new standards of treatment to examine, embrace and rejoice in.

There's no doubt that the "sickness" industry that has dominated our health consciousness especially for the last 100 years. Now, the technology of "wellness" has come of age, and its implications are so far reaching that many world economists believe it will become its own $1 trillion industry. By a consensus of predictions, it will do so within the next decade.

• Beyond traditional focus on vitamins, minerals, massage, subtle body healing and ancient Chinese and Indian (ayurvedic) methods of treatment, the practitioners of the "new wellness awareness" have compiled entirely new spectrums of treatment choices—some of them timeless, others very high tech. Today various magnetic therapies, including complete magnetic sleep systems, are being used to treat everything from athletic injuries to chronic fatigue syndrome.

• *Hormone replacement therapy* (HRT) has now found its way to many physicians' panoply of recommendation for women going through menopause and as a possible preventive against breast cancer, heart disease and even Alzheimer's syndrome. For these women compounds that include such hormones as estrogen and progestin have been found to markedly improve the systemic ping-pong and frequent pathologies that accompany this critical change of life.

•*Organotherapy*, using desiccated liver, kidney, spleen, heart and stomach glands from free-range cattle, has found support among some health professionals for treating many forms of male complications. According to several case studies, men (and women) suffering from various conditions ranging from severe prostatitis to degenerative kidney diseases have been helped dramatically by regular daily doses of these bovine organ capsules, including kidney, liver, stomach, heart and spleen.

Of course, many of these treatments carry moral, philosophical, and medical complications of their own. (Even as of this writing, HRT is undergoing a critical reevaluation of its benefits in light of its potential side-effects.) And it is ideal but not often possible to find a modality of healing that does not defy someone's parameters of safe usage. Now, however, there are possible ways to determine both the need for and the impact of using alternative therapies.

• *Electrodermal screening* (or EDS) is a combination of electronic scanning technology with ancient techniques to create a diagnostic tool that, some medical practitioners claim, has a 98% accuracy rate. Originally designed in Germany over 50 years ago, EDS has been refined over the decades into a sophisticated measuring device that can identify pathogens, toxins and organ dysfunctions before the physical symptoms ever present themselves. And where it is able to pre-diagnose inevitable systemic diseases, it can also gauge the impact of such healing modalities that have, up to now, been highly difficult to measure. Through EDS, it is now possible to define the pre and post usage impact of such treatments as acupressure massage, acupuncture, magnetic therapy, natural herbal remedies, and even certain homeopathic treatments. It has also proven highly accurate in measuring the impact of supplements and herbal remedies whose bioavailability had been previously subject to question. In fact, EDS has proved so effective that it is now being used on a regular basis by more than 100,000 M.D.s worldwide. To date, the only nation slow to accept it as a preferred diagnostic tool has been the United States, and EDS has now begun to breach the gulf of skepticism here as well.

All these findings point more strongly than ever to two areas that continue to gain both emphasis and respectability: natural herbal remedies, and healants that are also "foods" high in bioavailability. And when it comes to a GRAS qualified food that is highest in both bioavailability and absorption into the human system, no healant continues to provide more breakthroughs than the "silent healer," Aloe Vera.

Thus far in this chapter, we have made mention of a number of new healing modalities that may change our approach to wellness forever. We applaud them. We welcome them. We also hasten to observe that most of them have a couple of things in common: They are either scheduled for common usage far into the future and, for that reason, face the labyrinth of official approvals, debate, and delay; or they already come with their own set of baggage in the form of concerns about side-effects or the incompleteness of what they offer. All of these modalities have another common denominator: They may either be helped or supplanted by the broad-spectrum potentials of Aloe Vera itself.

Aloe Vera. The Once and Future King.

Thus far in the brief life of this new millennium, Aloe Vera the Silent Healer has finally come to universal prominence as a viable powerful broad-spectrum alternative "therapy of choice." After decades of research, reporting and volumes of tests it has come to be embraced by the scientific community with consistent, if cautious, praise for its proven effectiveness.

What's more, even the community of allopaths, the M.D.s previously skeptical of Aloe folklore and word-of-mouth, have come to recognize the healing plant's benefits as being more than just a superficial "marquee" ingredient used in hundreds of commercial products. They come not from anecdotes and hearsay but from scientific reports. They can be measured from control group and double-blind studies that have increased exponentially in the last ten years. And it is in the strength of those numbers and the force of those studies that Aloe Vera has risen to new levels of respectability.

We're happy to say that we have either sponsored or been willing participants in a number of them.

In fact, breakthroughs in Aloe Vera research and development have taken such dimensions in just the last ten years, that we feel they merit a study of their own—this one. In areas such as dread disease, veterinary medicine, athletics, men's issues, women's issues, autoimmune diseases, and care for a world's creatures, Aloe Vera in its many presentations has proven yet again that this is a healant that is finally coming to some long overdue renown and as such into the fullness of its true potential.

The following instances offer some stunning examples:

• *HIV and AIDS.* Thus far, no approved treatment has been able to be called "a cure" for HIV. However, there are now several treatments that have shown remarkable results in reversing the effects of HIV and AIDS, so that people stricken with these deadly syndromes may lead normal lives.

In four different studies over the last ten years, Aloe Vera formulations have proven effective against HIV. One of them, begun by Terry Pulse, M.D. as early as 1990 revealed how Aloe Vera, when used in conjunction with a complete complex of omega-chain fatty acids and a potent protein powder supplement, was able to reverse the affects of HIV in two dozen patients to HIV +1 and HIV −1 within a matter of 90 days.

Another profound breakthrough against HIV and the AIDS virus involves the work of Dr. Robert McAnalley and Dr. H.R. McDaniel on the Aloe isolate molecule, Acemannan, and its profound impact on defending against the HIV pathogen. As early as 1986, Dr. McAnalley and Dr. McDaniel had been able to identify and sector off a mannose derivative of Aloe Vera called Acemannan and successfully test it against a number of viral pathogens. When these two doctors tested, the Acemannan molecule against such viral strains herpes simplex, measles, and FLV (Feline Leukemia Virus), the Acemannan—as part of the complete Aloe complex, and as an isolate—was able to reverse the effects of these diseases. It was also able to severely retard the progress of another virus as well—HIV. This triggered a series of tests under in which Doctors McAnalley McDaniel (as well as a separate series with Dr. Terry Pulse) found the Acemannan molecule to be highly effective in reversing the effects of HIV and fully developed AIDS. What's more, these effects were measurable within 90 days of initial treatments.

A third in vitro study at Texas A&M in 1997 revealed that a special concentrate of freeze-dried Aloe Vera was able to retard the AIDS virus upon contact within one's exposure—virtually nullifying its effect on HIV infected tissue samples offered it. Of course, cellular tissue does not constitute the body at large. So this leaves open to question the performance of this new Aloe concentrate freeze-dried compound when tested in the context of a living volunteer control group study.

Since the completion of all these studies, great strides have been made in reversing the effects of HIV. And yet Aloe's forum for acceptance in this area remains small. In order to expand the awareness of Aloe's impact in a number of areas, we intend to cover Aloe Vera's landmark laboratory findings in our Chapter 4—Major Milestones.

• *Autoimmune diseases.* No question. HIV is the summary autoimmune disease. And yet there are so many others with far reaching implications. Autoimmune diseases—although they too often manifest externally with trauma to the skin surface and other blood-bearing tissue—invariably have systemic origins, generally within either the endocrine glands or the central nervous system.

The human immune system functions in a very simple yet profound way through a process called *phagocytosis.* Essentially, whenever foreign particles, or antigens, invade the human system, they are engulfed by two kinds of white antibody blood cells called *macrophages* and *neutrophils.* Engaging these foreign bodies in what amounts to a set of cellular handcuffs, they embrace and assimilate a potentially harmful bacteria or virus into a "good citizen." But sometimes the bad virus or bacteria overcomes the macrophage and neutrophil policemen, and then the immune system starts to short circuit in some expressive ways.

In an article written in 1999 on the effects of "Aloe Vera and the Human Immune System," Dr. Lawrence Plaskett noted a chain of positive results using Aloe Vera and a concentrated derivative in various types of *immunotherapy.* When applied against a number of conditions, including Bronchial Asthma, tumor growth and Candidiasis (a rampant growth of *Candida albicans* in the mucous membranes of the human system, with particular implications in the intestine), the Aloe tested showed uniform abilities to dramatically slow tumor growth, and to completely retard the effects of the candida fungus as well as the bronchial asthma.

In his review of many tests that had been run previously and as a result of some tests of his own, Dr. Plaskett was able to conclude that the Aloe Vera, as well as its Acemannan derivative, did indeed measurably improve the body's immune functions against a broad range of autoimmune diseases. And he reconfirmed something else as well: Aloe Vera seems to have a secret sense of the immune system's regulatory needs.

In some autoimmune conditions such as Crohn's disease and type 1 diabetes, the body's white cells—the macrophages and neutrophils—underperform and are in need of stimulation. In others such as lupus erythemasosus and psoriasis, the same players overplay their parts during the process of phagocytosis. As a result, they overproduce themselves so that the system and its skin over express the desire to heal themselves.

In both instances, Dr. Plaskett suggested that the Aloe Vera seemed to be the perfect systemic "normalizer," in that it would be able to sense the immune system's needs and adapt accordingly.

Although Dr. Plaskett emphasized that he had not tested the Aloe against all of the above-mentioned syndromes, he expressed the conviction that it would work well. In these cases, his conviction is supported in a number of case histories for each of these conditions, many of them from our own archive dramatic cases, as well as a number of laboratory findings.

• *Staphylococcus aureus.* Although it has more benign presentations, *Staph aureus* has also come to be known as "the flesh-eating" bacteria. Primarily a disease that attacks the skin, it invariably chews its way through all epidermal layers down into the dermis, and doesn't seem willing to stop there. And the mere hint of its presence in a given area of the world strikes chords of terror among health practitioners.

As a disease it is the medical equivalent of Godzilla. It is deadly. It's rapacious. It's highly contagious. (So anyone exposed to it at any level is required to use extreme caution!) It is so carnivorous in its expression, one can almost visibly track its progress with the naked eye. Worst of all, no commonly used allopathic treatment modality seems to be able to stop it.

Although there have been isolated instances of it in what we refer to as the "developed world," outbreaks of it in the developing nations of Africa, Asia and South America have been violent and widespread. Broad-spectrum antibiotics, steroids (applied topically and taken internally), and a number of experimental washes, ointments, and systemic solutions have been found impotent against this particular strain of Staph aureus.

There is, however, one exception: Stabilized Aloe Vera. In challenge tests in vitro, our own formulations of Aloe Vera, when introduced to strains of this pernicious flesh-eating bacteria, were able to stop Staph Aureus dead in its tracks within two to four hours. All other modalities, even though they attained shadow results for brief periods of time, failed on every occasion to reverse the effects of this deadly bacterial strain.

Yet it is not merely against the Staph aureus, AIDS, or the laundry list of autoimmune diseases we have mentioned that Aloe Vera is once again proving to be the redoubtable treatment of choice of so many newly aware health practitioners. Its potential for broad-spectrum use continues to be endless. And Aloe lists among its advocates some pre-eminent names in science, medicine and biotechnology research. Because of their interest and their involvement, new vistas for the healing plant have opened up in just the last ten years. With them, comes an entire orchestration of new findings and research breakthroughs.

This then begins a new story in the healing plant's long but certain journey into the light. And it is that to which this book is dedicated.

Summary.

It might be said that we are currently at a tipping point in our global consciousness about what the meaning of true wellness is. And we are at choice about whether we pursue the darkness or the light.

Those of us who are at least aware of this can do one of two things: We can do little or nothing and hope that the new health technology—approved and available to all—will come charging in like some ersatz cavalry to save us at the last minute. Or we can take command of our wellness potential and realize that it is now, as it has always been, a matter of taking charge of our lives.

With 70 million plus Baby Boomers in America now crossing the threshold through the downside of middle age, health awareness has never been more in demand. This generation that has always possessed the activist muscle to shake the foundations of this world's political, economic, and environmental structure, is now addressing the issue of its own mortality. It wants answers about its health alternatives, its longevity, and its future quality of life.

Known more for its intensity purpose than its patience, this highly vocal demographic group is already bringing its influence to bear. And wellness alternatives for "the boomers" have come to be their particular cause celébre. They're looking for answers, and they will brook no compromise in doing so. As such, they are the spearhead of the "new healthocracy" we mentioned earlier—one that not only quests for longevity and quality of life, it insists upon them.

For that, this newly wellness-driven power base will have its alternatives. And, from all signals we get, they show a willingness to include Aloe Vera among them. This is not only a credulous decision, it is also a wise one. What is about to follow leads the way to all the new inroads of discovery, if you so choose.

Chapter 2

Aloe Vera: Q&A.

This chapter makes it easy and fun to learn about this amazing plant. Featured in this chapter are direct Questions and clear, concise Answers for what most people would like to know about Aloe Vera.

As a commodity, Aloe Vera is a plant that's full of surprises. Mass marketing and "junk cosmetic" exploitation of the Aloe Vera name have to some extent trivialized its significance. And yet its credibility persists. Because of striking research breakthroughs in just the last five years, Aloe continues to grow in prestige among learned clinicians and health professionals everywhere.

Since it now shows up in everything from shaving creams and shampoos to health drinks and toothpaste, it is broadly recognized by the general public but little understood. (In a private survey we ran of a small but reliable sample market, we found that, although over 56% of the people we interviewed knew the name Aloe Vera, less than half of those had any idea what it was or even that it was a plant.)

Frankly we're not sure that the mass market will ever totally comprehend the depth and scope of a plant such as Aloe Vera. The important issue is to make sure that everyone will be able to benefit from it. And to that end we press on with the process of education.

Beyond universal commercialization, Aloe has for a long time been sold in direct sales and network markets, either as the masthead product of large international companies or as one of their featured products. It is in this dynamically growing market that it still receives its most serious consideration by an educated distributor, wellness consultant and end user. And it is here that Aloe Vera still comes to us in a number of more sophisticated presentations from "pure aloe" tonics to skin crème, therapeutic lotions, balms and liniments.

Yet even among this select group, product efficacy and the quality of the Aloe Vera that is used invariably comes into question. Since the redoubtable popularity of the product has come into its fullest form of expression, there are many manufacturers and purveyors of the Aloe who claim to have original and effective formulations when they in truth do not. And the perennial questions invariably arise: How much pure Aloe Vera is being used? Have the Aloe products in question been properly stabilized? If they have, do they work? And if they work, have they proven themselves in a professional scientific context?

To all these questions, there is only one answer. Only laboratory tests and proof of numbers will validate any Aloe product.

William Faulkner once wrote that "facts and the truth have very little to do with each other."

Today, the fact is that there are more stabilized Aloe Vera products than ever before. The truth is that they must all be submitted to rigorous examination before they can be granted credibility for pharmaceutical grading and professional respectability.

For that, laboratory research, in vitro and in vivo studies, and the force of numbers from acknowledged scientists and health professionals are the only processes that serve the purpose.

The truth is that this is a process that takes time, money, patience and persistence. And yet our intention has robbed us of shortcuts. It is the path I have, with all my heart, endeavored to take for over 40 years. It is where I began my journey, and it is where I place the thrust of all my effort to legitimize this exceptional healing plant, even to this moment in time. So it has been my firm conviction that for any Aloe Vera formulation to be used at any level, it must first be able to prove itself in scientific test, and submit the results of that testing to public scrutiny.

Having accomplished that necessary step, we proceed to the next important issue—educating the reader, including both the professional public and the public at large. Since we've also spent the last 40 years or so figuring out how to do that, we've arrived at a very workable Aloe Vera primer. It involves 18 straightforward questions most commonly asked and answers them as simply and directly as possible.

Question #1. What is Aloe Vera? Aloe Vera is a plant that has been on this earth for millennia. (Its flawless chemical composition and versatility would lead one to conclude it had to have been one of the primal flora in the Garden of Eden.)

Because it has thorny ridges that protect the soft leaf, it is often confused for a kind of cactus. Actually it is a member of the Lily family, the plant family, *Liliaceae,* along with tulips, daffodils, onions, asparagus and about 200 other species of aloe. (In fact, a mature Aloe Vera plant will produce beautiful, fragrant lily-like blooms every spring and fall.)

Like all members of the lily family, Aloe is in its various forms is a leaf succulent. Its plump juicy leaves grow in a triangular shape and have thorny ridges along the edges. Their shape has given them the nickname "crocodile's tongue," no doubt an idiomatic peculiarity of the area of the world from which they came to be best known. The plant grows in a rosette pattern around a stalk, which gives forth a rich saffron-colored bloom only about twice a year.

With Aloe, as with so many things in nature, size does matter. And it is close to axiomatic to say that the larger the plant, the greater its potential for healing. And since Aloe Vera is known as a leaf succulent, it tends to thrive in dry arid climates where you find a generosity of wind and a paucity of water.

The True Aloe is a sturdy plant, known for being able to flourish just about anywhere and survive all but two things: hard freezes and too much water. In that regard, they're not unlike many plants that thrive in the tropics, deserts and prairies of the world.

Question #2. Where does Aloe Vera come from? Aloe Vera is a plant that has historical references dating back over 5000 years where it can be seen on the tombs of the pharaohs. Apparently it was an herbal remedy used in embalming mummies, both as a superb preservative but also as an excellent preventive agent against tuberculosis and other respiratory complications innate to that kind of work. The earliest recorded pharmacological usage was recorded in ancient Sumeria about 1750 B.C. where it was considered an excellent treatment for stomach irritations and nausea. Yes, in answer to the inevitable question, it was a favorite of the Hebrew king Solomon as well as Alexander the Great. The conqueror's physicians purportedly used it wherever they found it growing indigenously. And its primary use among them was as a healant for combat wounds and as a systemic stabilizer.

In the ancient *De Materia Medica* of the Greek physician Dioscordes, as well as that of the Roman Pliny the Elder about three centuries later, Aloe Vera is listed as a treatment of choice for scores of pathologies.

By all indications, its earliest and most intelligent recorded use was in and around all the nations of the Mediterranean Sea. Since that climate would be perfectly conducive to the growth and culturing of Aloe, these earliest references make sense.

Later, in the 13th Century, the explorer Marco Polo was said to have taken Aloe plants to China, only to find it growing there indigenously. It is also believed to have possibly been native to some of the islands of the Caribbean as well. In fact, the two most perfectly represented examples of Aloe Vera come from China (as *Aloe Chinensis)* and as *Aloe Barbadensis* based in large plants from the

Caribbean island of Barbados. It is also known as Cape Aloe (from the Cape Horn region of Africa) but can be found in very few other variations.

Although it may have had its origins of greatest recognition in the Mediterranean nations of Africa, Asia Minor and southern Europe, Aloe Vera is now found in profound patches of growth in such areas as all the islands of the Caribbean, South America, and the Netherland Antilles, Hawaii, Fiji numerous nations in Asia, and the continental United States. Plantations today may be found in the various states in the southwestern U.S., Mexico, Central America, Barbados, Malaysia, Indonesia, Israel and many other countries.

Whether Aloe Vera was native to the soil of many of these nations or not, much credit for the spread of Aloe can be credited to the travels of such explorers as Marco Polo, and to the work of the Jesuit priests who accompanied the Conquistadors to the nations of the New World. In the case of the Jesuits, they brought education along with conquest, and part of the education taught to indigenous peoples everywhere seems to have been exposure to the benefits of this silent healer. (Those priests brought baby plants in sacks and planted in the areas where they could grow.)

This custom of carrying the benefits of Aloe Vera from one culture to ennoble it to another seemed to have carried on even into this century. In fact, in the sub-text of modern commerce, we are doing it even now in the new millennium by working with foreign nations for its cultivation, development and refinement.

Question #3. Are all Aloes created equal? One of the most frustrating aspects of Aloe Vera is the fact that its often confused with other kinds of Aloes. In fact there are over 200 varieties of Aloe, and only a handful of them qualify as being the "true aloe." In fact, Aloe Vera is a Latin term for "true Aloe."

Although there is some healing power in some forms of Aloe such as the tree-like *Aloe ferox* and *Aloe perryi* (both African varieties), many forms of Aloe offer little in the way of curative potency. So one is well advised to be able to identify the "true aloe" on sight. Or, when in doubt, refer to photos like the one shown here.

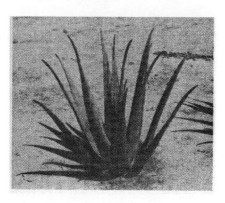

The True Aloe: Aloe Barbadensis, Miller.

Question #4. What makes Aloe Vera so effective? And how can one plant do so many different things? Aloe Vera is often recognized to be the most versatile plant in this garden of a planet called Earth. But it needs to be pointed out as well that versatility is not exclusive to this silent healer. There are estimated to be over 250,000 species of plants, and yet only about 6,000 of them are used in any way for commercial purposes by the tribe of humankind. There are a number of other plants that have multifarious uses. *Hemp,* for example, has over 40 different listed uses—from building materials to lip balm. *Eucalyptus* can be used as a respiratory adjunct, a healing salve or a very special kind of wallpaper. The *Yucca* plant can provide a number of different salves and medications. And flowers such as the *Madagascar periwinkle* and the *evening primrose* provide us with curatives that range from a treatment for juvenile leukemia to oils and foods that are reputed to help rebuild our immune systems.

Among the healing plants of Earth's garden, Aloe Vera is reputed to be the most complete in range. It carries a laundry list of uses that climbs into the scores of applications, sending unchallenged to #1 atop the alternative therapists hit parade.

Without naming all of the therapeutic uses assigned to Aloe Vera, we would feel remiss if we were not to name a few at least by category.

Still, hard pressed to answer the question, we point to three characteristics that Aloe possesses to which most experts agree are the keys to its universal effectiveness.

First, its sublime chemistry creates composition that few other plants can match. Not only does it contain over 21 key vitamins and minerals, it also possesses all 22 amino acids, plus lignin, saponins, a long list of anthraquinones, and a potent complex of enzymes.

Second, a profoundly active presence of Aloe polysaccharides act synergistically as triggering agents for Aloe's already expressive enzymatic activity. We'll discuss in more detail just how important these plant sugars are when we examine the polysaccharide factor and its relation to Aloe's complex composition. But for now, it is important to understand their role in the uncanny chemistry of this unique botanical phenomenon.

Third, is something we can only define as divine sensibility. And it does so in a number of ways. In every toxicology test to which it has been submitted, Aloe Vera has shown absolutely no measurable level of toxicity. Even in LD50s required by the FDA, Aloe Vera—even when megadoses were administered to test animals—left them unharmed and often in improved health. So, no lab animal ever died from taking even excessive amounts of Aloe. This places it in a category of one—a profound healer with a toxicity ratio that is lower than that of tap water.

Accompanying this unprecedented lack of toxicity is the fact that Aloe Vera also seems to generate its own rhythm that flawlessly flows into the process of healing. It senses what the body needs and supplies the missing factor. And nothing expresses this ability more eloquently than the role it plays in the treatment and amelioration of autoimmune diseases. As we mentioned in chapter one, autoimmune diseases express themselves in a number of ways. When the body's endocrine system malfunctions, the immune system short circuits. Its prostaglandins miscommunicate, either creating too few healing white blood cells or too many of them. Aloe Vera seems to be able to communicate perfectly with the endocrine system and enhance the process of *phagocytosis* so that it is able to place it back in balance.

In that sense, some research analysts believe that Aloe Vera is something like a cosmic thermos or the chemical equivalent of far-infrared technology. Just as these technologies balance the laws of thermal-dynamics and sense the animal body's needs for heat and cold, Aloe Vera somehow catalyzes the intricate process of helping the human system heal itself.

As a means of summarizing, we can only point to what might be referred to as *the synergy factor*. And that has to do with a hypothesis that we will cover momentarily. For now, it is important to know that any plant with the kind of intricate chemistry Aloe Vera is reputed to have is not necessarily going to offer a simple answer to any questions about how it functions.

Its synergistic potentials do, however, hold many of the secrets to its remarkable history of performance. And, no matter how many "secret ingredients" we manage to uncover, that synergy will remain a quality unique to Aloe.

Question #5. Is it better to use the plant itself or products formulated from the plant? To be sure, the native plant is remarkable on its own. And it's not at all a bad thing to have one on hand, provided it's large enough and is actually Aloe Vera. It's good for topical use—for cuts, burns, abrasions, and bites of various kinds (even spider and snake bites).

The challenge that comes with having an Aloe Vera plant exclusively lies in the fact that you are limited in the ways you can use it, both in terms of variety and intensity of usage.

At least half of Aloe's curative potential rests in its systemic applications, those that require oral or injected intake of the product. Since the native plant is not what we might call "flavor-friendly," we might want to recommend properly stabilized non-flavored liquid or fruit-flavored gels. Not only do they come already prepared and purified, they also add an improvement in taste.

Even applied topically, a properly stabilized Aloe Vera gel, gelly, cream, lotion or liniment provides a complete and versatile family of specialized usage that offers up to 9o% of the potency of the native plant. Properly formulated, these refined, stabilized Aloe products also provide Aloe in a form that is pure, efficacious, varied and convenient with state-of-the-art potency and variety of presentations. This provides a spectrum of usage and adaptation that no plant in its native state can equal.

In fact, today in the new millennium there are virtually dozens of presentations of commercially prepared, pharmaceutical grade Aloe Vera products now available for consideration. Formulated into creams, lotions, gellies, and gels for topical use, they also come in combination with eucalyptus and menthol and used as splendid counterirritants. We have personally been responsible for the introduction of Aloe mouthwashes, douches, toothpastes, and drinking gels introduced for the marketplace—each one of them accompanied by the appropriate clinical data to verify their efficacious use as a pharmaceutical grade product.

The challenge for all commercially offered Aloe Vera products then comes in making sure that the presentations you do select are pharmaceutical grade aloes that have passed professional scrutiny and enjoy some kind of institutional approval.

It is a code of presentation we live by. It is a standard we challenge other processors, manufacturers, and marketers to meet.

Question #6. Why is Aloe Vera's reputation still somewhat controversial? Aloe Vera's reputation has been controversial for three very good reasons. First, it simply does so many things so well that, in the last ten years in particular, everyone has embraced it as their own. However, almost none of mass marketers have truly understood the challenges that accompany its enormous potential.

It is an unfortunate truth of the marketplace that, today there are simply too many people formulating Aloe Vera products. Their processes are either inadequate or purchased from mass-market middlemen who are just milking the popularity. So the products that are being put out are often watered down, improperly formulated, or just commercially mongrelized. So, by and large, Aloe products used are either inert or contain doses that come in such absurdly small amounts that they offer no impact at all. So in the new millennium, more than ever before, Aloe Vera has been victimized by its own popularity. There are not so many proliferations of it that its hand has been virtually overplayed, and the results achieved—commercially at least—have been disappointing.

The second reason for the controversy surrounding it is the mixed blessing of word-of-mouth "mythology" for what it can do. Whether it comes in the form of a layman's praise for a usage experience or the casual evaluation of a health professional based on one or two instances of use, anecdotes can often become a poison in the pot of its credibility. Certainly, fantastic tales build interest in Aloe and products derived from it. But, improperly related or overblown, they can do more harm than good. Most health professionals will shrug them off, and institutional bodies such as the FDA actually frown upon them as sensationalism.

We have learned that it is only through research and force of numbers in professionally supervised clinical evaluation that one can prove Aloe Vera's true worth. It is the only way medical health professionals, and health-governing bodies such as the FDA are even allowed to take them seriously.

We have spent hundreds of thousands of dollars to achieve that kind of credibility for our formulations. At this point, we feel obligated to point out that there is great disparity in the Aloe Vera products that are currently available. It is only pharmaceutical grade Aloe Vera, that which has met rigid scientific testing criteria, that can be taken seriously as a broad-spectrum healant. And we challenge anyone who seriously intends to manufacture products from this plant to submit it to testing, They, and all of us, will only benefit further from the process.

The third reason Aloe Vera remains controversial lies in the difficulty surrounding many attempts to stabilize it. Today, safely stabilizing Aloe Vera is not the volatile issue it once was, and yet the proper stabilization of Aloe Vera remains a concern as well as an issue for debate. Still, there is in the uncertain science of stabilization the need to modify Aloe's delicate chemistry without rendering it useless at the same time.

Question #7: Are challenges to Aloe Vera's stability justified? And what has been done to make it more stable? Even though great strides have been taken in the last ten years when it comes to stabilizing Aloe Vera, a great deal more remains to be done.

In that regard Aloe's greatest strength, its profound enzymatic activity, has traditionally proved to be its greatest weakness. Originally, in fact for decades, any transferal of the Aloe from leaf-gel to product form resulted in accelerated degradation and contamination. Old attempts stabilize it by such processes as pasteurization rendered the Aloe product virtually inert. Just as canned foods and jarred foods have little nutritional value relative to the original fruit or vegetable, Aloe products cooked in the same way net a similar result. In such instances, the Aloe Vera formulations with such a personality will be of negligible curative value.

Today, claimants to the proper stabilization of Aloe Vera number in legion. And by now everything has been tried. Boiling, freezing, distilling, freeze-drying, desiccating, pasteurization of various kinds, molecule-trimming with preservatives, cold-processing, concentration-extraction and combinations thereof— everything within the realm of possibility has been done to stabilize Aloe Vera (and we've probably tried them all ourselves). And by now, many attempts to achieve that end have succeeded.

The questions, however, still remain: Is a stable product necessarily an effective one? And once the stabilization has been achieved, has it been properly put to the test? Do its efficacy, purity, and broad-spectrum healing potentials maintain their integrity?

As co-originator of the world's first effective stabilized Aloe formulation, and as co-creator of what many believe is its most universally acknowledged effective formulation today, I offer this simple suggestion to anyone investigating the potentials of a product: Ask to see the proof.

Laboratory tests, clinical data, double-blind studies, control group studies— all these and others should not only show the efficacy of Aloe Vera in general but also serve to validate any specific brand of Aloe Vera specifically placed under scrutiny.

Any company with true integrity will take the time and trouble to do so. And unless they do, you're gambling with the choices you make.

Question #8. How can I tell what Aloe Vera products actually possess the potential to do this? How can I be sure? There are four pretty good ways but none of them foolproof. First, ask to see the data. Any Aloe Vera company that is serious about what it's doing should be able to provide viable clinical data, either in its literature, on its website, or in professional references. Since this kind of information is often proprietary, some companies may be reluctant to share it. But the right kind of company will happily provide you with references.

A second way to determine a product's efficacy is to consult with a health professional—an M.D., N.D., D.O., Chiropractor or herbalist. Because of the dramatic strides Aloe Vera has made in recent years, there are increasing numbers of mainstream health professionals who now use it routinely as an effective treatment for a number of conditions. And these practitioners often have either variations of Aloe or specific brands that they have found to be effective in their patient or client applications.

Interestingly enough, price might also prove to be a third effective indicator of product potency and efficacy. Although there are unscrupulous vendors of Aloe who will charge a small fortune for a watered down, impotent Aloe product, we can attest to the truth that no one can sell a cut rate efficacious, pharmaceutical grade Aloe Vera product. There is simply too much cost involved in properly processing and formulating a sound, potent, sterile, stable product to ever sell it at bargain retail prices.

So, if you see a so-called "Aloe" gel, drink, lotion or salve that is a fraction of the cost of others, there is a reason for it. Potency comes at a price. And though it is by no means a guarantee of product efficacy to buy a more expensive product, price offers another, albeit imprecise, way to cull the pretenders.

Finally, word of mouth is perhaps a viable means of determining the value of a truly effective Aloe Vera product. But frankly that word-of-mouth recommendation should come from a health professional or someone professionally qualified in the business of networking wellness products. At least, if challenged to do so, they might at least be able to provide you with appropriate data to reinforce the products they recommend.

Question # 9. Should Aloe Vera be sold by prescription? The term "prescription" is often misinterpreted. A physician or licensed health professional may "prescribe" anything, including aspirin if he or she feels that is the proper modality to help the patient. The only drugs that are required to be sold by prescription are placed in the category of "prescription drug" because they carry a set of side effects (or contraindications) that require their sale to be restricted. What that means is that, after undergoing rigorous and necessary testing, it has been found that drug carries a level of relative toxicity that in excessive quantities makes it either dangerous or addictive. So people taking certain drugs can experience possible harmful side effects if taken in unrestricted dosages or for a protracted period of time.

As we have noted earlier in this chapter, the only means by which Aloe Vera needs to be sold by prescription might be in concentrated isolates or extractions distilled from the product. Although we have not experienced any measurable relative toxicity from the concentrates we have derived from our formulations, there may be individual formulations that achieve a different result. And those, at all times will require testing against all acknowledged criteria of toxicology.

As far as the individual plant is concerned, the products that we derive from our whole leaf extraction formula follow in Aloe Vera's tradition of GRAS qualification. As such, it is safe for any sensible use, without the need of a doctor's permission.

Question # 10. What does GRAS mean? What is its significance to the public? The term GRAS (pronounced "grass") is issued by the FDA and stands for Generally Regarded As Safe.

This means that, in testing, a product shows so little relative toxicity that it is deemed "safe" for use in the human system or as a topical agent. This classification is predominantly given to foods, plants, and nutrients that might also be pressed into service for health, medical, or scientific purposes. Such general usage acknowledgment is coveted by any plant, herb, food or nutrient, or any family of products derived from it.

Such qualifications, however, are tenuous at best. They are constantly under review by the FDA. And a plant's or nutrient derivative's GRAS rating can be pulled at any time for reevaluation and reclassification.

Question # 11. What is the secret of Aloe Vera's complex chemistry that makes it so effective? This is a simple question that requires a complex answer, but bear with us on this one. With improved methods of testing and evaluation we believe we have been able to define Aloe Vera's extraordinary composition and now put it into a language that anyone can understand.

Even now, there has come to be more acceptance for the notion that there are botanical complements to the physical needs of the animal body. Perhaps no plant underscores this belief better than Aloe Vera. We already know that the native plant reveals a botanical matrix that is rich in lignin, saponins, anthraquinones, vitamins, minerals, amino acids, enzymes, and polysaccharides.

Generally, it is acknowledged that both amino acids and enzymes carry the stuff of life in any living organism. These form the proteins that make up the life-giving fiber of any animal body. They are agents of life: and for that reason, the higher and more active the content, the greater the life potential in the organism. Aloe Vera, in its native plant form, contains the entire family of 22 amino acids. These amino acids are strung together in a seemingly infinite number of ways that help to promote the body's health, to give it the energy to function effectively, and to stave off oxidation, disease, and the effects of aging.

There are also constituents of the body's proteins called enzymes. All enzymes work to regulate the delicate chemistry of the body. Not surprisingly, in numerous laboratory tests over the years Aloe Vera has shown itself to have a very active enzymatic complex. These enzymes actually catalyze its efficient use of water and oxygen that are introduced to it in a process called hydrolysis. In that regard, they are referred to as *hydrolyzing enzymes*—or what is more familiarly known in scientific circles as proteolytic enzymes. These proteolytic (or protein bonding) enzymes enable the body to reform into amino acids, the life extending, antioxidant characteristics that the human body needs to fight disease, improve energy, and extend the cell life of the human system itself.

But it is paradoxical in the nature of these proteolytic enzymes that they are as fragile as they are energetic. So, they need the appropriate sugars to help them carry through the human system and go about their business as quickly and efficiently as possible.

And, befitting the chemistry of this very sophisticated creation of nature, it also offers the appropriate complement of complex natural plant sugars called *polysaccharides* to carry this intricate process of penetration, regeneration, and healing through to completion. Since they are presented in a mucous-like gel form, they are more commonly known as *Aloe polysaccharides*.

As we've just pointed out, the possibilities for Aloe Vera's varied chemical and nutritional complex seem unlimited. So the logical question arises: What if it innately sensed what to provide the human/animal system what it needed, when it needed it, and in just the right amounts? What if there were this divine phytochemical communication system between the *corpus humanis* and the plant itself that enabled it to rush healants and nutrients to that system whenever it was troubled or traumatized?

To open our minds to this possibility, we must at least be willing to accept that these elements germane to the plant needed for healing and revitalization may not be measurable in isolation but are instead rushed to the diseased or traumatized area *vis a vis* a triggering agent or a series of them. This would be an act of divine synergy indeed. So, to summarize we can only point to what might be referred to as *the synergy factor*. In fact, there are still many theories about the healing potentials of Aloe Vera and what gives it such curative versatility. And yet, no matter what proof is brought forth, the question of its synergistic capabilities invariably becomes a relentless contender.

Granted, this necessarily descends into hypothesis. But beyond hypothesis it is comes with its own brand of logic. All it requires is a little understanding of body language and a dash of common sense logic. It's based on the belief that the body contains within itself the power to heal if given the proper signals, the right phytochemical message to do so.

It has long been our belief that the true active ingredient in the Aloe Vera complex is in fact that kind of synergism. A synergism is of course the occurrence that takes place when the whole of any entity is greater than the sum of its parts. And there is little doubt in my mind at least that the synergistic activity in the Aloe complex is profound; perhaps more effective than any naturally occurring complex since the beginning of creation. Because of the interactive chemistry that naturally occurs between the enzymes, amino acids, vitamins, minerals, anthraquinones, lignin, saponins and all the other elements present in the plant, it has finally inched its way toward a solution.

Today, with more sophisticated means of testing, Aloe Vera is still a difficult plant to fingerprint. Nevertheless, it does the job. Perhaps better than any other healant from God's vast botanical pharmacy, Aloe most closely senses the body's needs and answers them.

The question remains, however, what triggers it to do so? What is the signaling mechanism? If the "active" ingredient in this complex serves a purpose, it is perhaps as a messenger from the traumatized entity to the Aloe's healing control center and back again, defining the need and acting as a conduit to speed the healants and nutrients to the area under assault. Mindful of that function, it is here that we try to put in place the final piece of the puzzle of Aloe Vera's mysterious chemistry.

Question #12. Where does Aloe Vera's curative potency really lie? At first, we'll answer this question as simply as possible. But the answer comes in two parts. The first part deals with the actual focus of potency for its maximum healing effect. The second attempts to identify its actual curative potency and the "key ingredients" that drive it.

The reputed healing power of the plant was originally believed to have been in the rind or outer layer. Later findings showed the soft pulp-like gel to hold a great deal of the plant's uncanny healing potential. Finally, sophisticated research has revealed that Aloe's greatest potency is almost invariably achieved through a combination of the two.

Understanding this, it is also important to realize that the way Aloe Vera is extracted processed and refined has a great deal of bearing upon its potential effectiveness.

Just as we believe the true potency of Aloe Vera lies in the synergism of all its components, we believe that using the whole leaf in a uniquely processed formulation is the most effective way to blend it into versatile compounds and prepare it for market. What's more, our research and findings indicate that this is the most effective presentation of Aloe discovered to date. As such it is, perhaps justifiably, the summary expression of its infinite potential.

The "combination" makes sense, because it not only echoes the concept of the plant's divine synergy, it also points to the activity of the plant's most active carrying agents, the Aloe polysaccharides.

Of course, in the mad soup of laboratory research, there have been individual contenders over the years—personal favorites of one research group or another. And they deserve mention if for no other reason than to emphasize the individual and collective potency of the plant.

In fact, many theories surrounding the mystery of the elusive triggering element that gives the Aloe Vera its remarkable powers. The theories, stemming from extensive experimentation by some eminent research groups, have varied over the years.

In 1938 and 1939, research scientists Tom D. Rowe and Lloyd Parks initiated the most extensive chemical breakdown of Aloe Vera to that time, and in a published study voiced their belief not only that the true power of the plant lay in the rind but also that the *anthraquinone* complex held the true secret of Aloe's healing powers.

Anthraquinones such as *aloin, emodin,* and *chrysophanic acid* have been credited with certain antibiotic powers but are also known for their reputations as potent agents to intestinal catharsis; in other words, strong laxatives. This is particularly true of aloin.

In a study on "The Bacteriostatic Properties of Aloe" in 1964, an American group headed by Lorna Lorenzetti found freeze-dried Aloe formulations be particularly effective against such pernicious organisms as various Staph infections, strep pyogenes, and typhus infections. As did Rowe and Parks before them, the Lorenzetti group believed the key ingredients in the Aloe Vera chemical matrix to come from the anthraquinones. Yet, when they tested *Aloe emodin, emodin,* and *chrysophanic acid* individually, they found these individual anthraquinones exhibited no semblance of the innate curative power that seemed to reside in the freeze-dried Aloe.

Other studies such as those by a research group headed by Myoshi Ikawa and Carl Niemann in 1951, as well as a research group headed by a group of Egyptian physicians, El Zawahry, Hegazy and Helal, in 1973, pointed to their independent beliefs that the true healing power and tissue building properties of the plant could be found in the mucilage (gel) of the plant—especially in the *mono and polysaccharides.* The Ikawa and Niemann group found that the mucilage (or pulp) of Aloe Vera consisted of the polysaccharides, *glucose, mannose, and (hexo)uronic acid,* along with some traces of *rhamnose,* and found them to be especially effective for their tissue-building properties and for their abilities as bactericidal agents.

And though they found the enzymatic activity of the plant highly contributory to its success as a healant, they too believed it was the *Aloe polysaccharides* that contained the active healing ingredient.

Drs. Ruth Sims and Eugene Zimmermann furthered the "enzyme axiom" in the early 1970s. Two research Ph.D.s studying the effects of an 80% Aloe Vera solution (our original stabilized formula), doctors Sims and Zimmermann found our Aloe to be remarkably effective in its antipruritic and fungicidal effects against a number of common maladies such as sunburn, skin rashes, poison ivy, and pruritus ani and pruritus vulvae. (An effective antipruritic stops itching and irritation. A fungicide as the name implies effectively kills fungus.) In the Sims-Zimmermann findings, a concentrated Coats Aloe solution accomplished both tasks to maximum positive effect. As a result of this study, however, both Sims and Zimmermann advanced the belief that it was the *proteolytic enzymes* that held the true healing power of the Aloe complex.

A few years ago, a research team of West German scientists came to conclusions similar to those of El Zawahry, Hegazy, and Helal, and added a few theories of their own. One of the theories, strongly held in some other scientific circles, is that the Aloe polysaccharides serve as the protective mechanism for the plant, that whenever the plant is traumatized in any way (such as the dismembering of a leaf from the plant) these polysaccharides instantaneously begin emitting an exudate. This exudate comes in the form of a thick gelatinous coating which naturally accomplishes two things: First, it stops the flow of gel from the leaf. Second, it seals the leaf from further exposure to the atmosphere, enabling it to throw up a natural protective barrier to against the invasion of bacteria, mold, yeast, or insect infestation that might otherwise assault the plant.

These findings confirmed what many have suspected all along—that the largest concentration of Aloe polysaccharides can be found just under the Aloe leaf surface. The German research group has consistently embraced the belief that there is a direct corollary between the harvesting of the leaf and the action of the Aloe polysaccharides. Their hypothesis states in effect that the moment the leaf is harvested from the mother plant, it will start diffusing a polysaccharide-rich exudate from the entire subsurface directly under the outer leaf, or what we see to be the green portion of the leaf. Additionally, it has been found that leaves harvested from the plant and left in storage, even for a short time, not only seal shut very quickly, but also emit polysaccharides into the gel in far greater quantities than those that commonly occur in a freshly harvested leaf.

This finding is highly significant. Since the Aloe polysaccharides act quickly as agents to rush healing and cell division not only to the wounded portion of the plant, there is every indication that they act in the same way to rush healants in the plant complex to other organisms as well. Second, it has been found that the

Aloe polysaccharides are at their most potent and most prolific directly under the outer leaf. Third, under previous methods of processing, if you kept leaves in storage for a time—even for a few hours—it is possible to dramatically increase the quantity and potency of the Aloe polysaccharides present in the Aloe's inner-gel fillet.

Still, one has to ask the question: Is a carrying agent, in this case the Aloe polysaccharide complex, the sole driving force in the intricate curative network of Aloe Vera. Some people prefer to go to an even more specific (muco)polysaccharide in the form of acemannan.

Acemannan, though isolated as a polysaccharide nearly thirty years ago was heavily researched for its curative potentials by Dr. T.H. McAnalley in the mid '80s, and later by his associate, Dr. H.R. McDaniel. The work of these two men in the late 1980s and early 90s sparked a virtual Acemannan revolution among researchers, clinicians, medical practitioners and biochemists. And we are personally delighted with the inroads Acemannan has made toward gaining both scientific respectability and acceptance by governing medical bodies. In fact, it has not only worked wonders for its own credibility as the "pivotal molecule" and for its recombinant capabilities within animal/human systems, it has also revived interest in its mother plant—Aloe Vera.

Specifically, Acemannan is a molecule isolated from a long chain complex mannose sugar in Aloe that does one heck of a job of helping the body's immune system fight disease.

For a time in the late 1990s, Acemannan was viewed by many clinicians to be the probable "magic bullet," the key ingredient in the Aloe Vera complex. By now volumes of research and clinical studies point unequivocally to its profound impact as an anti-bacterial anti-viral agent against a number of the world's Top Ten public enemy pathogens, specifically HIV, cancer, tumors, colitis and Crohn's disease in humans as well as FLV (or Feline Leukemia Virus) in cats. What's more the Acemannan long-chain polysaccharide molecule has shown the same promising absence of toxicity for which the matrix plant is so renowned.

As we mentioned earlier, Acemannan is remarkable but not without its limitations. In our findings there are certain things that Acemannan—miraculous element though it is—does not yet do that Aloe Vera, the whole plant, does in terms of the following:

• *Wound-healing and tissue regeneration:* Although Acemannan has shown tremendous potential to thwart the PGE-2 antigen and has shown in at least one clinical trial to offer superior wound-healing abilities, Aloe Vera in the full context of its natural presentation has proven in tests, to be a superior healant. Additionally, as we will soon show in a number of instances, both in the debridement stages and tissue repair stages, Aloe Vera offers a tissue regeneration factor that is superior to the point of being dramatic.

• *Pain relief:* Our laboratory findings have shown that such conditions as rheumatoid arthritis, athletic injuries, thermal burns, and ulcers of various kinds have all been seen their pain alleviated through treatment with stabilized Aloe Vera and whole plant gels from it.

• *Penetration:* Because of its proteolytic enzymes and lignin, Aloe Vera is one of the most explicitly tissue-penetrative healants known to modern science. This is particularly significant in the healing process, especially in the treatment of wounds, hematoma, injuries and areas not easily penetrated by normal topical medication.

• *Broad-spectrum germ killing:* Although Acemannan has shown some potent antiviral and antibacterial potentials, with possible positive effects in helping to destroy fungus in the human system, Aloe Vera has exhibited virucidal, bactericidal, moniliacidal and fungicidal capabilities against an extremely broad range of pernicious organisms. And its potentials for application offer a variety unequalled, that we know of, in modern science.

Although much research on Acemannan has been done, and though its list of potentials seems impressive indeed, the best opportunity for complete treatment we see is to combine Acemannan with Aloe Vera in many forms of treatment. This maximizes the opportunities for effective overall treatment, especially in instances of complex pathologies. In combating diseases such as HIV and diabetes where the innate disease interacts with opportunistic infections to create a hydra-headed monster, one must be willing to try any and all possible combinations. And one can, with Aloe, expect results that are both synergistic and beneficial.

Once again, despite all the contenders (and some pretenders) for the title of "key ingredient," we have to point again to the symphonic synergy of everything working together—the splendid chemistry of amino acids, enzymes, vitamins, minerals, anthraquinones, lignin, saponins, and mono and polysaccharides (including Acemannan) working in concert.

Just as one knows the heart is the power plant of the human body, it cannot complete its intended function without interacting with the other organs—the liver, spleen, kidney, lungs and digestive system. It is the synergy of their sublime and often mysterious cooperation that brings to bear the miracle of life.

The same then must be said for the complex chemistry of Aloe Vera. It best completes the body of its work with its divine synergy intact.

Question #13. Is Aloe Vera more potent as a topical treatment, or when used internally? There are scores of clinical studies, independent lab findings and physician's reports that reveal a seemingly limitless number of uses for Aloe Vera both as a topical agent and for internal applications. In fact we have written volumes on both subjects. And though this is not our intention in this section to list all the pathologies positively treated by stabilized Aloe Vera and the research findings that support them, it is at least a good indicator to name a list of each here, if for no other reason than to provide a clearer picture of the scope of this silent healer:

External conditions that have been treated topically for pain, exudation, and dysfunctional rate of healing include the following: thermal, chemical and friction burns; scalding, sunburn, turf burns, and wind burn; radium, x-ray and radiation burns; skin ulcers, blisters, rashes, prickly heat, razor burn, and abrasions; wasp, bee, scorpion and spider stings; snake bites, mosquito bites, and bot fly infestation; poison oak poison ivy, and poison sumac; allergic skin reactions, psoriasis, eczema, seborrhea, and impetigo; dandruff, alopecia aereata, uriticaria and bed sores; cracked nipples, moles, pedunculated fibromas and warts; cuts, contusions, lacerations, wet lesions, dry lesions, boils and abscesses; fever blisters, cold sores, herpes simplex, herpes zoster and Herpes II; contusions, bruises, hematomas and hyperextensions; groin pulls, "Charley horses," athlete's foot, ringworm and other fungi; muscle sores cramps, strains, sprains, and joint separations; tendonitis, vaginitis, venereal sores, canker sores, gingivitis and aphthous ulcers; corneal ulcers, conjunctivitis and sties.

Aloe Vera and properly formulated products derived from it have been taken internally to successfully treat the following conditions: headache, insomnia, chronic fatigue syndrome, fibromyalgia and multiple sclerosis; heart conditions, hypertension, stress, anxiety, anger, rage, and angina pectoris; indigestion, heartburn, hyperacidity, acid reflux, gastritis, and duodenal and peptic ulcers; hemorrhoids, urinary tract infections, prostatitis, vaginitis, inflamed cysts and various types of STDs; systemic cancer, heart disease, tension, stress, depression and manic depression; various autoimmune diseases (systemic diseases with topical or visible physical manifestations) such as diabetes mellitus, lupus, lupus erythematosus, scleroderma, bilateral scleroderma, multiple sclerosis, and rheumatoid arthritis; global pandemics such as HIV, Staph aureus, Ebola, and tuberculosis have also shown in challenge tests to respond positively to treatments of Aloe Vera.

Granted these lists are long and challenge professional credulity. In fact, we are the first to acknowledge that any self-respecting health professional who scans this laundry list of curative claims for the first time is going to respond with complete skepticism. All we ask is that you look at the evidence, review our landmark laboratory findings, and then decide. (We also hasten to note that these lists, however extensive, are also incomplete.)

By the way, we haven't forgotten the question originally put before us: Given the nature of disease and the way that cures can be measured, Aloe Vera's impact may be more readily evident in terms of its dramatic cures of topical ailments, if for no other reason than the fact that improvements are measurable on a daily basis. So the edge would probably go there.

Although we have volumes of records and physicians' reports that show systemic and autoimmune diseases treated successfully with Aloe Vera, these pathologies by their very nature are often viewed as largely indeterminate as to cause and effect. So many of them are reliant upon patient feedback and as such are subject to second-guessing.

You can see the visible traces of a burn being healed. A healed heart, no matter how completely recovered, is always a mystery left to conjecture and the possibility of relapse.

Question #14. If Aloe Vera speeds up a person's rate of recovery, is it effective for sports injuries and for people in professional performance athletics? One of the healing plant's most extensive records of successful usage resides in its chronicles of usage by world class athletes. Collegiate, Olympic, and professional athletes in virtually every field of sport have reported remarkable results from using our Aloe Vera products. Since many of our products were specially formulated to meet the specific needs of athletes and trainers everywhere, we are happy to be able to share our experiences, as well as their successes, with you. In fact, we will do so in our Chapter 3: "Aloe Vera All Stars."

Performance athletes at high levels of competition share two common passions. First, they will do whatever is necessary to excel at their sport, game or contest. Second, once injured, they will take any reasonable means to get themselves back into action as soon as possible. In virtually hundreds of instances of use by major athletic organizations from the Dallas Cowboys to the Toronto Blue Jays, we will be happy to share the exceptional healing potentials that Aloe Vera offers to athletes everywhere.

Question #15. Can Aloe Vera be used on our animal companions and livestock? In all its expressions Aloe Vera offers dozens of presentations that help virtually hundreds of pathologies that plague the creatures in our care. And they are generally allowed to do so with impunity.

There are a couple of reasons for this. First, there are fewer restrictions against the kinds of healing modalities that are approved for animal use. Second, there is a seeming willingness on the part of many veterinary practitioners to take chances with new therapeutic alternatives that might help a dog, cat or barnyard animal. Often the owners are willing to try anything. And given the current economic challenges to commercial farming and ranching, failure to achieve healthy solutions can often be economically catastrophic.

The good news is that stabilized Aloe Vera products have long been a staple in veterinary use. And, even as we write this, they are continuing to provide genuine therapeutic breakthroughs especially in the cattle and dairy industry that might amount to billions of dollars in savings.

At this point, at least, the use of Aloe Vera in the treatment of our creature companions has proven to be one of its most prolific forms of expression. It's a trend we expect not only to continue but also to expand.

We will also cover this very prolific issue in ensuing chapters in this book.

Question #16. Is it safe to use for children and infants? Because Aloe Vera contains no measurable toxicity, it is an excellent product for infants and children. Provided it is conscientiously formulated in an appropriate presentation for use by children, Aloe is exceedingly gentle to the skin, and creates the same level of synergistic benefit that rushes both nutrients and healing elements to the skin surface. And pharmaceutically tested for internal use, it is a healthy, nutritious, safe, and often energizing drink. Remember, Aloe Vera enjoys a GRAS qualification. That means that it is technically a food. So, food standards for safe uses generally apply.

Nevertheless, we also point out that these are still children. So you should always check your product labels for appropriate recommended children's doses. (And by all means, consult a qualified health professional for advice and consent.)

Once again, we caution the user with our own personal *caveat emptor*. Be sure you check your sources and your products out before buying them. Use our four recommended criteria for making your product decision. And proceed accordingly.

Question # 17: Why is Aloe Vera used so frequently in cosmetics and personal care? Second only to food production, the cosmetic and personal care industry is, in terms of numbers, the second largest in the world. At the same time, its needs are so varied and its demands so challenging that only the most versatile and efficacious products will survive the scrutiny of this highly astute marketplace.

It is also true that in no other industry are there as many brands, pretenders, and prestigious expensive treatments to address human skin health. And though an increasing number of men interested in skin health and the appurtenance of appearance, personal care and cosmetics remains 89% the domain of women. And women know only too well that they are constantly being courted by purveyors of products, mostly water-based, that claim to be beneficial and yet accomplish nothing.

Since Aloe Vera products use Aloe rather than water as a base, and since properly formulated Aloe Vera products are pharmaceutical grade, Aloe Vera can provide what we often refer to as prescriptive skin care for its users.

In fact, one of our longest standing associations is with the American Society of Cosmetic Chemists. In uses for such treatments as dermabrasion and such conditions as acne and other afflictions of the skin, Aloe Vera has been praised for providing the ideal combination of therapeutic treatment potentials followed by soothing personal care regimen that is renown for its beneficial effects.

In truth, the cosmetic potentials for Aloe Vera are directly proportionate to the ethics and integrity of companies that purvey Aloe Vera based products. But from our experience and our working relationships with several of them, the viable choices now available to the health-conscious consumer are growing both in depth and range of use.

Question # 18. *What is the most promising aspect of Aloe's role in the future of world health?* It may well take the rest of this book to answer this question. But for now, we'll keep it simple.

Aloe's potentials for the 2000s are infinite for two very good reasons.

In the first place, we are entering a new era of understanding where our health and wellness are concerned. As we mentioned, the demands of global populations for affordable, safe, efficacious, and effective modalities of treatment have helped broaden the forum for acceptance of alternative means of treatment. Exploding populations, the increase of highly resistant strains of pandemics, and the rising cost of health care, demand that we explore all reasonable means of prevention, treatment and cure.

Second, and most important, is the fact that Aloe Vera has earned its place in the panoply of remarkable therapies. Not only have those of us dedicated to carrying the torch brought volumes of research and clinical studies in support of the healing plant's infinite potentials, the scientific community has at last opened its eyes to see what has always been before them. Now after decades, there is a renewed consciousness of institutional credulity that allows explorations to be made, reports to be heard, and actions to be taken.

In terms of animal disease pandemics and super viruses, the dynamics of the marketplace demand it, and immediately.

In other fields of medicine, personal care and athletics the silent healer is already in play, and universal usage on a global scale is only a matter of time, research and an enlightened acceptance of what is already there.

Chapter 3

Aloe Super Stars

It is widely known but little discussed that Stabilized Aloe Vera products have long been held in high regard in the world of professional, Olympic, and collegiate athletics. In fact, our own Aloe Vera formulations have been used to treat athletes in the NFL, NHL, the National and American Leagues of professional baseball, Olympic athletes, and a number of NCAA colleges and universities. At last, we offer Aloe Vera's brief but colorful journey through the world of competition athletics, and the impact it has made with thousands of athletes and dozens of sports organizations in the last three decades.

Dateline: New Orleans, January 1994. Super Bowl XXVII. Dallas Cowboy running back Emmitt Smith has just won the award for the championship's most valuable player in their 53-20 rout of the Buffalo Bills. It capped a brilliant year for the future Hall of Famer, including a 1993 season that saw him win the NFL rushing title and an NFL championship. It was both fitting and ironic that Emmitt had accomplished all this while enduring the effects of a shoulder separation that he had received in the fifth game of the regular season.

In the first half of a game against the New York Giants, Emmitt had taken a hard fall to the Astroturf after a 12-yard carry and felt the shattering tear and tingle in his rotator cup that usually comes with that kind of injury.

Ordinarily a shoulder separation of that magnitude would take a player anywhere from five to eight weeks to heal. And even then, there would be no assurance that the healing process would permit the kind of resistance and mobility he would need to complete the rigorous demands of an NFL season. But one can never underestimate either the determination of great athletes or the resourcefulness of experienced athletic trainers.

Characteristic of his grit and courage, Emmitt finished the game with a separated shoulder but was in considerable pain on the Monday following the game.

In this case, Emmitt's trainer was Kevin O'Neill. Not only was Kevin coach Jimmy Johnson's head trainer, he had also come over with him from the University of Miami. While at the university, Kevin had used our Aloe Action* products for his athletes in a number of sports, so he was familiar with Aloe Vera's remarkable capacity for healing even the most debilitating sports injuries. Still, Emmitt's condition was a major cause for concern. And since he was the Cowboy's franchise player, Kevin got in touch with me to find out (in his words) "how we can keep him on the field..."

Remembering what another Cowboy star, cornerback Charlie Waters had done for his injuries, I recommended for a night treatment that Kevin take a cotton pad, saturate it with the Aloe Vera liquid, put our Aloe Vera gelly on top of that, wrap it around Emmitt's shoulder with an Ace bandage and cover the entire area with Saran Wrap® to allow the healing compound to incubate. That would be the treatment before he went to bed.

During the daytime, Kevin would use Aloe liniment and whirlpool in a regular regimen for no less than 45 minutes at a time. Then he would saturate the Aloe gelly with a pad and (again) use the Saran Wrap® as a cover around it.

Kevin O'Neill and Emmitt Smith followed this regime on a daily basis for the remainder of the 1993 season. As a result, Emmitt not only played in every game, he also won league rushing honors rushing for 100 yards or more in nine of the Cowboy's remaining eleven games.

The Super Bowl victory was the capper. I have no doubt that a lesser man than Emmitt Smith still might not have made the comeback. And I'm equally certain that even Emmitt would not have made it back in action had it not been for the Aloe Vera treatments. That's a point upon which I'm certain Kevin O'Neill would agree.

---

* Aloe Action for Athletes was the name of a sports line we originally formulated and marketed in 1974 specifically for athletes at all levels of competition.

That season, I was delighted but not surprised by what I had seen that this great running back was able to do, despite his injuries. Granted it was an amazing feat, one in which Aloe Vera had played a major role. And yet it was one story among many that I had been able to witness and, in some small way be a part of, over the previous 20 years.**

The rest of this chapter is devoted to the story of Aloe Vera and its quiet but profound impact on the world of athletics, the dedication of the men and women who are willing to undertake any challenge in the pursuit of excellence, and the trainers and physicians who are determined to see them through the physical demands often made upon them.

It's a remarkable study of the higher aspects of human nature, and yet it says so much about what makes the human race such a miracle of creation.

The Natural Superiority of Who We Are.

"What a piece of work is man! How noble in reason! How infinite in faculty…"

—William Shakespeare
Hamlet, Act 4 Scene 2

Let's hear it for the creature *Homo sapiens*. Despite the misnomers about our physical shortcomings when compared to the other creatures of the world, we are exquisite pieces of natural design. In fact, we are flawlessly constructed to do what we do best—dominate this planet Earth.

We are endowed with legs innately designed to run down hunted animals for days on end, and imbued with the psychic stamina to so do. We have appendages that enable us to climb where no other creatures can and the wisdom to discern when to do so. We are the only creatures with an opposing thumb and forefinger that allows us to not only to envision great things but also to act upon that vision. We are the only creatures on this planet driven to the pursuit of excellence for its own sake.

** Later, Kevin O'Neill called me to let me know his perspectives from his experiences with using our Aloe Vera. "Bill," he told me, "I'm certain from our use of the product that the Aloe penetrates through the skin through all the tissue to the blood stream, stopping pain, irritation, inflammation, and swelling, removing swelling, blood clots, and acts as a hemostatic agent, and it does so without any side effects whatsoever."

When properly attuned, the human body is a celebration of its own natural heritage of dominion over this tiny planet. In toto, it is the most intricate neural and anatomical complex known to science. In terms of structure, it has a skeletal framework of 206 bones (give or take a few, depending upon the individual), a network of about 600 muscles, over 17 yards of viscera and intestine, more than 60,000 miles of venal, arterial, and capillary tubing just to carry the blood through the circulatory system, and nearly 20 billion nerve cells in the brain that carry more than 90,000 impressions to it for processing and assimilation every single day.

Yet if the human body's individual systems are phenomenal in design, their interaction is a miracle of precision and balance. For example, all the bones in the skeletal structure—for all their strength and elasticity—account for less than 18% of its total body weight, or about 30 pounds for the 175 pound man. That means most of the weight is accounted for in the muscle tissue. And yet it is that balance between the bone and muscle that creates the miracle of movement. The muscles are tied to one another and to the bones and cartilage in a series of opposing yet connective cables—about 600 of them in fact—tautly drawn and meshing in perfect synchronization.

All of this is triggered by a motor nerve system that enables it to make acutely quick responses. It has been estimated, for example, that the nerve system of the average athlete trips to a response movement rate of about 350 feet per second.

In the course of normal behavior, the body of even the sedentary human being performs miracles of moment and creates concentrations of stress that, purely in terms of structural engineering, tend to boggle the mind. So much so that even routine functions, when measured structurally, reveal themselves as marvels of divine engineering.,

A sedentary man riding his desk from nine to five each day will still pump from 5,000 to 6,000 quarts of blood through his heart. A woman walking down the street puts 1200 *pounds per square inch* (psi) of pressure on her ankle every time she takes a step. And a man who simply bends over to pick up his morning paper puts an average of 4,000 psi on his back.

One can only imagine the kind of stress a performance athlete experiences in the pursuit of peak performance. And it as it this point that we must demystify the process.

The Performance Athlete.

In following the sublime pursuits of the performance athlete, we are extending the demands of the physical body to its ultimate extreme. By the very nature of their training, conditioning and performance, the body of the well-conditioned athlete compares to those of the average person the same way a Formula 1 racer compares to the family SUV. The design and structure is not the same; nor are the demands. Performance athletes cannot just afford to get by; nor can they afford to be out of action.

For example, a 125 pound woman out for an evening walk may place about 1200 pounds per square inch on her ankles. The typical long distance runner places about 5000 psi on his ankles. And the competition sprinter will exert about 8000 psi on his or hers. A collegiate running back facing a wall of tacklers averaging 300 pounds apiece may exert as much as 12,000 psi on his legs and lower extremities; and a pole vaulter landing from a 19-foot vault may exert as much as 20,000 psi on his resilient, perfectly toned thighs.

In cases such as these, conditioning is everything. And even when these athletes are perfectly tuned, toned, and "ripped" to become living monuments to peak performance, a lot can go wrong—especially under the stress of competition.

Impact injuries, overuse, constant wear and tear, the stresses and strains of a very long season—all these work to tear down the athlete's perfectly tuned body. Sometimes these factors are debilitating but not crippling, and so the athlete becomes one of the "walking wounded," limited in his ability to perform at optimum levels. Either that, or they are actually taken out of action, sometimes for protracted periods of time.

When this takes place, there follows the dull, numbing, demoralizing process of recuperation. And with that comes the inevitable "down time'" that accompanies a loss of mobility, debilitation and lapses in conditioning. So the athlete loses the tonality, intention and emotional resiliency needed to get back into action. And the team loses an integral part of its championship aspirations. That costs both prestige and money to have these athletes out of commission. So, getting them back into action is paramount to the dynamics of survival.

Small wonder every major professional sports organization and every major NCAA college has an entire family of trainers and very often a team physician to keep these athletes healthy and performing at optimum levels.

Ordinarily, team physicians are only brought in for general physicals or when a sports injury is serious enough to require either surgery or extensive rehabilitation. That leaves the day-to-day monitoring of the athlete's well-being and rehabilitation to the athletic trainer.

So it is the athletic trainer's role, as much as those of the athletes themselves, to keep the teams under their supervision as fit, injury-free and event-ready as possible. This requires healthy fitness regimes and, more than that, a means of preventing injuries before they have a chance to occur. For an infinite number of uses as a "prep" for workouts, university and professional sports trainers find stabilized Aloe Vera to be the ideal therapeutic adjunct. In those uses it has worked remarkably well to forestall the onslaught of injuries.

When injuries do occur, those same trainers are dedicated to finding a treatment that will get their athletes back in action in the shortest period of time, functioning at optimum performance levels and with as little pain as is humanly possible. It is also a given that, when an athlete is sidelined, he or she will use any reasonable means available to get back in the game in the shortest time possible.

The Aloe Vera Connection.

In cases of both minor irritations and incapacitating injuries, stabilized Aloe Vera has proved to be an invaluable treatment of choice in the training room of some of America's largest sports franchises and collegiate organizati0ns.

Among them, we cite a number of major athletic organizations from our own client list. They include the following from the NFL: the Detroit Lions; the Arizona Cardinals; the Dallas Cowboys; the Miami Dolphins; the Buffalo Bills, the Chicago Bears; the Washington Redskins; the Tampa Bay Buccaneers; the San Francisco 49ers; the Minnesota Vikings; the Indianapolis Colts; the Denver Broncos; and the Seattle Seahawks.

From major league baseball, we list the following among our past clients: the Toronto Blue Jays; the Texas Rangers; the Cleveland Indians; the St. Louis Cardinals; the Atlanta Braves.

From the NBA; the Dallas Mavericks.

From the NCAA collegiate ranks we note the athletic departments of these universities: the University of Texas (Austin); the University of Louisville; Georgia Tech; Texas Tech; the University of Iowa; the University of Miami; the University of Florida; and Southwest Missouri.

In all our experiences, we have found that these clients all share a common set of challenges—a hit list of sports injuries—that seem to plague them most often. Taking a brief unofficial poll, we find them to be the following (in no particular order):

1). *Blisters, burns and turf burns*
2). *Scrapes, cuts, lacerations, contusions, and lesions*
3). *Groin pulls, hamstring pulls, and muscle pulls*
4). *Ankle sprains and strains*
5). *Wrist sprains*
6). *Hyperextnded elbows and knees*
7). *Tennis elbow and carpal tunnel syndrome*
8). *Muscle strains*

9). *Shoulder and collarbone separations*
10). *Lower back pains and injuries*
11). *Pulled Achilles tendons and tendonitis*
12). *Athlete's foot and jock itch*
13). *Hematoma, Charley horses, and bone bruises*
14). *Headaches, concussions, blurred vision*

No doubt the list could continue to include everybody's personal favorite added. And yet they all share one common need: to get their athletes back in action, and to undertake whatever safe, proven effective means is necessary to do so. They're also morally obligated to have those athletes performing, pain free, and at a level of comfort and rehabilitation that matches or exceeds their physical capacity prior to injury.

Needless to say, leading sports organizations such as the ones we have just mentioned are successful because they are constantly able to embrace health technologies that are ahead of the curve. What follows is a chronicle of how stabilized Aloe Vera became an unchallenged modality of treatment for injuries to some of the world's best athletes, and for the world famous sports organizations for which they played.

In a way, it reads like a good work of fiction. Yet as a string of facts and personal experiences, it perhaps makes for the most interesting story of all—a reality-based action adventure

From Orthopedics to Athletics. The Next Step.

Question: What do future NFL Hall of Fame running back Emmitt Smith, former Heisman Trophy winner Earl Campbell, and several Olympic medalists have in common?

Answer: Although injured, they were all kept in action at the top of their game with regular treatments of stabilized Aloe Vera.

The real beginning of Aloe Vera's longstanding relationship with major sports had its beginnings prior to 1976 with the work of a number of orthopedists, dermatologists and physicians in general practice with whom I had personally interacted in the early 1970s.

One of the most important moves we made toward establishing the professional credibility of stabilized Aloe Vera in those days had to do with the fact that, whenever possible, we always secured physicians' reports for all conditions treated with our stabilized Aloe Vera products.

Physicians' reports provide an excellent record of treatment(s) using a certain type of modality in a given number of cases. In these reports the performance of the therapy is checked off against specific criteria applicable to the pathology being treated.

In their ratings of our family of Aloe Vera gels, lotions, creams, oral solutions, and liniments, the physicians and trainers issued reports on their performance for 1) penetration, 2) wound healing, 3) relief of pain, 4) anti-inflammatory activity, 5) healing acceleration, 6) antiseptic qualities, 7) enzymatic debridement, 8) fungicidal activities, 9) improved mobility, and any other criterion as it applied.

In the prestructured reports of a number of physicians—orthopedists and dermatologists—our stabilized Aloe Vera products rated (G) as good as, (E) excellent or (S) superior to any other modality of treatment ever tried. The most encouraging aspect of these reports rests with their sheer numerical volume. In treating every condition from hematoma and sprains to severe lacerations and deep tissue trauma, our Aloe products received (S) superior and (E) excellent ratings not in dozens or hundreds but in thousands of instances of treatment.

Since the criteria for orthopedic and dermatological treatments directly parallel those of many standard athletic injuries, the next step in broad-spectrum application of usage was a logical one.

No one saw this more clearly than a physician and working associate of mine, Dr. Richard Russell. Not only was Dr. Russell an M.D. in family practice, he had also treated a number of athletes in his district and was in fact the team doctor for the Mesquite, Texas High School football team for a period of five years.

Given his success in hundreds of cases of using our Aloe Vera products on his patients, he documented his various Aloe treatments of athletes on the Mesquite football team in the following way:

"...These products have been used for strains, sprains, muscle aches, and tendonitis as well as cuts, bruises and burns.

"I have found them to be an excellent medication. They have also been frequently on burns from artificial turf, and in general for overall body massage...There is no drug effect or any other ill effect of medication, in my opinion, that would be a detriment to the athlete."[1]

Dr. Russell's report, made in the early 1970s, was passed on to the Texas Board of Education and subsequently left to languish into bureaucratic limbo for a time. But as truth is the persistent daughter of time, word-of-mouth and Dr. Russell's redoubtable reputation and constant advocacy enabled us to persist at least to the next step.

It is here that we emphasize a delicate truth. In the world of athletics, trainers and team physicians, intent upon scrutinizing all reasonable healing alternatives for their athletes, are often hit with every "miracle drug," radical therapy, and foolproof treatment modern quackery has to offer. The stakes are often high, and so the parameters for acceptability must also be high. So, although they are willing at least to give audience to a new kind of treatment, the burden of proof still rests with the manufacturer and marketer of the products.

Having spent years in research, study and application, we knew that our Aloe Vera would stand the test. All we needed was a major forum for presentation.

Fortunately, the opportunity came again in 1975.

This time it was in a manner that would change the way the functionaries in major athletics would perceive Aloe Vera from that day forward.

Just as there are prime movers who leverage shifts in consciousness that change the way we do things, in the world of athletics a man came forth to bring a great therapeutic alternative to light. The therapy was stabilized Aloe Vera. The man was Frank Medina, Head Trainer at the University of Texas in Austin.

A man of diminutive stature, Frank Medina stood no more than five feet tall in height. And yet he was a giant in his field of endeavor. In the world of college athletics no trainer had more professional credibility than Frank. He was acknowledged as a pioneer in various techniques of treating injured athletes.

"If Frank Medina thinks it works, chances are it does." That was the sentiment expressed by one trainer for a major NCAA university. And it was echoed often a loudly in colleges and universities everywhere. For that reason, Frank was understandably guarded when I first approached him about our stabilized Aloe Vera products. His reputation was on the line, and he wasn't about to compromise it.

Understandably, my first meeting with Frank Medina was brief and to the point. I presented the Aloe Vera products, explained the nature of each of our [Aloe Action] samples—the liquid, lotion, liniment, and gelly—showed him our documentation, and took my leave.

I didn't hear from Frank Medina for a month and wasn't really sure that anything would come of our get-together when he suddenly called to invite us to put up a display of our products at the upcoming Texas Relays.

The Texas Relays is a combination track meet that included the best high school and university teams in the southwestern United States, each competing in their own separate divisions. As such, it is a highly prestigious event, and not every pharmaceutical company was granted access to this body of physical therapy experts.

On the second day of the relays, Medina called a gathering of leading trainers into his office at the venue in central Texas and made an announcement.

"Gentlemen, you know me," he said. "I'm generally quite conservative in my practice. Normally, I don't recommend products of any kind. But today is a little different. Today, I'd like to share with you some of the results I've gotten working with Aloe Action Products."

His first story was one of a personal nature.

Apparently, Frank had been suffering from a badly inflamed foot that he hadn't been able to heal through conventional methods when he remembered the Aloe Vera product samples I had left with him. Applying generous portions of the lotion on his foot ankle, he found to his amazement that, within five minutes he was experiencing no pain whatsoever. By the time he had finished showering and dressing and had walked out to his car, he suddenly remembered he was experiencing no pain whatsoever.

Another story, he frequently related concerned Tim Campbell, a defensive standout and linebacker for the University of Texas from 1976-1979. The younger brother of Heismann Trophy winner and all-pro Houston Oiler running back Earl Campbell, Tim was on his way to an all-conference year himself when he got injured. On a Tuesday prior to a big game against Baylor University, Tim had been kicked above the knee and was suffering from a hematoma that was so painful he could barely walk. Frank Medina immediately saw to it that Campbell received frequent massages (about one an hour) with stabilized Aloe Vera and left both his assistant with orders that Campbell return the next morning for additional treatments. On the following day when Frank noticed that Tim had been missing from his scheduled therapy, he inquired around and found, to his amazement, that the young man was back at practice.

"My knee," Campbell told him, "isn't swollen any more. And it doesn't hurt."

Since this kind of injury, depending upon the severity, can take anywhere from three days to two weeks to heal, Frank Medina was surprised. He was also pragmatic and, after taking a quick check of Tim's knee, cleared him to go back into action.

When Frank Medina had given his personal accountings, he was both articulate and enthusiastic. And I thank heaven that he was also open-minded, particularly in view of what I found out after he gave us his unconditional endorsement. Apparently, prior to having put our Aloe Action products to the test, he and his staff at the University of Texas had been introduced to three or four other Aloe Vera companies whose products they had found wanting in every category of usage. This was not the case with our products, and Medina was emphatic in his support of them.

This kind of endorsement from a man so renowned for his professional integrity impressed his peers at the relays—except one trainer from Baylor University who continued to voice his skepticism. Later in the same day, one of his sprinters felt something in her ankle pop. Although she finished the sprint, the girl was in such agonizing pain that she had to be taken off on a stretcher. The acid test was to follow...

The trainer, seeing what condition his athlete was in, surprisingly turned to me and offered this challenge: "Well…what are you going to do for her?"

Surprised, but willing to work, I wrapped the young woman's ankle in a wrap soaked with Aloe Vera gel and let it soak-in for about half an hour. Then I rubbed it gently with Aloe Vera lotion for several minutes. Within 45 minutes of my doing so, the young athlete who had been on a stretcher an hour earlier was able to walk freely on the injured ankle.

Before long, Frank Medina became passionately committed to seeing to it that our Aloe Action products were represented in the elite sectors of world athletics. He began working in 1975 to get them accepted for use in the 1976 Montreal Olympic. Having been an official trainer for the Olympics since 1948, he could exert extraordinary leverage and did so on our behalf.

Before his first meeting with the Olympic committee to present our products for approval, Frank asked him to meet me at the Dallas-Fort Worth International Airport with nothing more than a 2 oz sample of our Aloe Action Lotion. Curious, I asked him why he'd requested such a small and (I thought) limited representation of our product, when he assured me it was all he'd need to get his point across with the committee.

"I'm sure you're wondering why I haven't charged you a dime for any of this, so I'll tell you," he said. "For all that your products have done for my athletes at the University (of Texas)—and for what I believe it can do for athletes everywhere—I'll promote it wherever I can. I personally feel that if I can make these products a household word, I could do no greater service for my profession."

Frank Medina was a man passionately disposed to his beliefs as well as to his profession. Small wonder that he was not only able to get Aloe Action Products approved for the 1976 Montreal Olympic but also provide some dramatic opportunities to put it to good use.

While in Montreal, Frank was asked to treat four Soviet athletes who were suffering from Achilles' tendonitis to such a degree that they were certain to be pulled from their events. After using Aloe Vera to treat the athletes for their conditions, Frank was able to get all four back into their events. Three of them medaled. As a result, Frank was later invited by the Soviet Olympic committee in 1977 to demonstrate the latest training techniques to their athletes and trainers.

Not surprisingly, Frank Medina's espousal of our Aloe Vera products prompted other trainers from all over the nation to give them serious consideration. The grapevine for modalities that work in the world of sports is both constant and relentless. And it wasn't long before trainers such as Larry Gardner began to embrace the concept of Aloe Vera and particularly this exceptional family of therapies. A trainer for the Dallas Cowboys for eight years, Gardner had come back at the request of Dr. Pat Evans to head the North Texas Sports Medical

Clinic. This clinic, only blocks of the Dallas Cowboys training facility, was a key center for aiding athletes in the repair and recovery of injuries in all fields of sports. Athletes from such professional organizations as the Dallas Cowboys, the Dallas Mavericks, North Texas University, Southern Methodist University and the Texas Rangers Baseball Club were among the many major sports groups that sent their athletes for treatment, rehabilitation and even surgeries.

As long as he was head of the clinic, Larry Gardner was an avid supporter of our Aloe Action products and even gave the following endorsement on a film he did for us back in 1981.

"We routinely use the aloe Action Lotion on our post-surgical knee patients. We give it to them to take home, and we use it here to apply to the incision area to keep it from becoming dry and flaky—and to help it blend in with normal skin so it won't be quite as obvious. Also, we use it as a conducting agent for Ultrasound® and massage.

"While we don't feel it is a panacea for all problems, it is of definite benefit as an adjunct to modalities we would normally use to help the patient to progress more quickly."[2]

While director of the North Texas Sports Medical clinic, Gardner routinely used our Aloe Vera for such conditions as muscle or ligament injuries, cuts, scrapes, and both cutaneous challenges and muscle tissue damage. Both Gardner and Frank Medina provided us with extensive trainers' reports on a number of uses in which our Aloe Vera rated superior to any other modality of use.

Physicians' and trainers' reports are often based in patient studies that number in the hundreds and even thousands of cases. They measure such important qualities such as penetration, rate of healing, recovery time, antiseptic qualities, wound repair, pain relief, bactericidal and fungicidal properties, anti-inflammatory capabilities, improved penetration and other comparative analyses.

In the case of trainers' reports, the trainers in question showed especially positive results in such areas as turf burns, contusions, abrasions, fractures, strains, sprains, dislocations, tendonitis, and secondary infections. In most cases of application, the Aloe Action products showed superior results when compared to any other modality of healing.

It is these reports that we are able to submit to health oversight bodies such as the FDA for their scrutiny and approval. Fortunately, over the years, we've been able to make use of reports by such professionals like Frank Medina and Larry Gardner, as well as those by scores of doctors and trainers in similar fields to achieve increased credibility for Aloe Vera. We have also been able to establish appropriate toxicology measurements for these products—professional yardsticks by which all approved means of treatment are measured before they can be considered viable pharmaceutical quality healants.

I was made aware of the necessity of these reports early in my attempts to offer these products to the world of athletics in 1968, when I first visited Southern Methodist University and met their head trainer Eddie Lane.

Even though Lane, had personally experienced a remarkable episode even as we were initially discussing the product, the presiding physician responsible for SMU's athletes still declined to approve our Aloe for use.***

"I know Mr. Lane would like to use these products. I know he believes they work. But I'm responsible for the health of these kids, and as far as I know you have no toxicity studies on them. Without those studies, I can't allow them to be used on this campus."

As there are tipping points in the progress of all things, this occasion provided me with the incentive to proceed at all costs to undertake whatever toxicity studies and laboratory studies necessary to see to it that our stabilized Aloe Vera products received the kind of validation it needed to be accepted as viable pharmaceutical grade broad-spectrum healants.

As we will soon show in our next Chapter, "Major Milestones," Aloe Vera not only exhibits low relative toxicity, it also possesses an LD50 (kill) ratio that is no more than that of tap water.†

Having gathered momentum for our Aloe Action products, we continued to work with trainers and physicians in all areas of the sports world. Some of our most enduring relationships came to be with a number of professional football teams in the NFL, notably the Dallas Cowboys, the (then) Baltimore Colts, and the Arizona Cardinals. Since the Dallas Cowboys are virtually in our backyard, we have particularly enjoyed a strong working relationship over the years with "America's Team,"

*** When I first met with Eddie Lane in 1968, he told me he'd just severely bruised his wrist cutting wood on the weekend. "As you can see, it's sore. It's inflamed. It's swollen." He demonstrated for me. I gave him some Aloe Vera lotion and showed him how to rub it into his hand and wrist. Later as we discussed the product line, he stopped me after three minutes and marveled. "I can't believe it, but the pain is going away!" So, I knew I had a convert in the making.

† LD50s are an unfortunate but necessary process of "animal" testing, in which rats or other lab animals are exposed to what are referred to as "kill-ratios." In other words, they're orally administered enough dosage of a product to kill them. In the case of Aloe Vera no kill ratio has ever been established. It is virtually harmless.

Without a doubt, our earliest exposure to the Cowboys over the years came when I was introduced to then Cowboy running back, Dan Reeves as early as 1968.

A star all-purpose offensive standout for the NFC East Champion Cowboys, Dan had been in one of my pharmacies at the time with a badly sprained ankle he had sprained while playing in a charity basketball game. In fact, when I first met him, he was in the doctor's lounge of my office building and was barely able to stand on his ankle. At the time, the only product I had that would match his needs was a product called Aloe 99 Cream. I showed him how to apply the cream to his ankle and left him in the doctors' lounge for a few minutes to take a call. When I returned ten minutes later, I found Dan bouncing up and down on the sprained ankle.

Reeves was elated and returned to practice a couple of days later. When he did, I supplied him with a jar of the cream with the request that he introduce it to the Cowboy training staff. He promised he would. But when I went out to the Cowboy's field house a few days later to follow up on my presentation, I found that none of them had ever heard either of the product or me. When I asked Dan about it, he quipped lightheartedly: "This stuff's too good. I'm not about to share it with any of those jokers." ††

More amused than taken aback by this experience, we pressed on in 1977 until our products finally became a treatment of choice inside the Cowboy's training regimen.

One of the most consistent proponents of stabilized Aloe Vera was longtime Cowboy trainer Ken Locker.

In the past, Ken had used our Aloe products for a number of conditions, including sprains, strains, turf burns, Achilles tendonitis, hyper-extended joints, muscle spasms, and to hasten recovery from a long list of injuries.

In 1982 when we decided to make a film defining the benefits of Aloe Vera in treating athletes, Ken volunteered a couple of Cowboy starters for the filming. To our surprise, one of the "starters" he brought us was four time pro-bowler, Charlie Waters.

---

†† After his playing career ended, Dan Reeves went into coaching and later became head coach of the Denver Broncos and the Atlanta Falcons. His record as a head coach has included 33 playoff appearances and ten Super Bowls (five as a Cowboy player and assistant coach).

There are a lot of fine athletes in the NFL and with the Cowboys, but few are as personable or have the movie-star good looks of Charlie Waters. Not only was a perennial all-star, he was also very well spoken, and in this case had chosen to bring his endorsement down on the side of our Aloe Action products.

I found this remarkable, because on the same field at the same time, a major soft drink company was paying a number of Cowboy players $2000 a person just to jump in front of the camera and drink their product.

Charlie Waters, who could have charged a nice fee for such an endorsement, had chosen instead to volunteer his time and bring his leverage to bear on our behalf. His reason? He had achieved such remarkable results from using our Aloe Vera product that he thought it was important to the sport and to his fellow athletes to share the news.

In the video Ken Locker and Charlie Waters showed how quickly they had brought Waters' injured thumb back from a severe sprain by using a very special Aloe Action regimen:

First, the thumb was wrapped with a pad of cotton gauze soaked in Aloe Action Gel, and applied in a way that enabled the whole area to be soaked in the gel. Then the thumb was wrapped in roller gauze, which accomplished two things: 1) it held the gel-soaked gauze pack directly on the injured areas; 2) it also assured some immobilization of the joint. The cotton gauze was then wrapped with some elastic to give further support to the area and allow the thumb the rest that it needed for more rapid recovery. Locker explained that he usually undertook this procedure just before he sent the player home at night. That way, he could leave the pack on until he removed it the following day.

By that time, Charlie Waters had become very innovative in his own use of the product for a number of functions, and had this to say:

"It's helped me in a number of ways—especially on places such as the finger and foot joints. Also I had some bruises and the Aloe Vera pack was quick to show results."

Even though Charlie's thumb injury had been severe, he was able to return to action before a knee injury in the team's final exhibition game of 1982 ended his career.

Keeping the athlete injury free and on the field is the primary objective of any trainer. And no episode emphasizes that more strongly than a call I received from the (then) Baltimore Colt's head trainer Mike O'Shea, regarding his kicker David Lee. Previously, Lee's leg had been so sore that he could not kick at all, and worse. He couldn't even work out. O'Shea reported that he had wrapped lee's leg with gauze saturated with our Aloe Vera liquid (gel) and followed it with gentle massages with our lotion. He repeated the therapy three times a day, and by game time on the following Sunday was able to clear David Lee to play. Lee responded not only by playing but also by clocking in one of his all—time best performances. The two men called me on the following Monday, and Lee was still in a state of amazement: "I wouldn't have believed it myself. But it was my leg!"

When we made our film promoting the importance of Aloe Vera in the treatment of Athletic injuries, Mike O'Shea was one of the first trainers to volunteer:

"I was introduced to Aloe Action Products…a couple of years ago, and was totally amazed by the effectiveness of these products. The gel is one of my favorites because it does so many things so well. I for one use it by saturating a gauze roll with the gel and putting it on the affected area two or three times a day. I give the athlete a small jar of Gel and a few gauze rolls and tell him to apply it at night…I have used this especially on the extremities—the toes and fingers. When a player has had a sprain or even a fracture, I'm amazed at the way the pain and discoloration are consistently reduced in a three to four day period…I can only say that I am a firm believer in these products. I truly believe that if he uses the products properly the athletic trainer will get the same results I have gotten in the past two years."[3]

Since this report and his enthusiastic endorsement of our Aloe Vera, Mike has moved on in his career and became head trainer for the University of Louisville in Kentucky where stabilized Aloe Vera continued to be one of the mainstay therapies he uses to treat his athletes. Now, as head trainer at the University of Houston, he still uses our Aloe products routinely to this day.

As we live in a world of virtual corporations and supra communications, it is possible to establish and maintain professional relationships all over the world without actually ever meeting people in person. So, in this era of the virtual corporation, electronic "friendship" become part of the stew of technology.

This had been the case with Mike O'Shea. I've never met Mike personally. But were I to do so, I would have to thank him beyond all measure for the work he has done to promote Aloe Vera in the world of professional football and other sports. I hope this retrospective can extend yet another verbal handshake to replace the personal one we've not quite made…at least not yet.

Sometimes, contrary popular to Biblical cliché, a prophet is heard in his own land. And I'm happy to say that many of the longest term relationships we've enjoyed in the world of sports have been with organizations in the southwestern United States. This is particularly true of the University of Texas.

After Frank Medina retired as Head Trainer at the University of Texas, his successor Spanky Stephens carried on the tradition of cutting-edge therapies and modalities of healing that were definitely ahead of the curve of health technology.

As passionate a proponent of Aloe Vera therapy for his athletes, Spanky, like Frank Medina, provided us with trainer's reports on hundreds of cases of athletes in more than a dozen sports at the University of Texas, all of whom benefited from extensive applications of the Aloe products that we were able to provide.

In summarizing his many positive experiences from using the silent healer, Spanky Stephens wrote us with the following observations:

> Aloe Action Products get fantastic and fast results on sprains and strains of muscles and tendons. These products are also great for turf burns, infections such as ingrown toenails, athlete's foot, and jock irritation. I use the gel in both my cold and hot whirlpools. I put it on all strains and sprains immediately. I have found that the Gel when used properly can take away swelling almost immediately. The 100% gel is a deeply penetrating solution that will draw any kind of substance that you want in to all affected areas. This is what is so great about the whole Aloe Action line—that these products and treatments derived from them are all deeply penetrating. By all the evidence we have, they will take anything into the area and heal it faster.
>
> These products are particularly good for massage and Ultrasound. They fight all kinds of fungus infections without burning the tissue involved. The lotion is also great as a sun screen. It also takes away the peeling and pain of sunburn.
>
> I feel that these are the best set of products ever to come out on the market in the athletic training and physical therapy field.[4]

Trainers like Spanky Stephens are hard pressed week in, week-out during all the seasons of sports to get their top athletes back into action, and yet to do so with the health and well-being of the athlete as a primary consideration.

A good friend, working associate, and co-author on our book *Healing Winners,* Spanky related one episode to me that underscores the broad-spectrum effectiveness of these products.

It was the week before the Texas/Oklahoma game in 1979. One of the longest standing rivalries in college athletics, the Texas/OU classic was a clash of Titans. Both teams had identical 3-0 records and a high national ranking in the polls. And both knew that a loss to the other would almost certainly strip the prospect of a national championship from their horizons.

By all appearances both teams were equally matched, except in one area—injuries. Oklahoma was relatively healthy. In relative terms, the University of Texas was not.

In the previous weeks' game, six starters for the University of Texas had been hurt and, given normal treatment regimes, were certain to be out for the contest with Oklahoma. All conference defensive back Johnny Johnson had suffered a deep thigh bruise. Starting offensive lineman Lawrence Sampleton had sustained a shoulder injury, as had starting guard Les Studdard. Two other players had severe groin pulls. A sixth had what has commonly become known as "turf toe." (Turf toe is a funny name for a very painful hyperextension of the ball of the foot, a peculiarity of playing on artificial turf; hence the name.)

Ordinarily these injuries, though routine, would take anywhere from ten days to three weeks to heal. This, however, was not an ordinary game. And fortunately for them, Spanky Stephens was able to resort to some extraordinary means of getting them back into action—our Aloe Action products.

No question, each injury presented its own set of unique challenges, and yet many of the same kind of injuries share a common ground of application. Since most of these were deep tissue injuries, Spanky came up with a special treatment using stabilized Aloe Vera frozen in an eight-ounce paper cup. He and his staff would apply the cup-frozen Aloe on the affected area, tearing away the cup to the Aloe ice level until the contents had melted entirely. After allowing the "aloe ice" to penetrate deeply into the tissue, the training staff would follow with a massage of Aloe Vera Lotion or Liniment, rubbing gently for minutes at a time. Finally, they would follow with a regimen of Aloe Vera wraps.

They followed this procedure several times a day for the first three days of the week, with the anticipation that they would have to continue it up to game day, reviewing each condition on a day-to-day basis. But by Wednesday of the same week, Spanky Stephens and his staff of trainers knew they could cut back on the therapy sessions. By that time, all six starters had been able to return to full contact practice.

As a final testament to the success of that treatment, Texas beat Oklahoma 16 to 7 in what many described as the game of the decade.

In fact, it was a marvelous accomplishment. In truth, Spanky Stephens was delighted, but not all that surprised with the result. Frankly, neither was I. By then, we had been through a history of healing that went back for years and would continue for years to come.

It was another example, albeit a striking one, of what can be accomplished through the miracle of Aloe Vera.

It is important to emphasize here that our Aloe Action line of products, viable though they were, were developed in the early 1970s. Certainly, we stand by the efficacy and potency of all our products and acknowledge these formulations for all their remarkable contributions to the world of sports at the time. But in terms of product research, development, and refinement, we've risen considerably on the evolutionary scale since then.

All the more reason that, today, more than ever before, our whole-leaf process is a bona fide alternative to any other treatment or therapy offered to athletes in all fields of sports. Whether they are Olympic medalists or weekend joggers, they can benefit from using properly presented Aloe Vera products such as the ones we have just discussed.

Summary. The Sports World of 2020.

What we have hoped to unfold in this chapter is a journey—one that has neither begun nor ended. It is in process and, in a way, at a crossroads.

Today, public expectations for peak performance from world class athletes are at levels that are almost ballistic. We have created a super race of super heroes that almost beggar description to contemplate. Seven foot NBA basketball players are now expected to run the floor and knock down at least 40 points a game. A lineman in the NFL who weighs 300 pounds is considered average, and the median height for a pro quarterback is now six foot four. Women Olympic runners are on the verge of breaking the 4 minute mile, and our distaff tennis professionals are routinely slamming down 100 mph serves at Wimbledon and the U.S. Open. In baseball, growth hormone enhanced multimillionaire ball players are jacking juiced balls over shortened fences and creating home-run records that are now beginning to seem routine. Weight rooms are filled with athletes of all kinds who will undertake any nutrient, drug or oral stimulant to keep them at the top of their game.

These athletes are being paid astronomical salaries and are being watched by a public that is neither particularly sympathetic nor tolerant of their shortcomings. Excellence in performance is not expected, it is now demanded. And heaven help the professional or college athlete who falls short of the demands now placed on them.

In such cases, injuries and incapacitation are not only feared, they are dreaded as death knells to an athlete's career.

There is an irony in this, because much of that need for personal bests and the supreme sacrifice that accompanies them has trickled down into the world of the weekend athlete. Little League soccer and basketball games have become venues for fierce competitions, parental fist fights, and muggings of officials who make bad calls. Pre-teen children are being treated for injury and gotten back onto the field of play with the same ruthless efficiency as one might find in a college training room.

Joggers and flag footballers are putting themselves back into action, playing even when hurt. And the recreational weekend athletes in America—all 68 million of them!—are now more intent than ever upon keeping fit, no matter what the cost.

This kind of obsession with excellence pleads for both perspective and understanding. It also cries out for help. And it brings an issue into focus, at least for me, that more than ever before, we need a safe, broad-spectrum, universally reliable healant. It should be a family of products that all athletes, whether they're NBA forwards or in local recreational leagues, can use and benefit from.

We have created these products—specially formulated whole leaf Aloe Vera gels, gellies, lotions, liniments and creams—and yet realize that the challenge that now remains is one of education. We have to work harder to heighten the awareness of sports professionals and amateurs alike regarding the need for the right kind of Aloe Vera in their lives.

After forty years in the business, one of the most poignant recollections I have is in the time I've shared with friends in the sports field. Men like Ken Locker, Eddie Lane, Kevin O'Neill, Mike O'Shea and Spanky Stephens still work to serve in their relative fields of expertise.

Old friends like Frank Medina and Dr. Richard Russell—giants in their respective profession of sports medicine and medical practice—are no longer with us. And yet their words still echo home to me like truth itself.

"If I can make these (Aloe Vera) products a household word, no other act would help my profession more." Frank's words, repeated here, still place upon me the welcome burden of completion. What others did to help begin, it is our intention to finish in our lifetime. So it is our pledge to help make Aloe Vera a commonly embraced term, "the treatment of choice" for athletes everywhere. Considering the fact that millions will benefit from that decision, we could do no less.

Chapter 4

Major Milestones

It is an inviolate truth where medications of any kind are concerned: Validation can only come through the labyrinth of scientific approval. The progress of Aloe Vera can best be charted through the clinical tests that have helped validate the healing plant either through in vitro studies or sheer force of numbers. The following are our "Magnificent Seven" Major Milestones in the growth and development of the plant many scientific proponents still refer to as "Nature's Pharmacy."

It has been said of the world of science that what often begins as heresy ends as superstition. When you think about it, the observation is a paradox that makes absolute sense.

So much of what we accomplish in the way of discovery is usually due to the work of a handful of visionaries who are willing to wade through a sea of indifference to prove what they already know in their hearts to be true. This requires experiment, but experiment with a purpose—that which can be justified both by force of numbers and an intensity of correctness.

Proof positive! By its own description that means proof acquired by unimpeachable means that can be accepted by all bodies of review. The secret lies in finding the unimpeachable means. And that is often easier said than done.

In so many ways throughout the history of Aloe Vera's growth and development, it has been victimized by anecdotes. Dramatic, sensationalist, seemingly outrageous at times, they seem to come in droves (and we've been guilty of our fair share of them). Even though most of them are true, and even though we've experienced many of them firsthand ourselves, they all fall short in light of the disciplined laboratory tests that have served the truth so well.

What we intend to do in this chapter is to underscore Aloe Vera's remarkable range and curative depth of character by picking what we believe are the seven most significant breakthroughs for the healing plant.

It is important to note here that these breakthroughs have all been accomplished in established, detailed examinations either in the laboratories or in clinical studies with volunteer groups of patients. Most of them carry sufficient force of numbers to rate as qualifying studies in themselves. Others have led us to what clinicians refer to as "meriting further study." But in all cases, the verdicts come clearly and unequivocally.

Although the majority of the breakthroughs can be found to have been in areas of treatment and cure or application against a specific pathogen, we also felt it necessary to address issues such as toxicology, tissue penetration, absorption and the process of stabilization itself. Without having made progress in these three areas, the curative results achieved would have been rendered moot, and we'd all be fighting a losing battle to establish the plant's identity.

With all this in mind, we now offer our "Magnificent Seven" all time Aloe Vera breakthroughs. We do so by leading with the end result as our headline for each category. We also list them, though not necessarily in order of importance, in logical sequence. As such, we refer to our first three breakthroughs not so much as those of curative phenomena as a necessary legitimization of all that Aloe Vera is.

1) Proof positive: Aloe Vera is virtually non-toxic.

We address this as the most significant issue regarding Aloe Vera, or any healant for that matter. It addresses itself to the "Prime Directive" of the Hippocratic Oath: *First, do no harm.*

Against this resounding echo of integrity all measures of treatment must be taken. It is curative Genesis. It is the physician's first commandment. And unfortunately, it has become the one that is most frequently broken, often despite all attempts to do otherwise.

In our Chapter 1, "The New Face of World Health," we touched upon the breach that was forming between patient trust and the ability of both medical practitioners and medications to continue to hold their confidence. And it has been a timeless concern that often—too often—the purported cure has been more dangerous than the disease itself.

The fact that modern pharmacology is now under fire is best illustrated by the fact that over 30% of all patients on prescription drugs have reported unpleasant side effects from minor nausea to violent trauma and allergic reactions. This level is unacceptably high, and has caused justifiable alarm among major health organizations.

Despite all the toxicology tests that major pharmaceutical companies conduct, allegedly to prevent these kinds of occurrences, they seem to be on the increase. And yet they've always been with us. Some drugs such as Thalidomide and Fen fen have proven to be so deleterious as to have been forcibly been removed from production. Others such as Valium and AZT continue to be administered despite volumes of study and patient reports showing them to be addictive, ultimately debilitative, or excessively toxic to those who use them over protracted periods of time.

Unfortunately, there persists in the mindset of "traditional medicine" that, in order for a drug to be effective, it must carry with it high degrees of relative toxicity. This bias is not only flawed, it is becoming increasingly disastrous. More and more health professionals have now come to accept a more nutritive approach to treating disease, one that rebuilds immune systems rather than tearing them down. For that reason, alternative therapies like Aloe Vera are now beginning to look more attractive than ever to allopaths, osteopaths, and holistic practitioners alike partly because the healing plant is, above all else, perceived as both effective and harmless.

Whatever else in this book we are able to illustrate about Aloe Vera, we believe we will be able to show, unequivocally, that both Aloe Vera and properly stabilized products from the plant exhibit no relative toxicity. And we like to believe we have played our small part in establishing that very important aspect of its credibility.

It is important to note that some elements in Aloe Vera such as the anthraquinones and even some enzymes can be toxic if isolated and used in excessive quantities. And yet in the symphony of synergism that takes place inside the complex chemistry of Aloe Vera, they exhibit no such toxicity. There is data to support this, and it has come to us in a number of ways.

We explained briefly in Chapter 2, "Aloe Vera: Q &A," about what are referred to in research circles as LD50s or animal kill ratios in laboratories and their impact on the measurable toxicity of Aloe Vera. And it is here that we have to express our philosophy about (necessary) lab experiments on our animal friends. Personally, we dislike them. We feel no creature on earth should be subjected to unnecessary tests just to satisfy someone's intellectual curiosity.

Whenever possible, we will undertake *in vitro* (test tube or Petri dish) tests to establish our findings about an aspect of Aloe Vera. At least 90% of the time, they work as well as *in vivo* (live subject) studies.

Having made this point, we also acknowledge that there are bodies of tests, dictated by government health agencies, that require us to test on laboratory animals such as rats, hamsters, rabbits, dogs, and small primates such as monkeys. Invariably, toxicology tests require kill ratio animal sacrifice. Those are the rules of the game. The FDA sets them, and we must all play or risk disenfranchisement for our products.

That's the bad news.

The good news where Aloe Vera is concerned is that they're virtually never killed because apparently Aloe Vera only knows how to heal.

Basically, there are two kinds of LD50 kill ratios. One is internal. The other is topical. Taken internally, the test animals are fed oral doses often up to as high as 200 times the normal daily dosage. In instances where topical applications are to be tested, the test animals are exposed to dosage ratios high enough to induce advanced levels of irritation or, when applicable, death from irritation. In view of these criteria, the enumerations of Aloe Vera's non-toxicity are exceptional and, at this point, unfailing.

A number of tests in modern history examined the apparent lack of toxicity in Aloe Vera. But three tests in particular went a long way in helping to establish the relative lack of toxicity of the healing plant, as well as a number of products derived from it.

The first toxicology tests of which are aware were conducted by Lakeland Laboratories of Dallas, Texas in 1966. Under our sponsorship, Lakeland conducted dermal tissue experiments as well as oral dosage tests on 20 test rabbits. After thorough testing, Drs. Henry Cobble and Mervin Grossman found no toxicity in the vital organs, muscle tissue or skin of any of the animals subjected to testing. There was some minimal weight loss incurred upon the rabbits subjected to oral doses, but even that was considered normal due to a lack of other nutrients necessarily denied the subjects during the course of the test. Most important to note is that, even in extremely high doses, the toxicity was too insignificant even to record.

Another independent study in 1968 was conducted simultaneously at Brooke General Hospital in Fort Sam Houston, Texas and at the well-known Baylor University College of Dentistry in Dallas. In this study, Eugene Zimmermann, D.D.S. (chief pathologist at Baylor), Dr. James Brasher, and Dr. C.K. Collings studied the effects of Aloe Vera gel on tissue culture cells. In this case, the tissue cells were extracted from what are called rabbit kidney fibroblasts and were highly sensitive to irritation of any kind.

In these Brasher, Zimmermann and Collings tests stabilized Aloe Vera was tested against two potent medicants—*Indomethacin* and *Prednisolone*. Indomethacin, like Aloe Vera, was purported to possess strong analgesic properties, as well as being an effective antipruritic. (In other words, it stopped itching and irritations from itching.) Prednisolone was the pilot designation for what has come to be known as Prednisone, a potent corticosteroid still prevalent as a pre-scription anti-inflammatory 35 years later.

Not surprisingly, Aloe Vera showed itself to be a far better analgesic and antipruritic than Indomethacin, and a superior anti-inflammatory to Prednisolone while proving unilaterally better than either.

Additionally when tested against special cell cultures, Aloe Vera revealed a capacity for stimulating reproduction of healthy tissue that, in a 72-hour period, proved to be nearly twelve times that of Indomethacin and more than seven times that of Prednisolone.

More important for our purposes here, is the lack of toxicity the Aloe also dis-played. When tested for toxicity in tissue culture studies, the Aloe Vera showed none whatsoever. At the same time both the Indomethacin and (especially) the Prednisolone proved highly toxic to the test animals subjected to the necessary megadoses of the drugs.

These tests not only confirmed our findings in 1966, but finally prompted what we feel to be a landmark study in 1968. At our behest and under our spon-sorship, Hazelton Laboratories in Falls Church, Virginia conducted a series of animal tests at three levels. Supervised and coordinated by Hazelton's Chief Pathologist, William M. Busey, M.D. over 80 test animals were subjected extreme LD50s according to the following criteria:

1). Acute oral administrations on 60 test rats. These were given more than 21.5 g/kg, an extremely high dose.

2). Acute oral administrations to eight test dogs—acute oral doses administered by stomach tube at 31 g/kg, also an extremely high dose.

3). Acute dermal administrations to 12 test (white) rabbits at 10 g/kg of body weight, also considered a maximum level for dermal appli-cations of this kind.

All three groups were exposed to extremely high dose levels for fourteen days and then evaluated at that time. In all three cases, the ensuing results were unequivocally benign:

• In the acute oral application to the rats, there were no recorded deaths or even severe reactions to the administrations.

• In the acute oral administrations to the dogs, there were no LD50s or kill-ratios achieved.

• In the acute dermal tests of the rabbits, dermal irritation was min-imal and non-progressive; in other words, easily healed.

What's more, the Aloe Vera products tested were determined to be of very high quality and free of any kind of detractive bacteria.

There have been other toxicology studies made since our original reports in the late 1960s, notably a series of independent Acute Oral Toxicity Studies conducted by Dawson Research Corporation in 1977 and again in 1981. Those were followed by acute dermal studies and further acute oral studies in 1982 and 1983. And though their results were slightly less emphatic (we feel partly due to the Aloe samples used), these like others have been largely supportive of our findings. But none have been more definitive than the ones in which we participated. None show the clear force of numbers. Nor do any more clearly define the resolute potential of Aloe Vera to help generate the perfect curative environment for whatever pathology it is brought in to treat.

We have often compared it in levels of toxicity to common tap water. At this point, we might even be so bold as to say that it ranks even higher on the scale than that. Given some of the failing grades some municipal water systems have been given in recent years, we might have to make our comparisons on a city by city basis.

As regards the future of Aloe Vera in a pharmaceutical context, the implications for this are extraordinary. Ordinarily, prescription and OTC drugs carry warnings not to exceed dosage limits. Especially in the case of prescription drugs, exceeding recommended dosage can bring on severe toxic reactions, especially over extended use.

With a GRAS qualification (Generally Regarded As Safe) for pharmaceutical grade Aloe Vera, our dosage levels are recommended. They are not bracketed with warnings, because even at higher levels of use, the products are virtually nontoxic. Purely in terms of addressing all the uses soon to be put to it, nothing could proffer a brighter future for the healing plant than the kind of validation found in these tests. If nothing else, they helped construct a platform for acceptability that would last for the next 35 years and that, even in this new millennium, provides us all with a safe field upon which to play.

Having laid this groundwork, we also add a caveat. We must all play by the rules. Just slapping the name "Aloe Vera" on a product neither guarantees its efficacy nor its relative lack of toxicity. All products that claim 50% or more Aloe Vera content should adhere to the strictest testing criteria for toxicity. They should be willing to submit to toxicology tests and to present them with their other data for approval both by governing bodies and by the public at large. It is then, and only then, that Aloe will continue to sustain the professional credibility it is at last beginning to enjoy.

2) The Power of Penetration.

Perhaps the most important aspect of any drug, healant, or nutritional element lies in its ability to penetrate tissue and get to the core of the trauma where primary healing takes place. Its power of penetration presages proper cell division. It speeds up the healing process and accelerates wound repair.

Although, after forty years of intense research and discovery, we still stand in awe of Aloe Vera's complex chemistry, we do understand that its enzymatic activity carries much of its healing potential. We also now realize that the Aloe polysaccharides carry so much of the penetrating power in the plant and products formed from it—that they are the phytochemical messengers carrying with them the cellular "news" of nutrition and healing to the body that cries out for it.

We also know that, along with them, there resides a super messenger—a bullet train—as it were that speeds the message along its way. That element is *lignin.*

Very early studies in the modern history of Aloe Vera, such as those of Chopia and Gosh in 1938, expressed their conclusion that the lignin in the Aloe Vera complex was the carrying agent for the plant's complex chemistry. Since on its own lignin exhibits an uncanny ability to penetrate the human skin, the opinion was a sound one. Subsequent findings, including many by Ivan Danhof in the 1990s have borne this out, but none delivered penetrative potency to the extent to which the lignin plays its role in the "sweet symphony" of Aloe Vera's complex chemistry. And the question constantly arises: Is it a virtuoso performer? Or is it merely another piece in the harmony.

It is a matter of intelligent extrapolation that tissue that responds rapidly to a healant is going to be the beneficiary of remarkable penetration, and Aloe's penetrative powers have long been a given. With both the enzymatic activity and the Aloe polysaccharides being credited as carrying agents for the plants curative powers, there has long remained the unanswered issue of laboratory proof. Just how potent is the presence of lignin in the plant? And can this kind of penetration be measured empirically?

(Unofficially, in 1969 I ran an empirical test with four of my staff members to test Aloe Vera's powers of penetration. Using a bitter compound called glycerol glycolate in combination with our own Aloe Vera gelly, we rubbed a paste onto our wrists and were able to taste the bitter substance in our mouths within ten minutes. Ordinarily, this substance will not reveal its presence in anything less than an hour, if it shows itself at all.)

A large measure of clinical proof of Aloe's penetrating power came in a laboratory study in 1997 conducted by Robert H. Davis, Ph.D. While he lived, Dr. Davis was inarguably one of Aloe Vera's most articulate and respected apologists.

No one did more to espouse the cause of the healing plant or more to establish its credibility. His tests number in legion. Virtually all of them have great merit. And every one of them deserves serious consideration.

Professor of Physiology at the Pennsylvania School of Podiatric Medicine, Dr. Davis led a series of laboratory tests in which he helped validate Aloe Vera's abilities as a major factor in wound healing, anti-inflammatory activity, and power of penetration.

In a book he authored in 2000, *Aloe Vera/A Scientific Approach*, Dr. Davis devoted a very pivotal chapter entitled "Aloe Vera and Aspirin" to report a schedule of tests in which he administered oral doses of Aloe Vera in combination with a single aspirin in order to see how quickly it would penetrate the cellular linings of the stomach and get into the system.

Aspirin is and probably always will be the number one OTC drug in the world, simply because it is so effective. It has often been observed that, were aspirin brought into the pharmaceutical marketplace today, it would probably have to be sold by prescription. As an analgesic it has already proven its worth as a broad-spectrum painkiller. As an anti-inflammatory it is a reasonable short term palliative. And tests in recent years have proven that, taken in a very small daily dose, it does seem to help reduce arterial plaque and limit the user's susceptibility to heart attack.

Originally formulated from willow bark (in a much purer expression of its potency), aspirin is now mass-produced from simple inexpensive salicylate solution.

Traditionally, simple aspirin it its native form can be highly effective, provided it is given the proper forum for absorption and can be administered in ways that precludes its potentials for repercussive toxicity, especially when used at high doses.

Since aspirin, like all analgesics, must pass through the (GI) gastrointestinal tract, it is often late getting into the human system and works as a vasoconstrictor. Sometimes the effect of the aspirin can take as much as half an hour to an hour to take effect. And since both absorption and relative toxicity can become an issue, the more quickly aspirin can be blood-booted into the system, the less wear and tear there will be on the liver. (The liver is the body's principal disburser of toxins. All medications carry certain toxic implications. Usually the stronger the medication, the greater the toxicity. So, the wages of frequent aspirin usage can take a toll on the liver.)

> If Aloe Vera was additive or synergistic with aspirin on inflammation or analgesia, we could use Aloe as a 'biological vehicle' for aspirin. The dosage of aspirin could be reduced to eliminate the side effects as well as increase the absorption of aspirin.[5]

With that in mind, Dr. Davis set up a series of control group tests to establish a number of criteria to prove the efficacy of aspirin and Aloe Vera's positive effect on it.

Focusing on that set of objectives, Robert Davis set up a series of tests to determine the following:

a) Cardiovascular disease, aspirin and Aloe. In a Foot Blood Flow test with 5 male subjects, four out of the five showed improved blood flow with the Aloe Vera and aspirin combination, as opposed to 5 men in pre-test controls. (The subjects showed nearly double the foot blood flow and vasodilation than the pre-test controls using only aspirin.)

b) Inflammation, whole leaf aloe vera and aspirin. Topical tests of whole leaf Aloe Vera and aspirin revealed that the Aloe Vera had an additive and synergistic effect on reducing inflammation in 10 test mice, which showed that Aloe Vera was nearly 75% more effective than the aspirin when used on its own, and more than 80% more effective than the Aloe Vera when used on its own.

c) Anti-inflammatory Activity of Whole Leaf Aloe Vera and Aspirin on 2% Carrageenan-induced Paw Edema. (Paw edemas are laboratory-induced inflammations of tissue.) In this test, 10 male rats with inflammation were injected with subcutaneous doses of 1)Aloe, 2) aspirin, and 3) an Aloe-aspirin combined solution. The combination of the Aloe Vera and aspirin solution proved nearly 60% better as an anti-inflammatory than the aspirin when used on its own, and more than twice as effective as the Aloe used on its own.

d) A Test of Aspirin's Analgesic Effects "when combined with Whole Leaf Aloe." A test group of 12 test rats showed a pain-relief response that was 300 times more effective than the placebo (saline) control group of mice, and 50% more effective than the group treated with aspirin alone.

In his conclusions, Dr. Davis figuratively tipped his hat to aspirin by noting that aspirin can help to prevent strokes, heart attacks, blockage of blood vessels, inflammation and cascades of negative (PGE2) prostaglandins to reduce pain. He also concluded unequivocally that, in his tests he was convinced that Aloe Vera given with aspirin increases the biological activity and absorption of the aspirin in ways that enable the doses of aspirin can be reduced, and with it the relative toxicity.[8]

No question, these findings were a milestone of discovery, one of many in which Dr. Robert Davis was a functionary.

And it has now been given further validation through a study by a group of noted research scientists from the University of Scranton in Pennsylvania. In a test recently reporting the "Effect of Aloe Vera preparations on the human bioavailability of Vitamins C and E," Doctors Joe A. Vinson, Hassan Al Kharrat and Lori Andreoli selected "the two most popular vitamins found in supplements" as subjects for their test.

Whether this was intentional or not, we note that this team of doctors also selected both vitamin C and vitamin E in forms that have long been determined to be their least bioavailable—ascorbic acid (for vitamin C) and alpha tocopherol acetate (for vitamin E). Both are synthetic forms of the vitamins as opposed to natural presentations such as Ester C and natural extractions of alpha tocopherol from plant sources.

In the test the "plasma bioavailablity" for the two vitamins was determined in eight fasting subjects for the vitamin C and ten fasting subjects for the vitamin E. In what is referred to as a *random crossover design* two test groups were subjected to two different presentations of Aloe—a whole leaf Aloe Vera preparation and a gel pulp Aloe preparation. The control group was fed doses of the (synthetic) vitamins only.

Although the two types of Aloe Vera scored mixed results in the degree of impact of their presentation, both showed score curves that were significantly higher than those of the vitamins when administered solely on their own. And in the research team concluded without reservation that both Aloes had a salutary effect on the absorption of these vitamins. Their conclusion in reviewing both types of Aloe Vera was uniform and complete:

"Aloe is unique in its ability to improve the absorption of both of these vitamins and should be considered as an adjunct for people who take these vitamins."[7]

Often due to the vagaries of different criteria for testing, the nuances of findings regarding the use of Aloe Vera may vary from test to test. But the bottom line is almost invariable. Aloe Vera's contributions to absorption are invaluable. Its function in an adjunctive role to other kinds of both nutrient and medication remains unimpeached. In purely therapeutic terms, Aloe may prove to be the ultimate team player—one that facilitates the process of healing, repair, and the elevation of potential for good.

3) The Secrets of Stabilization.

It has become an irrefutable quality in dealing with Aloe Vera that products derived from it are only going to be as effective as proper stabilization will permit. Because of the powerful enzymatic activity of the plant, and because of the presence of highly potent but proportionately perishable Aloe polysaccharides in the native plant, proper stabilization has been an ongoing challenge. No one is more aware of that paradox than I. Ever since original attempts to commercially process and market Aloe Vera in this country took place in the 1930s, manufacturers have been hard-pressed to come up with a stabilization formula that could capture Aloe Vera's intricate balance and keep its potency intact.*

In the 1960s, both billionaire H.L. Hunt and entrepreneur and former owner of Braniff Airlines, Troy Post, paid millions to formulate and market their own separate brands of stabilized Aloe Vera products for the mass market. Both failed miserably in the attempt. Add their names to a long list of wealthy, well-intended individuals and investment groups who have attempted to come up with efficacious, effective, and stable Aloe Products for the mass market. They often try but seldom succeed, and soon go out of business. We have a list of names that would make a Who's Who of American business. Usually this is due to the fact that both the research labs and the manufacturers who often sponsor them address themselves to the wrong set of criteria. And if we have learned anything in trying to solve Aloe's complex chemistry over the last four decades we have arrived at a least two conclusions:

a. When it comes to capturing its complex chemistry, Aloe Vera is a "paradox, wrapped in a puzzlement, cloaked in an enigma."**

b. Even when you leverage your efforts against the wrong criteria, you still are able to create a product that works.

We have faced both prospects, and still manage to be amazed. Because after forty years of working to master the perfect formulation for a commercially processed pharmaceutical grade Aloe Vera, we still find ourselves in a constant state of discovery.

The issue of challenge lies in its delicate chemistry and the fact that it can be so easily violated. Boiling the gel kills the potency. Even pasteurization severely inhibits its potency. Improper cold processing often introduces an agent that is not approved by the FDA for oral consumption. All of these processes render a product that is of marginal potency, much in the way canned vegetables are of marginal potency. There are very few enzymes left unkilled to do their job, and Aloe Vera without enzymatic activity is a gun without bullets.

---

* In most early attempts at formulating commercial Aloe, the live bacteria that were not neutralized during an improper stabilization process often caused the product to explode on the shelves.

** We're paraphrasing here. The specific description matches what Winston Churchill once said when attempting to describe the Soviet Union—that it was a "paradox wrapped in a puzzlement cloaked in an enigma." The description always seemed to fit Aloe Vera, though for far less sinister reasons.

Despite what appears to be a maze of complication, there is a bright side to all of this. And that is that there are ways to successfully stabilize Aloe Vera. At times, I wondered if any formula we conceived could ever match the almost mystical eloquence of the plant itself. And I remember one instance in particular when I was visiting a well-to-do rancher and farmer in northern Mexico to inquire about using his Aloe Vera harvest as a source for our product. The rancher was showing me his magnificent acreage when one of his hands informed us that his prize registered bull had just been bitten by an enormous rattlesnake. Without wasting a moment, the rancher cut a large leaf from one of the Aloe Vera plants, split the leaf lengthwise, wrapped it in cloth, using the entire leaf, gel face to the wound, as a poultice. He left the poultice on the bull's foreleg overnight, and by the next morning when he removed the Aloe poultice, the creature's bite had healed. I remembered the severity of the snakebite and marveled at the curative power the Aloe poultice had shown when the leaf and gel were left in context.

Still, I continued to press on with my search for the right kind of stabilization formula that would help put Aloe Vera at least in some measure of credibility in the pharmaceutical marketplace.

To my everlasting gratitude, I was able to be a part of the first team to ever hit upon an effective, safe stabilization process for Aloe Vera in 1964. Working with a brilliant biochemist named Henry Cobble, we were able to create a low heat, molecule-trimming process that enabled the plant to keep a significant portion of its healing potency intact. Even though this process only worked to develop the mucilage or pulp in the plant itself, it still came to be a formula that, in test after test for the next 10 years, proved highly effective in killing the pathogens against which it was tested. It also managed to keep much of the plant's powers of penetration, anti-inflammatory activity, wound healing, and antiseptic capabilities at measurable levels of potency.

At the time, we believed that the curative potential in the Aloe Vera plant resided primarily, if not entirely, in the pulp or gel of the plant. We were wrong, and yet I never cease to be amazed that, even as flawed as our reasoning was during that period, we still managed to create an effective formula that is still in use by some major world marketers of Aloe Vera.

But our knowledge of the plant and how to make a better product from it has evolved to newer heights over the years. It has been accompanied by increased clinical scrutiny and new international standards for acceptability that have been set over the years. Although our formulation for stabilized Aloe Vera set the standard for nearly two decades, too many things had happened in the meantime to convince us that this was the ultimate formulation.

First, it had been determined by a number of researchers both in the U.S. and Japan that the anthraquinones aloin, Aloe emodin and emodin, although non-toxic in the complex chemistry of Aloe Vera, were indeed toxic on their own. Second, it was determined in one Japanese study that Aloin (already noted as an effective if violent purgative) was sufficiently toxic to prompt a severe restriction by the Health Ministry of Japan: that no Aloe Vera product containing more than 50 ppm of Aloin would be allowed for market in that country, even if sold under prescription.

Meanwhile, in 1987, I had begun work with another biochemist, Charlie Queen, to develop what appeared to be the first successful cold process formulation for stabilized Aloe Vera. Without revealing the innermost secrets of this successful formulation, I can tell you that it involved a unique combination of antioxidants and preservatives that worked synergistically to stop the oxidation and to kill the bacteria without destroying the enzymatic activity of the gel.

At the time, we believed the cold process to be infallible for a couple of reasons: It was our belief at the time that this cold process enabled us to work on a formulation that kept the potency of the Aloe polysaccharides at maximum levels of integrity. We also believed with some degree of justification that cooking at any level destroyed a great deal of the Aloe's nutritional potency.

Although this cold process has been copied by dozens of formulators since then, we eventually found the formula to be incomplete for a couple of reasons. First, it still addressed the curative powers as having been located in the gel. Although we now looked to a segment of the gel that was much closer to the rind, we were still committed to the gel as the primary carrier of Aloe's healing power. Second, no cold stabilization process that we could develop was able to properly extract the anthraquinones (specifically the now controversial aloin) from the gel. Third, we still had not learned all there was to know about the role the Aloe polysaccharides played in our activity mix and just how far the implications of their role as a carrying agent went.

Throughout the brief modern history of Aloe Vera, many eminent researchers who had delved into the plant's healing powers stated their belief that the secret of the true healing potency in the plant lies in the Aloe polysaccharides. And in 1994, a research group in Düsseldorf, Germany hit upon a set of findings that changed the way we would perceive the functionability of the plant from that day forward.

Up to that point, we had always been led to believe that fresh gel harvested and extracted directly from the plant and its meaty leaves would offer the most chemical potency, the highest level of enzymatic activity and presence of potently active Aloe polysaccharides. So, perhaps understandably, logic would dictate that the fresher the gel from the plant, the better the Aloe product. Such reasoning seemed irrefutable. In Nature, the laws of freshness invariably apply, and the healing plant, of all entities, should bear our that iron dogma. But as usual, we were about to be surprised. It was the Düsseldorf testing group's hypothesis that the largest concentrate of Aloe polysaccharides lay just under the outer portion of the leaf. It was further believed that there was a direct corollary between harvesting the leaf and the activity of the Aloe polysaccharides.

After several tests in which the whole leaf was removed from the plant and allowed to reseal, it was found that a remarkable process took place. In tests on scores of leaves, it was found that the moment the leaf is harvested from the mother plant, it will start diffusing a polysaccharide rich exudate from the entire surface directly under the leaf. In other words, the dismembered leaf in an attempt to seal itself (and therefore heal itself) will actually generate a quantity of Aloe polysaccharides that far exceeds the number found in the original leaf immediately after harvesting.

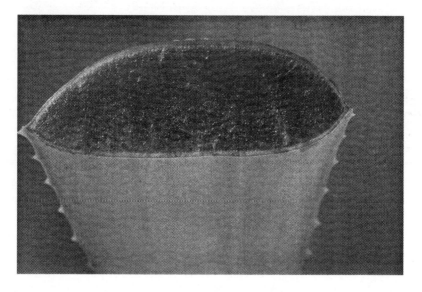

An Aloe Vera leaf approximately 3 hours after it has been harvested. Note: The leaf is already being sealed by the exudate and is beginning to "heal." It has now been recorded that, in this detached condition, the whole leaf is redistributing its Aloe polysaccharide content to work more synergistically.

The benefit in all of this is directly related to a process called *cell division*. And it is through cell division that all effective healing takes place. The more quickly and effectively cells divide, the more rapidly such natural body occurrences as wound healing, reduction of swelling, and tissue rebuilding take place. In truth the detached leaf that rushes healing to its own body of mucilage becomes the catalyst to the same healing process when it is introduced to the body of the human being or creature being treated. So, in the case of Aloe Vera, the plant that accelerates the healing process in itself has also learned to match that process when introduced to animal systems to which it is introduced.

This "detached leaf" phenomenon prompted some rethinking on our part. So, we decided to reexamine the issue. In the meantime, however, the issue was redressed for us. A number of clinical evaluations in the 1990s focused upon testing the plant's potency in the context of the whole leaf versus the gel from the leaf.

Some of the more significant ones were undertaken by a dear friend and working associate, Ivan Danhof, Ph.D. One paper in particular, "Aloe Vera. The Whole Leaf Advantage," written in 1995 underscored the remarkable curative potential that the whole leaf showed when used intact—leaf gel, rind, and exudate left unaltered and applied in kind actually optimized the healing potential of the plant.

In Dr. Danhof's studies, not only were tests conducted on detached Aloe Vera leaves that corroborated the findings of the Düsseldorf group's (1994) discoveries, his analysis of the curative potentials in the whole leaf also proved exceptional, if not infallible.

This prompted us to reintensify our efforts and to perfect what we now call a "whole-leaf stabilization process" for Aloe Vera. Given the sensitive nature of these new laboratory findings, we have to plead the cause of sensible secrecy in choosing not to disclose all the intricacies of this new method. There are simply too many important steps to the whole leaf stabilization process. Most of them entail an intricate balance that must be achieved to bring Aloe Vera its fullest level of expression in a product form. It is a balance we have achieved with past formulations. And yet in the current rise in emphasis on the healing plant, we bring our own formulations to a new level of curative potential.

Milestones are meted out with such rarity that occasionally we have to reevaluate our interpretation of what they truly mean. In the matter of stabilization, we feel there have been three. And we're happy to say that at some level we've been a part of them all.

We're even appreciative of the fact that a number of presentations of stabilized Aloe Vera today come from products that have either mimicked our own past formulas or copied them outright. We don't deny their potential for doing good work, however attenuated might be the potency they offer. Oftentimes, there is no limit to what this silent healer can do, even when limited in both quantity and potency.

What we do believe is that there should be no limitations to Aloe's potential. There is simply too much at stake. And in the evolution in the growth and development of the plant, there also resides the need for an evolution in consciousness. One can use old technologies to address new challenges in the new millennium wellness marketplace. But is that the best answer?

In an age where super viruses mutate and immunities build against outmoded antibiotics and untested palliatives, in our opinion we need all we can get. That means a new kind of Aloe Vera—a superhero curative made just for the new millennium and all the complex challenges that come with it.

From time to time, I remember my episode with the Mexican rancher, the prize bull and the poultice, and it is then that I realize that there are no accidents. That moment, in its way, was the message that I'd always been looking for: "It's in the leaf," it seemed to cry out. Finally, we got it. Once again, the whole is greater than the sum of its parts, just as God intended.

4) Healing the Heart.

By now we've learned in spades that heart health is 90% a matter of prevention. Proper diet, exercise, reduction of stress, the elimination of toxins, the regulating of LDL cholesterol, and (most of all) the lowering of triglycerides all play their part in creating a platform for a healthy heart.

Still, one can neither discount the perversities of genetics nor the cost of life in the high stress, high fat, fast track of modern times. With high-tension schedules, working moms, fast food restaurants, microwave meals and an annual intake of sugar that exceeds the weight of the average sized family golden retriever, we place leverage against our already overworked hearts that often boggle the mind to contemplate.

It's a terrifying truth: 63% of all deaths list heart failure as the primary cause. Knowing that heart disease, along with the atherosclerosis that often precedes it, is our number one killer, we as a nation are in constant pursuit of any corrective therapy, treatment or drug that will help combat it.

That's why we are delighted by a series of tests that will show how remarkable Aloe Vera has proven to be in its ability to lower LDL cholesterol and triglycerides as well as arterial plaque. And even though will also be able to show how this has helped many sufferers from the effects of angina pectoris and post-operative cardiovascular complications, we emphasize that not even Aloe Vera can make up for the excesses of an immoderate lifestyle.

We cannot emphasize strongly enough that the test we are about to reveal— impressive though it is—cannot be viewed as the ultimate cure-all for heart disease. Still, it can give hope to millions who are willing to embrace a healthy, sensible approach to living.

In an ambitious test that spanned five years from 1980 to 1985 an Indian physician, O.P. Agarwal of Uttar Pradesh, India set about establishing a test group study of 5,000 patients all of whom were suffering from varying degrees of *atheromatous heart disease.*

Atheromatous heart disease is a pronounced formation of plaque in the arteries, and is often initially expressed in the form of *angina pectoris*, a temporary but often painful throbbing in the chest accompanied by numbness in the extremities.

Atheromatous heart disease can be caused from a number of conditions, and many of the forms in which it presents itself are self-induced. Smoking, excessive intake of saturated fatty acids, obesity, lack of exercise and type 2 diabetes mellitus (often lifestyle induced) all wreak havoc with genetic predispositions toward this sort of disease, So do inclinations toward gout and hypertension, although both are alarm bell syndromes that can be immediately remedied by dramatic moderations in lifestyle.

Aware that atheromatous heart disease was on the rise worldwide, Dr. Agarwal began his study in 1980, using 5,000 test patients ranging from 35 to 65 years of age. All patients had clear-cut evidence of *ischemic heart disease* from angina and unequivocal readings on electro-cardiograph tests (ECG). What's more, all patients had been subjected to serum chemistry and were screened for fasting blood sugar, post parandial blood sugars, total cholesterol, serum triglycerides, and total lipids.

Of the 5,000 patients, 3,167 were diabetics, 2,572 had a history of smoking 10 to 15 cigarettes per day for about five years, and 2,151 patients had evidence of hypertension. (Patients with severe hypertension, severe type 1 diabetes, and anyone on insulin therapy were excluded from the test.) All 5,000 patients were instructed not to consume alcohol in any form during the study, and smoking of any kind was also expressly forbidden.

In testing the Aloe Vera gel, Agarwal combined it with another Indian folk remedy, the husk of *Isabgol* a very high fiber plant indigenous to India. All 5,000 patients were instructed to take 100 grams of fresh flesh gelatin from the plant Aloe Vera along with 20 grams of the Husk of Isabgol mixed with wheat flour and lightly baked in a kind of bread. Strict diets were also enforced, and varying regimens of regular drug therapies were allowed to continue. All patients were asked to report weekly at which time they were assessed clinically and biochemically. And they were to do this for five years—from 1980 to 1985.

According to the report from Dr. Agarwal's study group, most of the patients started responding from the second week after the therapy was introduced with almost immediate disappearance of the symptoms from the angina pectoris. ECG changes started improving dramatically after three months, and in one year all but 348 of the patients had normal tracing "even after [using a] treadmill."

After the first year the report quoted the following:

"None of the patients suffered from myocardial infarction during the study. The lipid profile also started improving after three months of institution of therapy.

"Out of 5,000 patients, 4,652 had their normal levels of serum cholesterol ranging from 160 Milligrams to 240 milligrams, serum triglycerides from 50-90 milligrams%...Total lipids from 500 milligrams to 800%, HDL cholesterol ranging from 50 milligrams% to 75 milligrams%."[8]

The regularly prescribed medications, during the five-year course of the study, were never entirely discontinued, though it was noted that in the vast majority of the cases the dosages were greatly reduced.

After the full five years, Dr. Agarwal noted substantial improvement in 95% of the 5,000 patients in the study and was able to conclude the following:

"The plant, Aloe Vera, when mixed with the husk of Isabgol and given to the patients of atherosclerotic heart disease, prompted a definite and substantial improvement (about 95%) in their clinical profile apart from bio-chemical changes and ECG tracings." [9]

It must also be noted that bio-chemical changes and ECG tracings were uniformly excellent. And, significantly but not surprisingly, Dr. Agarwal remarked with some amazement that, "the most interesting aspect of the study was that no untoward side-effect was noted, and all the five thousand patients are surviving to date."

By all systems of measurement, the O.P. Agarwal study must be considered a milestone for several reasons. First, it was the first mass patient study of any kind that had been conducted using Aloe Vera as a medium to test against heart disease and atherosclerosis. Second, it was a conscientious long-term study during which time 95% of the patients showed an unequivocal improvement in all areas against which the study was judged. Third, it is most surprising that nowhere in the western world at least has this study been duplicated or (to this author's knowledge) attempted. Fourth, this study had a couple of subtexts. Those included the fact that the remedies under discussion—Aloe Vera and Isabgol—were both very high-fiber non-fat natural foods, and the important element that this regimen was combined with moderate behavior free of alcohol and tobacco and combined with a sensible low-fat diet.

The results of this study also serve to corroborate the fact that moderation and a proven effective plan of healthy living, consistent exercise, and avoidance of toxins and stress are essential in eliminating cardiovascular problems and heart disease in the future. Without them, even the most pronouncedly effective therapy will eventually prove inadequate.

Nevertheless, we do note two other important aspect of this study, One is the fact that if Aloe Vera was so pronouncedly effective in the lowering of the circulatory system's danger signs—high LDL and triglyceride fat levels in the arteries—then it also makes exceptional sense to use it in one's daily regimen, as a part of the high-fiber cholesterol controlling properties that it already offers.

The other is the fact that the Aloe Vera used in the study was not one of maximum potency. It was a cut-down version of one of our original formulations that, in our professional opinion, offered less than optimum potentials for good result.

Still, within just a few weeks, the Aloe Vera/Isabgol combination began to work to a positive effect on the vast majority of the patients in the study.

What's more this reinforces in greater numbers a simultaneous group of tests run by another research group of scientists at the University of Rajasthan in Japer, India. In this series, doctors V.P. Dixit and Suresh Joshi ran a series of blood samples on a test group of primates—Presbytis Monkeys in this case. In this test, two groups of five monkeys were captured, weighed and fed a chemical stimulant) as a means of increasing blood level cholesterol. After 72 hours, the blood was then withdrawn to determine what is referred to as "Zero H" sampling. After another 48 hours, another sample was taken and both were exposed to centrifuge testing to determine the levels of both HDL, LDL and VLDL (Very Low Density Lipoprotein) cholesterol.

Then, Aloe Vera and Clofibrate (basic tissue extracts) were introduced separately to the respective test groups and blood samples again were taken. All five animals tested with the Aloe Vera showed remarkable reductions in both the dangerous types of cholesterol, as well as triglycerides—a rate that was more than twice that of the Clofibrate treatment. In the test, Dixit and Joshi also noted a significant rise in the level of HDL (or good cholesterol) in the Aloe test group.

Three years later in 1986, doctors Dixit and Joshi ran a second set of tests, this time with two test groups of white rats. One group was fed a high fat, high cholesterol diet. The other was fed Aloe polysaccharide constituents from the native Aloe Vera plant. In subsequent readings, the Aloe test group showed decreased total cholesterol, decreased total triglyceride levels, decreased non-esterified fatty acid levels, and increased HDL cholesterol levels.

In both tests, Dixit and Joshi proved to their satisfaction that the Aloe Vera did lower lipid fat metabolism and would very likely decrease the risk of cardiac problems, especially if taken on a regular basis.

Although the two tests are both significant in their way, the Agarwal test on 5000 human volunteer patients proved by far the most conclusive. In the first place, it won by force of numbers and by virtue of time. Second, it revealed a distinct focus on long term results—the kind that are required to shift entire bodies of thought and cause serious health professionals to reconsider their approach to the range and scope of this remarkable healing plant. A third issue was the undeniable power of the "human factor" in any scientific equation. Both tests were remarkable. But at the end of the day numbers and the human element prevail in any comparison of equals.

5) Modern Breakthroughs in Wound Healing.

If any aspect of Aloe Vera's profound curative power could qualify as a milestone in itself, its ability to heal wounds would visibly surpass all the others. We emphasized the term "visibly" because all trauma against the body wounds it in some way. And yet it is those eternal trauma to the skin surface that give us the most immediate evidence of violation and healing. Wounds we can see are vivid. We can experience them, even vicariously, and we can behold the level of their repair and amelioration.

By primary definition, a wound is "an injury to an organism, usually a rupture of tissue of the integument or mucous membrane…"

When completed, the definition implies that the wound comes from a blow or external violent force. And yet the manifestation is often no different than a lesion, sore, burn or ulcer. Whether it is a blow from a violent hit in a football game or a mouth ulcer from an allergy, the surface must be treated with the same kind of constant caressive care and go through the same step-by-step healing process.

In our 40 years of experience with Aloe Vera and its ability to heal any kind of wound, laceration lesion, sore, hematoma, burn, or ulcer, we have found that it does three things exceedingly well.

First, it rapidly tears down necrotic (or dead) tissue. Second, it promotes the rapid cell division that leads to accelerated healing and repair. Third, it blocks thromboxane. In brief, thromboxane is what is seen visibly as the process of scabbing. And though scabbing is seen as a necessary part of the process of healing, it is not necessarily so. In the first place, scabbing often leads to scarring. Second, the tears that scabbing forms often shred the healing skin and slow it in the later stages. Aloe Vera has shown us another way by eliminating scabbing from the healing process and allowing tissue to heal in a normal but accelerated process that minimizes both the time and disfigurement that often accompanies scarring.

Aloe Vera's positive effects on the healing of all skin conditions is given added emphasis by virtue of physician's reports on its treatments of burns, abrasions, cuts, lacerations, contusions, ulcers and infections. Between the years of 1967 and 1981 alone, we received hundreds of physician's reports on thousands of patients that listed our stabilized Aloe Vera formula's superiority in the following:

1). Healing acceleration—excellent to superior to all other treatments

2). Reduction of swelling—superior to all other modalities of treatment

3). Anti-inflammatory—superior to all other treatments

4). Enzymatic debridement—excellent to superior to all other treatments

5). Relief of pain—superior all other treatments.

6). Antiseptic—equal or superior to all other treatments.

7). Antipruritic—superior to all other levels of treatment.

Since not everyone is aware of some of the terms, we'll define a couple: Enzymatic debridement refers to the time in which it takes tissue to tear down. In other words for a true healing to take place, the dead or damaged tissue has to go through a kind of cellular death. The quicker the damaged (or necrotic) tissue dies away, the more rapidly cell division and healing can commence. It is also a cardinal rule of healing that all injuries, wounds, burns—any disease in fact—must go through a cyclical process in which it gets worse before it gets better. The sooner it does so, the better for the healing process. According to all tests and practitioners' reports (some of which we will show) Aloe Vera helps that process along perhaps better than any other healant in history.

Pruritus is a constant state of itching. It is a dangerous part of the healing process, in that the skin virtually screams out irresistibly for relief. And the inclination to answer it (or scratch) is an unconscious one. The term, *antipruritic,* means the healant stops itching and therefore the scratching that succeeds it.

What we will follow with in this section are three clinical studies on wounds, burns and other violations to the skin that redefined Aloe Vera's role in cutaneous treatments and the world opinion that followed.

It cannot escape truism. To have skin, one will inevitably in the course of one's life experience a wound of some kind. From a paper cut to third degree burns to disfiguring trauma, nobody on this earth gets through life without experiencing them. The first best hope is that those wounds or burns will be kept at a minimum; or, if they are more traumatic, that they will be easily healed.

By broad definition, a wound is a disruption of the skin's normal anatomical stasis resulting from some extrinsic injury—a cut, a gash, a burn. The wound can be intentional (as one inflicted during surgery). Or it can be accidental through the introduction of some trauma or other.

The immediate response to wounding or burning is an inflammation response (the body's way of trying to compensate for the trauma) that includes swelling, heat, pain, bleeding, redness, and the possible loss of function of the area affected.

On a physiological or subcutaneous level, this kind of trauma is responded to by the body's sending out a host of helper cells including leukocytes, phagocytes and the release of what are known as eicosanoids. Basically there are three stages of wound healing: *the acute stage,* or what is known as traumatic anesthesia, when the wound needs immediate response and help (this is usually triggered by the body's defense mechanisms); *the chronic stage* when the wound progresses with the normal healing process; and *the repair stage* when actual healing and rebuilding occur.

With these challenges in mind, it is obvious that the ideal healant would be one that helps the body's response systems to heal the wound at every stage of development. We do this with a tip of the hat to the past, but with the bulk of our focus on some landmark studies that have been conducted in recent years.

Not only for his studies in Aloe Vera but also for his work in wound healing and healing of ulcers in general Dr. John Heggers, Ph.D. is one of modern science's most scrupulous and dedicated researchers. A staff member at the Shriners' Burn Institute & Chief Division of Plastic Surgery at the University of Texas, Galveston's medical branch, Dr. Heggers, along with his research partner, Dr. Martin C. Robson has made burn studies and wound healing his cause celébre; small wonder he has taken Aloe Vera into serious consideration.

In one study, "Eicosanoids in Wound Healing," Dr. Heggers and Dr. Robson examined the role of eicosanoids and their role in stable prostaglandin formation to heal wounds. Prostaglandin research is a highly complex issue and one that takes knowledgeable scientists years of research to grasp totally.

For the sake of simplification, we observe that there are helpful and harmful prostaglandins in the human system—or more accurately, stable and unstable prostaglandins.

Stable prostaglandins comprise the building blocks of the body's immune system. It is in that system's best interest to cultivate as many stable prostaglandins as possible to participate in the healing process and to strengthen the output of the eicosanoid agents in the process of healing itself. It must also be noted clearly that in the normal process of an average wound, the normally functioning human system possesses tremendous wisdom to heal itself, to balance its stable and unstable prostaglandins and to phase into repair.

In their research in the role of eicosanoids in the wound healing process, Heggers and Robson set up a series of fibroblast tissue samples and through those samples noted the wound healing process.

In order to skip through the technical jargon and cut to the chase, we observe that in order for the body to heal itself in its initial stages proper histamine production has to be generated. Histamines are the healing agents that come from the histidine complex. Histidine is an essential amino acid as well as a building block for others. Again there is a balancing act, here. Too few histamines and healing is inadequate. Too much histamine production and the system overproduces *thromboxane*. We know by now that thromboxane is that coagulant that prompts rapid healing but also increases formation of scab and scar tissue. Too much of it can bring about unnecessary exudation, pussing, and fluid generation. So the balance has to be just right in order for the tissue to heal properly.

Naturally, the greater the trauma, the more severe the threat to the delicate balance that needs to be maintained in healing the body. When this occurs, it has to be noted that in order to maintain that balance and aid in the healing, certain healing agents often need to be introduced to the body in order for it to heal properly.

In their report on the healing process, Heggers and Robson concluded that some of the body's responses to standard inflammatory agents offered to relieve pain and inflammation in early stages of wound-healing may actually impair wound-healing during the course of the repair. This particularly applied to such known therapies as *aspirin, Indomethacin, ibuprofen, and corticosteroids, particularly cortisone.* Particularly in the case of cortisone, if it is introduced after 48 hours of the wound trauma itself, it shows absolutely no positive anti-inflammatory effect and over the long course of the healing process actually retards it in direct proportion to the degree of its use.

As alternatives, Heggers and Robson proposed the consideration of vitamins A and E for their known nutritive and tissue-building abilities and as compatible agents to eicosanoids in the wound-healing process. (We never miss an opportunity to note that both vitamin E and vitamin A appear in synergistic profusion in the chemical composition of Aloe Vera.)

Although these gentlemen do not attempt to take credit for all the conclusions at which they arrived, through their findings and synthesis of others' findings they were able to determine the value of some healthy natural alternatives to aid in the wound-healing process.

This next step led Dr. Heggers at least down a new path to seek answers, not the least of which was the Aloe path.

In 1992 John Heggers published a private paper entitled "Wound-healing Potential of Aloe and Other Chemotherapeutic Agents," based on his group's study of Aloe Vera and five other topical therapeutic agents for their performance as healants.

In a large test sample of five test groups and one (1) control group, Aloe Vera along with four other topical agents, were tested for their ability to heal wounds during the short term or acute stage of healing all the way through long-term (reparative healing) stage.

The elements tested were
  1) Aloe Vera
  2) Mupirocin ointment
  3) Clindamycin phosphate
  4) Silver sulfadiazine (plus an Aloe/Silver sulfadiazine combination)
  5) Untreated controls.

The tests were taken from four wound models (1.5 cm each) on groups of test rats. The rats were anesthetized. The acute wounds were then created on their backs and then tested with treatments over a 14-day period of time. Wound healing was monitored at intervals ranging from acute or early stages all the way through the final stages of the test. Wound half-lives (or progressions) as well as overall healing rates were then calculated over the test period.

During the acute healing stage, the first three-day period, the Aloe group showed the shortest half-life of all test groups excluding the control group. The Aloe showed a healing rate equal to that of the control group (which, remember, receives no medication). The aloe plus silver sulfadiazine increased the breaking strength of the healed wound and actually helped overcome the negative or wound retardant effect of the silver sulfadiazine.

At the end of the 14-day period, the groups were again measured for overall healing, and the Aloe Vera test group showed the greatest rate of healing over all other groups, including the control group. It showed the greatest level of wound reduction and the shortest half-life, or required time of healing over all the test groups, and the only one that was in fact better than the untreated control group.***

*** *To explain the nature of them as simply as possible, test groups are broken down into two groups: the "test group" that is given the actual drug to be tested, and the "control group" that is given a placebo. It is often surprising to note that the control group often wins these tests. This has never been the case when it has been tested against Aloe Vera.*

The bottom line: In a normal circumstance of healing with the group tested Aloe Vera has shown itself to be by far the preferred treatment. What's more, in lieu of a properly stabilized Aloe Vera compound, it is often better to let the wound heal itself than to attempt many of the commercial preparations available today. Or, if you are going to embrace one, be sure you have checked out its track record for healing and amelioration of the wound, burn, lesion or ulcer.

Sometimes it's helpful to understand that the body does have considerable wisdom to heal itself. Aloe Vera seems to understand that simple communication naturally. It's also important to recognize that, especially in this new millennium where healing and challenges to healing have come to a point of critical mass, there is such a thing as patient responsibility. In today's complex tapestry of wellness versus sickness, we owe it to ourselves to be both well-informed and proactive where our personal health is concerned. As knowledge is indeed power, we offer this additional precaution: When in doubt about your health issues, due diligence is not only suggested but also essential to survival. When you are, help will inevitably come. And you will be secure in your choice of it.

Milestones in health are often matters of individuals as much as events. Since these significant reports, Dr. Heggers has continued spearheading reports on Aloe Vera and wound healing. One of his more recent papers in 1996 was entitled "Beneficial Effect of Aloe on Wound Healing in an Excisional Wound Model." Leading a large group of associates, including Dr. Robson and Wendell D. Winters, Dr. Heggers et al. conducted a control group study on test groups of 50 fibroblasts broken into five groups of ten. In the five groups, Aloe Vera and sodium hypochloride were tested against four other topical healants for effectiveness and toxicity over a fourteen day period of intense application. In every instance the Aloe Vera and sodium hypochlorite (NaOCl) tested far superior in non-toxicity and nearly 30% better in rapid tissue cell growth than any other test product, including the NaOCl solution when tested by itself. It also showed that Aloe Vera when combined with any of the other healants showed better rates of healing and cell tissue growth than those elements when tested on their own. Ultimately milestones are a matter of constants. When, in test after test over decades, one healant emerges as the pivotal ingredient in wound healing, cell regeneration, and a lack of toxicity, there are conclusion to be drawn. The studies of Dr. John Heggers and associates, like so many before them and so many yet to come, arrive at the same destination. Aloe Vera is the ultimate healer. It has always been. And when formulated with integrity and awareness, it always will be.

6) "Natural Born Killers." The Broad Spectrum Story of Aloe Vera.

We'll be brief in this section and to the point at the outset. Aloe Vera has proven to be the most effective broad-spectrum bactericidal agent ever put to the test. It has also proven to be virucidal, fungicidal, and moniliacidal.

If the terms seem too technical then we will simplify. In test after test, Aloe Vera kills germs or bacteria of just about every imaginable description. It also kills a broad range of viruses, fungi and monilia (a particularly active fungus that attacks the mucous membranes).

To the man on the street this might not make much impact. To the man of science or the health professional who lives in a world of pathologies it is nothing short of astounding. More than a milestone, it offers all the potentials of a Force 4 event. And because it does, it is certain to push the envelope of credibility beyond containment.

At the outset, it is important to emphasize that there are major drugs in legion, almost all of them highly toxic and therefore sold by prescription, that flood the marketplace annually and thrust against one pathogen—one family of bacteria, one virus, one fungus. And, just by addressing one challenge, they make fortunes for their manufacturer, create new franchises, and launch pharmaceutical stocks and drug companies into the rarefied air of the darlings of Wall Street.

And yet by their very nature, they are limited as to what they can do. So called "broad-spectrum" antibiotics, however many bacteria they may kill, are ineffective against viruses, fungi, monilia, or allergies. Steroids and penicillin based derivatives, especially in today's broad-spectrum overdose environment, often run up against strains of microbes that become quickly if not immediately resistant to them.

Aloe Vera, on the other hand, effectively kills a broader range of pathogens than any other curative known to science. And yet it does so (see Item #1 in this chapter) with virtually no relative toxicity. This, to the allopathic mindset, is tantamount to heresy. It is fit sacrifice for the skeptic, and a challenge to the seeker of truth. For the caustic minions of disbelief, we offer no rebuttal beyond the truth of the following findings.

As you will soon see, they are as timeless as studies in the healing nature of the plant itself. They are as up-to-date as the last study we sponsored in 2002.

What you will note are a number of findings that reveal Aloe Vera's broad spectrum healing potentials not only against every imaginable pathogen but also against diseases that seem to number in legion. And one thing it is important to remember that for every pathogen—every bacteria, virus, fungus, protozoan, and other pernicious microbe that Aloe Vera has proved effective in killing—brings with it a score of diseases well-known to the average person on the street.

One of the first tests in modern history was a test in 1950 in which a research team headed by R.Y. Gottshall and J.R. Jennings found Aloe Vera gel to be bactericidal against *tubercule bacilli, Staphylococcus aureus, and E. coli bacteria.* It is interesting to note that tuberculosis in 1950 was still considered a pervasive, deadly, and often incurable disease. Thought to have been eradicated by the 1960s, it has reemerged with a vengeance in the new millennium and yet drugs now created to combat it are few and far between. And none, it seems, has ever been able to match the curative powers of Aloe Vera. Staph aureus, originally manifested in boils, carbuncles and numerous skin infections, has now mutated into a gram positive strain (the "flesh eater") that has become the scourge of the developing world. And E. coli is that strange pathogen that behaves itself in our own elimination system, but becomes the ravager of worlds once released outside the body on its own. It is oddly well behaved in that singular context inside the colon and rectum. And yet once it is released to outside air it can wreak absolute havoc especially when exposed to wounds, mucous membranes or adjacent to foodstuffs such as meat. Perhaps just as curiously, it has traditionally been tamed by Aloe Vera, and to great effect (often when no other modality tried will work).

The Gottshall, Lucas, Lickfield, and Jennings tests were among the first of their kind. And though they were crudely constructed and perhaps hit upon the wrong conclusions for Aloe's "active ingredient," they prompted us all to think a bit more deeply about the opportunities to help establish the healing plant's "germ killing" potentials.

For that reason, we sponsored a series of tests with Dr. Eugene Zimmermann, D.D.S., Chairman for the Department of Pathology for Baylor Dental School, and Ruth Sims, Ph.D., a virologist and research scientist in Dallas, Texas. Dr. Zimmermann had already spearheaded a successful series of tests on Aloe's anti-inflammatory capabilities and relative toxicity. And we had already established a research relationship with Dr. Sims at Dallas Microbe-Assay.

In an in vitro study sponsored by us in 1968, Doctors Sims and Zimmermann tested one of our earlier Aloe Vera formulations for their ability to kill four pervasive microorganisms—*Staphylococcus aureus, Streptococcus viridans, Candida albicans, and Corynebacterium xerosis.* And they did so at different percentages of Aloe Vera present in the compounds ranging from 25% Aloe Vera to 70% stabilized Aloe Vera.†

---

† At the time, we believed 70% would be a minimum effective base for stabilized Aloe Vera, though we recommend higher percentage levels for challenges against most strains of microbe.

Staph aureus we know only too well by now. *Strep viridans* is a curved genus of bacteria that is particularly infectious and often found in wounds that will not heal. *Corynebacterium xerosis* is a parasitic microbe that produces excessively dry skin and flaking such as that found in eczema and seborrhea, both nasty skin conditions.

Candida albicans is a monilial fungus that is in a class all its own. More commonly known to manifest in such conditions as sore throat, congestion, and (most prevalently) yeast infections, Candida albicans (more commonly referred to simply as Candida) is also believed to be the culprit behind such perennial systemic destabilizers as colds, bronchitis, and dozens of different strains of the flu. It is also found to be present in enormous quantities in such conditions as Chronic Fatigue Syndrome, Fibromyalgia, and even acute prostatitis. Although there are debates about the sources of these conditions—and surely specific immediate causes may differ—the Candida fungus is the natural seedbed for their growth and development. When you take a look at this handful of "bad guy" microbes and observe the diseases that stem from these alone you begin to realize the chain reaction these can create, as well as the phenomenon that a single herbal remedy may be able to destroy them all.

In this case, the Aloe Vera did so very well. According to the initial Sims/Zimmermann findings, Aloe Vera at a 70% level killed all the strains against which was tested within 24 hours. More important, it killed 100% of the Candida fungus in 24 hours at only a 50% level of potency.

Impressed but challenged to repeat the results, we commissioned another research group in 1978 led by Dr. Jean Setterstrom of the Walter Reed Army Research institute. In testing our stabilized Aloe Vera against the same strains of microbes. To our delight (but not surprise), Dr. Setterstrom achieved the same result, not in 24 hours, but in 16. And she had used a solution of 45% t0 50% Aloe Vera!

Granted, some Aloe can vary from batch to batch as to degrees of potency. Still, the preponderance of evidence in test after test points to the fact that Aloe Vera is a germ killer. Given appropriate levels of stabilization, it is unfailing and consistent.

Dr. Setterstrom's tests in 1978 did not end with the corroborative findings she rendered on the *Staph aureus, strep viridans,* and *Candida* group of pathogens. In fact, in terms of breaking new ground, her second series of tests on our Aloe Vera products proved to be even more of a milestone in terms of new pathways of discovery, and new areas of focus.

This time, the studies were made in terms of oral toxicity with particular focus on a group of bacteria known as *Streptococcus mutans.*

By this time, it would become apparent that there are virtually scores of malev-olent microbes that spin out of the Streptococcus and Staphylococcus strains of bacteria. Among them, Strep mutans form colonies of one of the most lightly regarded and most pervasively active bacteria known to modern pathology. In fact, they invade us all. In truth, winning over them is a lifetime struggle, because they are the nasty little germs that form plaque and eventually decay on our teeth and gums.

Whether it is in the mouth or the heart, plaque forms up totally as a matter of build-up. When it does, it must be ground away, scraped, brushed, and scrubbed—except when Aloe Vera is introduced to the pathogen.

In an in vitro experiment, Dr. Setterstrom used our Aloe Vera gel in only a 40% solution and then introduced it to a Strep mutans culture she had allowed to build in a row of test tubes. After just a few hours with a minimum (40%) solu-tion, all the S. mutans plaque formed in the test tubes had fallen to the bottom of the tubes—virtually detached from the host glass and enamel.

The implications of course are staggering. And even though we acknowledge that modern dentistry has evolved exponentially in the last 20 years, Aloe Vera is a player in the game of prevention that deserves further consideration—such is the role bacteriology plays in beholding the new frontiers of Wellness. Such is the role Aloe Vera plays potentially on so many fields of endeavor.

Doctors Sims and Zimmermann, for example, ran two bacteriology tests in 1970 against a number of different pathogenic strains.

The first was against common *Trichophyton* fungi that caused athlete's foot and ringworm and nail fungus. The Aloe (in an 80% solution for the athlete's foot fungus and a 90% solution for the ringworm fungus) killed both fungi within 24 hours.

Later in the same year, Sims and Zimmermann's research team tested for us once again, this time against two of the best known public enemies in the world of virology—*Herpes simplex and Herpes zoster*.

Herpes simplex is well known not only for its manifestation in fever blisters but also in its more infamous form as *Herpes II*, or the now pandemic genital Herpes. (In fact Herpes simplex and Herpes II are the same virus. They differ only in degrees, as pertains to location on the body.)

Herpes zoster expresses itself in two distinct ways: As chicken pox, and as a nasty autoimmune condition commonly referred to as shingles.

In two separate in vitro tests, the stabilized Aloe Vera in a 100% solution killed the very potent Herpes simplex virus in 72 hours. And it killed the less potent Herpes zoster virus in less than 24 hours.

When you consider the fact that, even 25 years later, they are just now finding drugs that can finally treat and control (not kill) these viral strains, it is both remarkable and sad that Aloe Vera has not been given further range of study in treating these two relentless viral strains.

At this point, we acknowledge that progress in the scientific context is a matter of stops and starts. We also recognize the fact that our bacteriological studies, however thorough, have been in vitro studies. To be sure, in vitro (test tube or Petri dish) tests are generally viewed as being 95% as effective as live patient or animal studies. Nevertheless, they are still relegated to the middle rungs on the ladder of research, because in the view of governing health bodies, they lack the impact live case studies and the force of numbers of double-blind live subject tests.

Still, we press on. We do so with each new formulation and for each new era, because old research is often held in the same regard as an old car: It's okay for its time. But what's new?

We have an answer for that: In the last ten years, a great deal.

It is part of the heritage validation that we have to constantly sponsor and conduct new laboratory studies. We have to update with each new formulation. And we have to justify ourselves to each new generation of skeptics.

At best, these tests arm us with further clinical armaments to face the professional naysayers we must face from time to time. At worst, they teach us something about this complex world of science and medicine, and in this vast universe one can never suffer from too much knowledge.

For that reason, and because of the fact that we never give up trying to make it better, we recently sponsored a pair of tests involving some of the newest formulations of stabilized Aloe Vera gel.

One of them in 1995 involved a bacteriological study conducted by Dr. Kathleen Shupe-Ricksecker, Ph.D. A biologist and assistant professor at the University of Dallas, Dr. Shupe-Ricksecker recently undertook a series of *in vitro* bacteriological examinations testing various percentages of Aloe Vera solutions against tissue cultures of four common pathogens—*Streptococcus pyogenes, Staph aureus, Pseudomonas aeruginosa (pseudomonas),* and *Eschericha coli* (more popularly known as E. coli). Strep pyogenes are particularly known to be present in cross-infections and side-infections from improper wound-healing, as are pseudomonas. *Pseudomonas aeruginosa* is also present in a number of secondary urinary tract infections in men and is commonly found as a second microorganism present in prostatitis. E. coli, as we know by now, can be one of the most dangerous bacteria known to medicine. Unchecked, it is a cause of pandemic food poisonings involving contaminated beef, poultry, and dairy.

In her findings, Dr. Shupe-Ricksecker noted that all these microorganisms were killed within 24 hours of exposure to high levels of stabilized Aloe Vera (85% or greater). The *Strep pyogenes* and *Staph aureus* strains were virtually killed (99.5%) within the 24-hour period. The more resistant strains, *E. Coli* and *pseudomonas* were killed upon an increase of Aloe percentages to 90%. And even though these strains are traditionally more resistant, the Aloe was 90% bactericidal against them even in a short period of time.

In any event of the findings, and given the new age of the mutant microbes in which we live, these findings were both reassuring and exceptional. Even though we had experienced similar results 25 years earlier against some of the pathogens tested, we remained aware that as our products evolve so do some of the viruses, bacteria, fungi, monilia, and parasites set up to oppose them. So, as the thermodynamics of the battle rise to fever pitch, we stand armed and ready to meet the new breed of " super strains" that come up against us.

In a separate test, Dr. Shupe-Ricksecker studied the germicidal effects of stabilized Aloe Vera on *Propionibacterium acnes* (ATCC strain 6919). The name is self-explanatory if you look at the second word, acne. This is a causal agent in the formation of acne, often resulting from the introduction of a comedogenic agent such as an improper oil-base ingredient to the skin. Since we have used Aloe Vera to successfully treat *acne vulgaris* (what is commonly referred to as "acne") for decades, there was little doubt that the tests would be favorable. What we needed to determine was the degree of intensity and the percentages at which our new formulation would be most effective.

Once more, one day's in vitro testing of samples using various percentages of Aloe Vera revealed that a 100% killing ratio against the bacteria could be achieved within that 24 hour period. Significantly the same or similar results could be achieved at concentrations of 75% Aloe Vera gel versus 90%. This is important to know for the simple reason of cost. If you can achieve the same beneficial results at lower percentages, why overkill? It is ultimately a cost savings to the manufacturer and the pharmaceutical marketplace to have this knowledge. The product becomes more affordable to the consumer, and ultimately every one benefits.

What we have offered in this brief section is only a sample of the seeming horde of microbes that the healing plant has met and conquered in the labs. From the most seemingly insignificant microbe to the deadly pernicious Human Immune Virus (HIV) and fully developed AIDS, Aloe Vera has proven time and again that it is a treatment of choice.

Oftentimes, it is the only treatment available, because it is brought in as a last resort when all others have failed.

In ensuing chapters, we will examine Aloe Vera's expanded role when pitted against some of the most pervasively difficult conditions known to modern science. In it, we will show Aloe's abilities to combat various types of cancer, AIDS, and an entire rogues gallery of autoimmune diseases.

These, however, require a level of study all their own. And chapters, full chapters, are needed to cover them properly.

7) The Last Days of Addiction?

Very often breakthroughs come in ways that ordinarily we might never consider. Much earlier in the development of Aloe Vera as a cogent pharmaceutical contender, we might never have considered leveraging its broad spectrum curative potentials against the challenges of personal behavioral pathologies. When you're dealing with the internal uses of any modality of healing, it's understood that you're often tripping through a minefield of conjecture. Oftentimes the answers are often clouded and rife with disagreement. And yet, in a way much of what amounts to behavioral disorders come back to issues of biochemistry. In some instances, the body does not produce enough endorphins or serotonin to help it to cope with the abnormalities of stress or abuse. Such pathologies as paranoid schizophrenia and bipolar disorder (manic depression) can trace their roots to biochemical imbalances. And often drug therapy of some kind is the only answer.

In terms of behavioral problems such as substance abuse, the abuse itself creates such a biochemical chain of reactions that it causes addicts to become convinced, even at a cellular level, that they can no longer carry on without the addiction. And in a way that addiction becomes the addict's sanctuary—his or her "safe house."

By the same token, since the addict's dependency is chemical, there opens the possibility the treatment, at least in part, might also be found in chemically rebalancing the sufferer. Much of the addict's pain of withdrawal comes with the concomitant psychological baggage that accompanies it. Such elements as anxiety, depression, and a thorough voidance of energy form the walls of a personal hell from which the sufferer beholds only one route of escape: a return to the substance itself.

The therapist is then challenged to find the right elements to replace it—self-esteem, improved health and proper changes in chemical balance.

What's more, ordinarily the road to recovery for substance abusers can be a long and arduous one. The good news is that along the way there are signposts in human behavior, some of the best of which entail the simple process of asking the subjects themselves whether or not they feel better, or if their spectrum of conduct has tilted toward the positive side.

One thing you're sure to get is immediate feedback, for better or worse. And though it may be subjective, it is often honest and readable.

Mindful of this challenge, Frank S. Burns a leading Substance Abuse Counselor in the state of Washington, undertook a contról group study in the Spokane Veterans Outreach Center, where he served as chief counselor. Patients at this center traditionally undertake a course of rehabilitation for various forms of drug and alcohol abuse and follow what amounts to a 26 week regimen of treatment.

In the Frank Burns study, he established a test group of 25 patients to whom he administered regular daily doses of two ounces of stabilized Aloe Vera drinking gel, a popular brand of bee pollen and a nutritional supplement. He also set up a control group who continued their regimen without the Aloe Vera/bee pollen, nutritional supplement tandem.

It is important to note that the substance abuse rehabilitation program set up by Frank Burns and his staff is highly successful. And over the full course of 26 weeks, his patients showed a remarkable rate of recovery. However, the journey to recovery is not often a pleasant one, and subjects undergoing treatment frequently experience severe and persistent alterations in mood that are both intense and debilitating.

Such pathological personality manifestations as *depression, anxiety, sleep disturbances, loss of appetite, lowered energy level, anger, withdrawal, and lowered self-esteem* are not only common but predictable obstacles to the success of any program of rehabilitation. It is with these pathologies in mind and against those standards that Mr. Burns set up the Aloe Vera Control Group study.

The 25 test group patients on Aloe Vera and the 25 control group patients given no Aloe were evaluated and queried against nine criteria, and their progress was charted over the 26 week period.

The tables on the following pages graphically illustrate those criteria and how Aloe tested against them. They were *1) Depression, 2) Anxiety, 3) Sleep disturbances, 4) Appetite, 5) Energy level, 6) Withdrawal, 7) Anger, 8) Self-esteem, and 9) Desire to drink or return to drug abuse.* The tables and the summations for each of them are generally self-descriptive, though we feel it is important to note that against all criteria tested, the test group partaking of the Aloe Vera drink showed marked, dramatic improvement within two to five weeks (usually two weeks), while the control group did not approach the same level of improvement until the 25th and 26th week in some cases. Still others in the control group did even not approach the same level during the entire course of the study.

This of course raises the question: Is Aloe Vera providing a crutch for these patients? Cynics could argue the point, but not for long. In terms of substance abuse, the road to recovery is long, arduous, and fraught with pitfalls. It's easy to backslide, especially in the first four to six weeks.

That was where Aloe Vera seemed to make its strongest impact on these recovering addicts—just at the point in their therapy when they need it most. That's always been the most remarkable aspect of the silent healer; it has a sense of what is needed, and it fills it.

TABLE 1
DEPRESSION

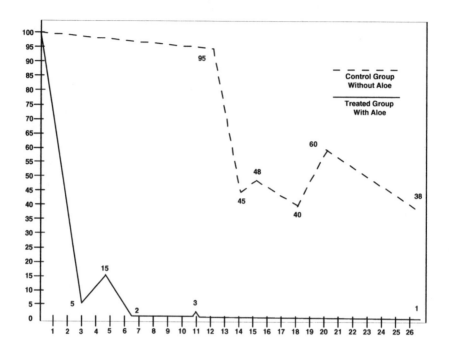

The severity or degree of depression, 100 = seven days plus with morbid thought, excessive sleep pattern, suicidal ideation, decrease in social interaction, and increase of guilt feelings over past behaviors.

Zero represents no existence of depression.

Time is estimated by week one through week twenty-six.

Table One—Depression—illustrates a significant decrease of depression by week three for those individuals using the Aloe Vera, bee pollen, nutritional supplement complex. Both groups received intensive individual and group therapy for substance abuse.

TABLE 2
ANXIETY

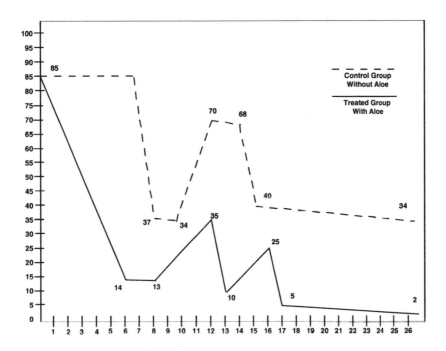

The severity or degree of anxiety, 100 = seven days plus with an intense state of apprehension, feeling uneasy, and fear.

Zero represents no existence of anxiety.

Time is estimated by week one through week twenty-six.

Table Two—Anxiety—illustrates a significant decrease in anxiety by week six for those 25 individuals using the Aloe Vera, bee pollen, nutritional complex bee pollen tandem vs. the control group not on the Aloe Vera, nutritional complex. Both groups received intensive individual and group therapy for substance abuse.

TABLE 3
SLEEP DISTURBANCES

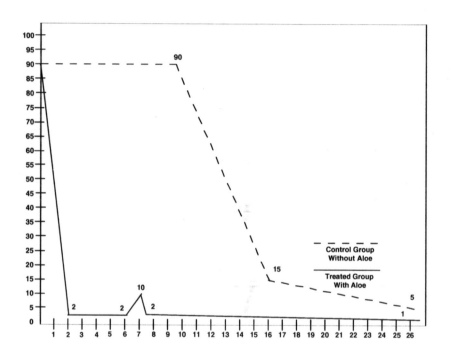

Zero represents six or more hours of restful sleep per night.

The severity or degree of sleep disturbance, 100 = seven days plus without six hours of continuous sleep per night.

Time is estimated by week one through week twenty-six.

Table Three—Sleep Disturbance—illustrates a significant decrease in sleep disturbance by week two for those 25 individuals using the Aloe Vera, bee pollen, nutritional complex vs. the control group not on the Aloe Vera nutritional complex. Both groups received intensive individual and group therapy for substance abuse.

TABLE 4
APPETITE

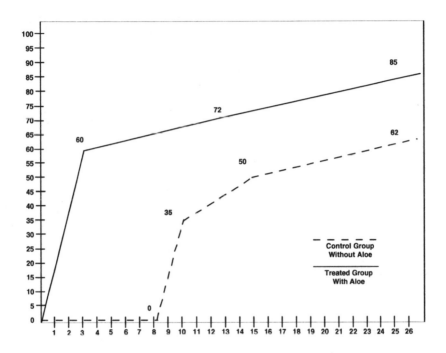

Zero represents no existence or a severe lack of appetite or improper nutritional intake.

The severity or degree of loss of appetite, 100 = seven days plus with malnutrition, and physical weakness due to improper diet and eating habits.

Time is estimated by week one through week twenty-six.

Table Four—Appetite—illustrates a significant gain in appetite and nutrition by week three for those 25 individuals using Aloe Vera, bee pollen, nutritional complex vs. the control group of 25 people not using the Aloe Vera nutritional complex. Both groups received intensive individual and group therapy for substance abuse.

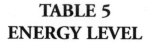

TABLE 5
ENERGY LEVEL

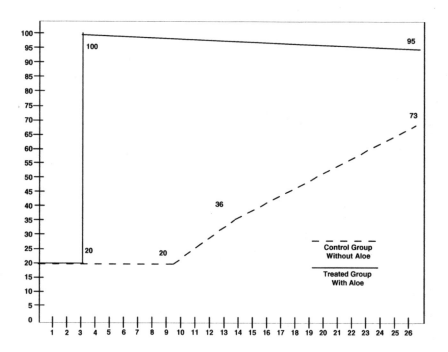

Zero represents no existence or a severe lack of energy.

The severity or degree of energy level, 100 = seven days plus with an increase of energy, i.e. improved work performance and increased recreational activities.

Time is estimated by week one through week twenty-six.

Table Five—Energy Level—illustrates a significant increase in energy by week three for those 25 individuals using the Aloe Vera, bee pollen, and nutritional complex vs. the control group not on the Aloe Vera nutritional complex. Both groups received intensive individual and group therapy for substance abuse.

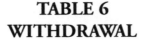

TABLE 6
WITHDRAWAL

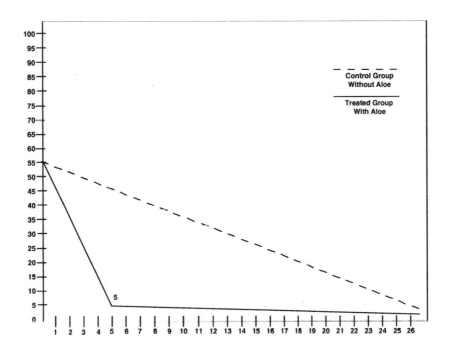

Zero represents no existence of withdrawal.

The severity or degrees of withdrawal range from moderate to severe. 100 = five days plus with a loss of appetite, confusion, nausea, mild shaking, diarrhea, and fever.

Time is estimated by week one through week twenty-six.

Table Six—Withdrawal—illustrates a marked decrease in withdrawal symptoms by week five for those 25 individuals using the Aloe Vera, bee pollen, nutritional complex vs. the control group of 25 people not on the Aloe Vera nutritional complex. Both groups received intensive individual and group therapy for substance abuse.

TABLE 7
ANGER

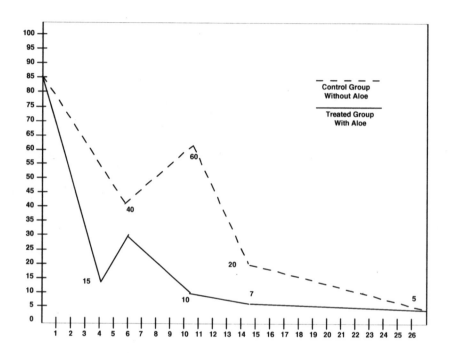

Zero represents no existence of anger.

The severity or degree of anger, 100 = seven days plus with argumentative behavior, overt hostility, and poor interpersonal relations.

Time is estimated by week one through week twenty-six.

Table Seven—Anger—illustrates a marked decrease in anger by week four for those 25 individuals using Aloe Vera, bee pollen, nutritional complex vs. the control group of 25 people not using the Aloe Vera nutritional complex. Both groups received intensive individual and group therapy for substance abuse.

TABLE 8
SELF ESTEEM

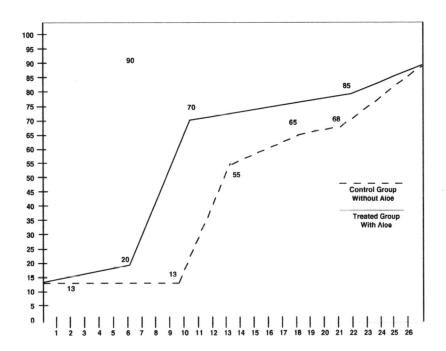

Zero represents little or no existence of self esteem.

The severity or degree of anger, 100 = seven days plus with increased self aware-ness, self worth, and the ability to resolve negative feelings (i.e. resentment, hate and fear).

Time is estimated by week one through week twenty-six.

Table Eight—Self Esteem—illustrates a significant increase in self esteem by week 5.5 for those 25 individuals using Aloe Vera, bee pollen, nutritional com-plex vs. the control group of 25 people not using the Aloe Vera nutritional com-plex. Both groups received intensive individual and group therapy for substance abuse.

TABLE 9
DESIRE TO DRINK
OR
USE OTHER DRUGS

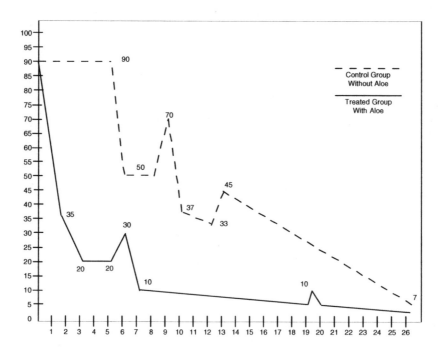

Zero represents no desire to use alcohol or other drugs.

The severity or degree to use alcohol or other drugs, 100—seven days plus with a strong desire to continue to use alcohol or other drugs.

Time is estimated by week one through week twenty-six.

Table Nine—The Desire to use Alcohol or Other Drugs—illustrates a marked decrease by week 2.5 for those 25 individuals using Aloe Vera, bee pollen, nutritional complex vs. the control group of 25 people not using Aloe Vera nutritional complex. Both groups received intensive individual and group therapy for substance abuse.

Many of the symptoms treated in rehabilitating addicts are some of the manifestations that are brought to the surface in cases of profound stress. However, although addiction can be the direct product of stress, it is often the cause of stress and is itself caused by a number of other factors, including the following: heredity; psycho-social factors including extreme peer pressure; asocial behavior; attention deficiency disease (ADD); alpha compulsive personality manifestations; any number of metabolic or biochemical imbalances such as hyperkinetic behavior, and even paranoid-schizophrenia.

Addiction itself is a complex tapestry. And though the means of curing it are as varied as the number of syndromes there are to treat, the addictive personality is a relative constant. People who express it are often beset by a small and even predictable list of behavioral patterns. And though the addict has to be guided through the perilous pathway to recovery, it is highly reassuring to discover that there are elements that are helpful, stable, predictably effective, non-toxic, and non-addictive in and of themselves.

A judicious review of these findings in the Frank Burns tests point quickly to a significant flaw in the criteria in that, for our purposes, Aloe Vera was not used exclusively. Bee pollen and a nutritional supplement were also a part of the mix, and that relegates the healing plant into the role a cofactor role in this reparatory collage.

Only a test using Aloe Vera exclusively would show results that could be considered conclusive. And yet, to answer that, we direct you to the preponderance of evidence in this chapter as well as those to follow. The Robert Davis aspirin tests were not only landmarks in themselves, but also emphasized the Aloe factor as making a difference. We will soon note tests in the arenas of both AIDS and cancer that point to the inextricable role Aloe Vera plays in the healing process.

One of Aloe Vera's finest aspects is its proven ability as an adjunct to other modalities in the healing process. Even when combined with antibiotics, steroids, and other potentially conflictive modalities of treatment, it does nothing to antidote and everything to synergize with the process of treatment and cure. Rather than conflict, it always contributes. And that is ultimately the best measure of a true healant.

Summary

We admit that any references we make to "milestones" can be both self-proclaimed and highly subjective. Truth be told, there are enough milestones in the annals of Aloe Vera to make this chapter 300 pages on its own. There are other landmark events both in the laboratories and in the various fields of application.

And each is so significant that it could easily merit chapters of its own—the ones that will follow this.

What we have done here is to emphasize breakthroughs on three levels: 1) the plant's emergence as a major alternative therapy in a number of areas; 2) a revelation of pivotal points of progress in which Aloe Vera has proven unsurpassed—its non-toxicity, its broad spectrum germ killing powers, and its powers of penetration; 3) some dramatic areas in which Aloe Vera alone has proved to be either the therapy of choice or the miraculous adjunct that seems to potentize a healing process that might otherwise not function at its optimum potential.

So, in the next chapters we continue on the journey that we have begun with Aloe Vera. Many of the reflections will be personal in nature. Some will be quite dramatic. Still others will involve some of the most challenging diseases of this modern era.

Chapter 5

Autoimmune Diseases Meet the Aloe Vera "Orchestra"

In this chapter we offer some seemingly radical notions on why only Aloe Vera seems to work on some of the most challenging diseases known to modern science. In it, you will be introduced to what is known as "The Conductor-Orchestra explanation for Aloe Vera's remarkable ability to synergize the healing process, and "The Thermos Theory," our own somewhat simplified version of what makes it perhaps the most inscrutable healant known to science. We'll also look at its success with what many believe to be the most difficult diseases of all to treat—Autoimmune Diseases. From type 1 diabetes mellitus to Lupus erythematosus, we will cite some dramatic case histories and how Aloe Vera has treated them with remarkable success.

There is a peculiar waltz of healing autoimmune diseases for which only Aloe Vera seems to have mastered the tempo. We make that observation with the firm understanding that we once again risk the damnable predisposition of overstatement. The truth is that autoimmune diseases are by their very natures so complex that they have proven all but impossible to treat with one modality, one drug, or one set of treatments. If they can be dealt with at all, the poor patient experiencing the bizarre rhythms of treatment and recovery is predestined to be assailed with an entire regimen of drugs, many of which are designed to work at cross-purposes with one another. So, at best we have a perilous path to recovery. At worst we have a deadly game of chemical ping-pong in which the attempted "cure" often becomes a part of the problem.

Autoimmune diseases always manifest in two directions at once. They begin with a systemic malfunction that almost unfailingly manifests itself in the form of physical symptoms that are invariably painful and often appear as unsightly sores, wounds, skin separations, and lesions. Or else, they are cripplers of such proportions that they virtually put an end to all mobility.

Many autoimmune diseases such as type 1 diabetes, pernicious anemia, rheumatoid arthritis, and multiple sclerosis are infamous and wide spread. Other such as systemic lupus, Lupus erythematosus, Myasthenia gravis, Addison's disease, colitis, Crohn's disease and bilateral scleroderma are lesser known but nonetheless hideously pervasive and distressingly on the rise.

In Chapter 1, we offered a concise description of how the immune system functions and what happens when it loses its points of reference. Here we offer a little more detail.

The Innate Human Immune System is regulated primarily through the endocrine glands. And though we are the first to admit the endocrine system is something of a mystery in itself, it provides a highly efficient means of guarding the body against disease, injury and pernicious microbes through what is called phagocytosis.

Through phagocytosis in its first line of defence, two kinds of white antibody blood cells (T-cells) called macrophages and neutrophils must engage in what amounts to an atomic identification check of every element in the human system. They must be able to reject and, if necessary, destroy any new ill-intended microbe that comes their way. But they do so more or less as a line of last defense. They are, in a way, the body's palace guard—or what is sometimes referred to as the innate immune system.

Initially, the immune system sends out an advance guard of white blood cells known as lymphocytes (or "B-cells). Lymphocytes are part of what amounts to an adaptive immune system that is rather like a police force. They not only run identification checks, handcuff and arrest "bad guy" germs called antigens, they also review and examine every new foreign particle that comes into the human system to decide whether or not it will be allowed to stay. Although these B-cells are very aggressive, they're occasionally not as discreet as they should be. Although they usually show good potentials for combination, sometimes, they throw out good new visitors along with the bad. (That's when you have a phenomenon like tissue rejection of a transplant or skin graft; or when you have tissue that doesn't heal as well as it should.)

When this occurs, lymphocytes are aided by new elements called leukocytes that try to help regulate the lymphocytes' decision-making ability. And they both send out helper cells called T-cells to round up the suspects and bring them in for processing.

Engaging these foreign bodies, these antigen terrorists, in what amounts to a set of cellular handcuffs, these white blood cells embrace and assimilate a potentially harmful bacteria or virus into a "good citizen," or just get rid of them. But sometimes in diseases such as cancer or pernicious, contagious diseases, the antigens find ways of hiding. They either cloak their identity or they carry what amounts to a cellular fake "I.D."

That's when it becomes a matter for the elite corps of the macrophage and neutrophil S.W.A.T. team to catch what remains. The word "macrophage" is Greek in origin and literally means "big eater." Essentially the macrophage and neutrophils envelope the antigens and either convert them into good citizens or simply devour them.

Usually, in the immune system, the macrophage and neutrophils do the job very well, and that's the end of the antigen gangsters. But sometimes the bad virus or bacteria or fungus has become too powerful. In fact, it has done such a good job of either hiding out or disguising itself as an acceptable life form that it has had time to reproduce its kind. That's when disease occurs. And the more powerful the antigen has become while it has been hiding out, the more complex will become the issue of combating it.

In most cases, some sort of drug therapy will suffice to rush an army of helpers to the immune system. Or in some cases a sudden nutritional boost to the immune system can strengthen it enough for it to recover its balance. The endocrine glands can send more macrophage and neutrophil troops into the fray. The bad guy antigens are routed. The cure takes effect, and the system normalizes.*

There are those instances, and too many of them, when the immune system isn't up to the task. It is either overwhelmed or it simply misfires and the process of phagocytosis is thrown into a welter of miscommunication and chaos. If the system is facing one powerful antigen such as that which exists in cancer, tuberculosis, or heart disease, the issue is one of knowing the depth and strength of the enemy and dealing with it directly, either with powerful drug therapy, surgery, and a rebuilding of the body's systems. Autoimmune diseases behave in a much more complex and sinister fashion in that they attack the host in not one but a number of ways. First, they all attack the body's regulatory system—the endocrine glands, often attacking more than one gland. Since the endocrine

---

*Allopaths are convinced that only powerful drug therapy, almost as severe as the disease itself, can do this. Homeopaths believe that a Judas goat like unto the disease itself can trick the pathogen into leaving and guide it out of the system. Aloe Vera, as we shall soon discover, offers another solution altogether.

glands—the pineal, pituitary, the thyroid, thymus, reproductive or spleen—regulate the body's immune system, they immediately get bad information about what kind of message they send to the macrophage and neutrophil S.W.A.T. teams. Those systems either over or under-react and, in turn, start over or under-producing helper cells. This prompts a series of manifestations either on the skin or throughout the skeletal structure that can prove painful and often unsightly.

A properly functioning immune system puts out something called prostaglandins. Basically, there are three kinds of prostaglandins—two good kinds of prostaglandins and one somewhat unfairly labeled as a bad prostaglandin. PGE-3 prostaglandins help build and fortify the immune responses for the heart and circulatory system. PGE-1 prostaglandins work to rebuild the rest of the body's immune system for the other glands, organs, and skin.

PGE-2 prostaglandins are labeled as bad prostaglandins because they're the ones that show symptoms. Pain, lesions, outbreaks on the skin, aches, throbbing, sores and cancers are all offshoots of the PGE 2 prostaglandins. This all sounds like a confederation of villains, unless you take into consideration the fact that PGE 2 prostaglandins are the body's alarm bells. They are the shadowy allies of prognosis. They tell the body when it is sick. They give it biochemical and symptomatic storm warnings of calamities yet to come. Were they not to function at all, the victim would not be able to determine that something was wrong, until it was very late in the came of diagnosis, treatment and cure. The individual would perish of a lack of symptoms.

So the only thing worse than PGE-2 prostaglandins becoming overactive is what occurs when they don't function at all. This is often the case with type 1 diabetes and some type 2 diabetes mellitus when the victim loses all feeling of pain, irritation or feeling in the extremities. Lesions, burns and scrapes are incurred from outside sources but are often neither felt nor observed. And because they are not felt the body sends no process of phagocytosis to deal with it.

When an autoimmune disease take hold on the system, it strikes in so many places that the body doesn't know how to respond intelligently. In syndromes such as (systemic) lupus erythematosus, the steroids and anti-inflammatory agents used treat the skin lesions may actually create addictions to the tissue they are trying to heal and damage the DNA that the endocrine system is trying to put back in balance. In multiple sclerosis, the broad-spectrum medications often used to repress the pain also short circuit the functions of the pineal and pituitary glands that are needed to rebuild and restore balance to the system.

Oftentimes medications such as steroids, antibiotics, and analgesics, which are administered to treat the symptoms, blunt the endocrine functions needed to build immune responses. Curatives rushed in to treat one manifestation of the syndrome often antidote other aspects of treatment. So the sour symphony of autoimmune disease and failed palliatives continues. There may be certain periods of temporary remission, especially when a new modality is introduced. But those are often punctuated by relapses that are even more severe. And as systemic immunities build to the new treatments introduced, the downward spiral worsens, often with catastrophic results.

To be sure, there are certain predispositions to autoimmune diseases. Many them are genetic. Many come cascading down through the gene pool, and some even seem to get worse with each generation. But autoimmune diseases are more and more perceived as a sinister by-product of life in modern times. Stress, emotional instability, and poor diet are contributory to the exacerbating of the autoimmune condition, if not to the onset of the disease itself.

Women tend to have more frequent instances of them (about 70% of autoimmune sufferers are women). And when women do get them, they seem to suffer more violent physical manifestations of the diseases. Some of this may be laid at the feet of estrogen production. But attempts to block overproduction of estrogen and other strogenics lead to complications of their own.

Attempts to treat some autoimmune diseases involves a series of treatments on two levels. The first involves the mimicking of the HLA molecules that act as self-sensitive antigens in the creation of multiple sclerosis and blocking them from further proliferation. Another comes in the form of feeding increased levels of ingested protein directly into the system of some autoimmune sufferers. Since it is protein that is needed to heal tissue, and since it is protein presented at the skin or cellular level that is often rejected by the system, this cellular trickery seems to be on the right track to rush healing to the immune system that is so badly in need of nourishment. Unfortunately, this is still in tests on laboratory animals and remains to be tested against human subjects.

If the music we've written for this unfortunate series of sour notes sounds a bit too measured and far away, rejoice.

We have some treatments that are working now. They may ring in a whole new kind of music. All of them involve Aloe Vera. And every one of them plays perfectly into the "Conductor-Orchestra" theory of Aloe Vera and its place in the sweet symphony of cure. Fortunately, at least according to initial findings, the Conductor-Orchestra ensemble of Aloe Vera has already found a way to get the protein messages to the depleted immune system and to do so at several levels.

The "Conductor-Orchestra" Theory of Aloe Vera.

Easily 75% of our getting well is dependent upon our immune system. 25% is doctors and medication.

—Bob Corbett, DVM

There have been many explanations for the remarkable ability that Aloe Vera has to synergize as it applies to treating and healing a laundry list of diseases that now seems endless. Nowhere does the healing plant shine more gloriously in all its applications than when placed against the most perplexing of all strains of pathologies—autoimmune diseases.

Autoimmune diseases are as hideous as they are frustrating, because in many ways they are the medical equivalent of the Hydra: the more heads you cut off, the more that seem to grow back. They never offer just one set of challenges, they offer pernicious outbreaks that seem ineradicable.

Such conditions as type 1 diabetes and multiple sclerosis are inevitable killers. Others such as Lupus erythematosus and bilateral scleroderma are cripplers that can ultimately be fatal. Other syndromes such as psoriasis and rheumatoid arthritis can lead sufferers to a life of disfigurement and pain. And more often than not, cases are written off as hopeless.

That is where Aloe Vera comes into its most eloquent form of expression.

In the early days of our research and development in stabilizing pharmaceutical grade Aloe Vera products either we or doctors working with us were brought in to consult in cases of autoimmune diseases for which "all other standard treatments had been tried and failed." In other words nothing else had worked. We were their last best hope.

In those years, it was often the only circumstance in which Aloe Vera would be allowed to be tried as a means of therapy, albeit alternative therapy. Although, at the time, we weren't altogether certain of the reasons why Aloe Vera worked so well against certain kinds of complex diseases (what we came to learn later were autoimmune diseases), we felt it was the synergy created inside the complex chemistry of the plant that led to its remarkable performance. At the time, some of those diseases such as bilateral scleroderma, lupus erythematosus and myasthenia gravis often mystified the average practitioner. Diagnosis was often exceedingly difficult, came tardy to the game, if it came at all, and misdiagnosis was common.

As long ago as the early 1970s, we believed we understood the sublime synergy of the Aloe Vera plant, thought we knew how it worked, and expressed our belief that the true conductive power rested with the Aloe polysaccharides. What we perhaps lacked was an ability to articulate the mysteries of the silent healer as well as it deserved.

That articulation eventually came in a magnificent form at the hands of Robert H. Davis, Ph.D. While he lived, Dr. Davis was perhaps the most ardent and well-versed proponent of Aloe Vera in the world of science. His work and studies on the healing plant comprise volumes of incisive well-developed Aloe research. His explanations of Aloe Vera's success as a healer have always been among the best defined in the annals of scientific study. And he has been responsible for many breakthroughs.

We speak of him in present tense because, even though he passed from us in 2002, his work lives on. One of his most eloquent legacies to us was what he appropriately named "The Conductor-Orchestra Concept" of Aloe Vera. It is the most depictive description of how Aloe Vera functions that we have ever read. And it is this hypothesis that we now recount for you on these pages.

"The Conductor-Orchestra Concept" was developed by Robert Davis in 1998 to define more completely the intricate tones and rhythms that enable the more than 200 biologically active components in the Aloe Vera plant matrix to function as they do.

We have devoted chapters in previous works to the scores of ingredients in the Aloe whole-leaf matrix. Even at 99% water and 1% solids, it is replete with entire complexes of vitamins, minerals, anthraquinones, lignin, saponins, enzymes, amino acids, essential oils, sterols, sugars and proteins, many of which make eloquent music on their own. When put together in a curative ensemble, they hold orchestral potential of great brilliance, provided they are set to task by a truly gifted conductor, one that can bring motivation, balance and direction to the music of healing. Properly conducted, the Aloe Vera orchestra can create therapeutic achievements of symphonic proportions. Were it not for the awareness and vision of the conductor the instruments, though melodic on their own, might easily create a cacophony of mixed results.

The conductor(s), we are now virtually certain, can be found in the Aloe polysaccharide complex. The nutrients work through protein leads (in the form of proteolytic enzymes) or what amount to first instruments in the sections. And it is through the proteolytic enzymes that we pass through the system to the Aloe polysaccharide conductor. The conductor reached in three stages of conductive sugars—glucose, mannose, and mannose 6-PO4. And it is here that we resist the temptation to get complicated and over-explain a very simple process.

What does take place inside the conductor complex of Aloe polysaccharides, however, is an ability to sense the curative rhythms that resonate with the body in need of healing and rush the particular curative strains to the affected area.

The important issue to note in this metaphor of pathology and treatment is the fact that the healing concerto is there. The instruments contain all the potential attributed to them. What they need is direction, composition, and a sense of movement. And only the conductor can provide those elements

In the Aloe Vera orchestra, the conductor can determine what is needed and direct the specific healing message to the area of specific involvement. Properly standardized and formulated, the Aloe orchestra can perform magnificent feats of healing, repair and physiological balance provided two things are appropriately in place.

First, the stabilized product applied to the pathology must be both efficacious and mimic all the healing potency of the plant. Second, the receptor from the orchestra and conductor has to be able to balance the syndrome it is facing. In other words, there has to be a sense of structure in the measures taken.

The beauty of the Conductor-Orchestra principle of Aloe Vera comes with the incredible intelligence that the plant offers to any autoimmune disease. Within the subtext of that cellular communication lies its ability to read what is needed and answer with almost perfect balance the curative potency that is required.

If autoimmune diseases have one perverse quality in common, it is their ability to confuse the body into making the wrong decisions about how to heal itself. Strong drug therapies often placed against them often deal with only one aspect of the syndrome, usually addressing the symptoms but not the deadly systemic that underlies the symptoms. Subsequently, the autoimmune disease worsens and more than occasionally becomes impossible to either treat or control. Oftentimes it will simply overwhelm all modalities placed against it, debilitate and finally destroy the living creature that hosts it.

Aloe Vera is not only difficult to fool, it seemingly has the answers for everything that comes with the taunting tango of cellular chemistry. It senses the body's aching need in the face of the disease and specifically rushes the healing agent to meet that need.

In certain diseases such as rheumatoid arthritis, for example, levels of vitamin C are exceedingly low, and the body seems either unable or unwilling to properly absorb it. By all indications, Aloe Vera aids in the assimilation of vitamin C by adding an "esterifying" agent that increases proper absorption.

In autoimmune diseases, this supersensing process is repeated time and time again with Aloe Vera answering the different challenges each of these terrible and often chronic syndromes present. In all its glorious application, the Conductor-Orchestra personality of Aloe Vera flies in the face of many long held theories that Aloe Vera is driven by a key ingredient or a "magic bullet." Although the concept is still hypothetical on its own, we now offer a series of case histories of different autoimmune diseases where Aloe Vera played its perfect part in the complicated process of healing. And oftentimes, it did so when all other treatments had been tried…and failed.

Some Dramatic Cases.

Psoriasis represents the classic autoimmune disease in that it betrays physical, very visible symptoms that reflect a serious systemic imbalance. And as such, it has to be treated aggressively at both levels. Mistakenly, many dermatologists only treat the skin lesions.

Psoriasis is a disease that effects more than 75 million people worldwide. It is chronic in that occurs frequently during the course of the year and, like many autoimmune diseases, is believed at least in part to be hereditary. Women tend to suffer from psoriasis more frequently than men, although the number of sufferers tends to be more evenly divided than other types of autoimmune diseases.

Psoriasis is characterized by scaly, shiny lesions that break out on what is known as the erythematous areas of the skin. In other words, they are found on skin areas that are affected by surface red corpuscles. Although unsightly and irritating, psoriasis is neither painful nor contagious. It can, however, be very unattractive and at times disfiguring to those who suffer from it at more extreme levels. Psoriatic skin lesions can break out on any part of the body, or they may cover the entire body area. They can appear as small, nascent flecks of dry skin no larger than a spec, or graduate to large sores that, at their worst stage, may begin to suppurate and form blankets over large portions of the skin surface such as the back, legs and even the abdominal area.

Like many autoimmune diseases, psoriasis is often described medically as etiology unknown. Yet it is curious to note that, with approximately 7.5 million sufferers, there are more victims of psoriasis per capita in the United States than in any other part of the world.

It is also interesting if not critical to note that incidences of psoriasis are higher in nations where there is an increased presence of convenience foods and "fast food" franchises.

Traditionally, this disease has been treated with some rather extreme and elaborate measures. Even as recently as 1990, coal tar and dithranol were still listed as major components in two out of every three pharmaceutical preparations used to treat this syndrome. More recently, reinoids, folic acid antagonists and corticosteroids have been used to treat psoriasis, all with limited success and some degree of addiction to tissue.

Among known practitioners who deal with the syndrome frequently, it is believed to be brought on by a combination of several factors, including diet, immediate environment, and a lack of vitamins A and D. In fact, psoriatic skin lesions respond well to sunshine, concentrations of ultraviolet rays, and more recently have been very well-affected by the saline rich mud of the Dead Sea.

In fact, pilgrimages by psoriasis victims to Dead Sea resorts and available spas in that area have become an annual ritual for those rich enough to afford them. In lieu of those, some Israeli pharmaceutical and cosmetic manufacturers are selling specially treated Dead Sea mud in pre-packaged allotment at a very hefty price indeed. And in truth, it seems to be the total immersion in the saline Dead Sea mud combined with the sun and warm climate of the Middle East that have a more measurable immediate benefit. The fact is that even this beneficial "topical" treatment seems to work well but not permanently when applied, unless it is used in combination with a radical change in diet and a schedule that includes a reduction of stress and overwork. And smart practitioners who apply this kind of radical therapy are at least beginning to get to the root causes of some of the problems that accompany psoriasis.

For those we have developed our own methods for treatment that, when put into practice and followed conscientiously, has worked for dozens of people to whom we have introduced it. The program includes an applied regimen of regular daily topical applications of Aloe Vera cream and large daily doses of Aloe drinking gel. Those applications are supplemented by a specific regimen of megavitamins and anti-oxidants and a strict all-natural whole food diet. This diet eliminates all processed foods, junk food, fast food meals, sugars, or foods heavy in animal fat or other high LDL cholesterol. We also find the more fresh fruits and vegetables one is inclined to eat, the better it will prove to be for the skin. Some practitioners we have worked with take this a step further.

Conscientiously applied and strictly regimented, this diet can and has worked exceedingly well, not only to address the symptoms of this unsightly disease but also to get to the systemic causes. At this point, we think it appropriate to show two sets of photos that illustrate just how well this Aloe Vera, altered diet and mega-dose nutrient package has worked on a number of individual cases.

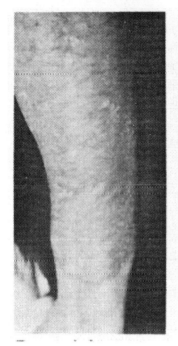 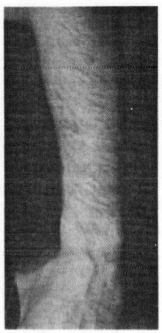

Exposed forearm of a psoriasis victim prior to treatment with stabilized Aloe Vera. Blotches and scaling cover a majority of the forearm.

Exposed forearm of the same psoriasis victim after 90 days treatment with stabilized Aloe Vera, a special diet and megavitamin therapy. Note: the area of the forearm is virtually without any trace of lesion.

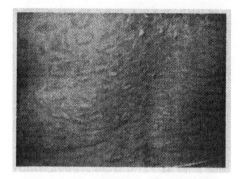 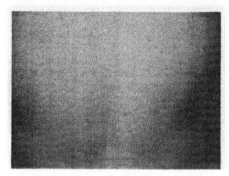

Exposed back of psoriasis victim after 90 days treatment with stabilized Aloe Vera, special "junk free" diet and megavitamin therapy. Once again, the entire skin area is virtually blemish free.

Final photo of psoriasis victim after she is fully recovered. Once adhered to, the Aloe Vera/ nutritional regimen can enable the sufferer to lead a normal life..

It was announced as recently as July 2002 that a number of major pharmaceutical companies such as Merck and Pfizer have about 30 drugs either pending examination by the FDA or under study that promise effective treatments for psoriasis. We applaud the good news but add the caveat that, from our experience, treating psoriasis is one issue. Getting rid of all evidence of it is another. And in our opinion, no single drug is ever going to do that. Psoriasis, like most autoimmune diseases, offers such sinister complexity that it can only be dealt with comprehensive, healthy remedies to bring it under control. Even Aloe Vera, as thoroughly as it works to answer the problem, is only part of the answer. The rest lies in a full program of diet, bioavailable nutrition, and effective Aloe supplementation.

Of course, we sincerely hope one of these "miracle drugs" does come along to eradicate the effects of psoriasis. But as is customary, their long awaited arrival may still be several years away. Meanwhile we offer a simpler remedy. Use the recommended Aloe drink, topical applications of Aloe Vera, and the regular regimen of nutritional supplements.

Systemic Lupus Erythematosus.

It is an unfortunate aspect of this pernicious and disfiguring disease that it is on the rise. It is even more disturbing to note that about 90% of all sufferers are women. There is little doubt that some of it has to do with estrogen production gone awry in the system of some women. But that only addresses one aspect of one of this volatile, intensely complicated disease.

Commonly referred to simply as *lupus,* this is one of the most insidious, systemically pervasive and hard-to-treat syndromes known to modern medicine. It manifests in two forms: *systemic lupus erythematosus (SLE)* and *discoid lupus erythematosus.* Of the two, systemic lupus is far more common and far more serious in that it completely pervades the human system.

Untreated, SLE is unwaveringly degenerative and can be fatal. In its more advanced manifestations it pervades most of the body's major organs. Although initially it presents itself through many of the symptoms that mimic those of rheumatoid arthritis (another autoimmune disease) it eventually makes its presence known on the skin in unsightly rashes and blemishes that often fester and spread. Usually it does this after the condition has advanced well beyond symptomatic confusion and into the horrid hydra-headed monster it will inevitably at last become.

By then, of course, most of the immune system's defenses have entirely short-circuited. The lupus is out of control on several levels. And, as is so often the case with advanced stages of many autoimmune diseases the body under assault is overproducing its own immune system responses. In fact, the process of phagocytosis has gone all haywire, and too many "good guys" from the macrophage and neutrophil "police" are now rushing to the rescue, creating a negative force all their own.

Lupus, like scleroderma, psoriasis, and *Pemphigus vulgaris,* appears to have no apparent causal parent. Genetics are occasionally a factor. But with SLE environment and lifestyle also seem to have a certain perverse impact. Certain medicines, excessive exposure to the sun, and high-fat, high-processed "junk food" diets seem to set it off.

Traditional drugs used to suppress the overactive immune system such as cyclosporine have had some positive effect on Lupus. But the detrimental side effects such as urinary tract problems and gastrointestinal blockages bring nearly as much toxic baggage as they do palliative influences.

In the last decade there has been some positive effect obtained from administering massive doses of high antioxidant complexes such as Vitamins C, E, A (especially beta-carotene), selenium, Coenzyme Q10, L-glutamine, and pygeum extract.

But the fact is also true that systemic lupus erythematosus is so dramatically on the rise among women over 35 in the last ten years that more and more time and effort have been devoted toward addressing the trauma it creates that several new treatments are now under study, some of them pretty radical.

One of them is the deadly sting of the scorpion. (And no we're not kidding!) It is called TRAM-34, and it's modeled on scorpion venom, because the bite from that deadly little arachnid apparently offers some immunosuppressive benefits. Another therapy happens to have come recently from our neighbors at the Southwestern Medical Center at the Dallas Center for Immunology. In 1999, a research team headed by Dr. Edward K. Wakeland found that at least two genes in an individual body's DNA had to be present for lupus to be able to form. By discovering four suppressor genes and introducing them to a test group of laboratory mice, the Wakeland research team found that it was able to stop all the effects of systemic lupus. This is great news and we applaud it. Unfortunately the findings, still being corroborated, will preclude a drug being brought to market for another three to five years.

Meanwhile, we offer positive point of reference in that we, and physicians we have worked with, have been able to use stabilized Aloe Vera to combat and defeat SLE in dozens of instances over the last few years. Much of this has to do with one courageous woman's fight for survival and her introduction to stabilized Aloe Vera in 1983. The woman's name is Rita Thompson. And in her way she is as much of a pioneer in lupus research as any of the doctors and scientists who worked to treat her.

When her symptoms began to appear in 1975, neither Rita Thompson nor any of the physicians treating her were privy to the information available today about autoimmune diseases. In fact, there was no such recognition of them as a family at the time. In fact in 1975, so little was known about lupus that Rita was originally misdiagnosed by her physician as having rheumatoid arthritis and was treated accordingly. For the next five years, the aches and pains continued, as did the incomplete treatment.

In fact, it wasn't until mid-year 1980 that the lupus appeared cutaneously, and it did so as a series of measle-like lesions. Appearing first on her legs as slight irritations, they lasted only about two weeks and appeared to get better. Unfortunately one of the most insidious qualities of lupus is its apparent capacity to mimic spontaneous remission. So often the symptoms disappear and the lesions lessen only to reappear a few days later in an even graver expression. Such was the case with Rita Thompson.

Within a few days of appearing to get better, more lesions appeared—on her legs, to be sure, and on the rest of her body as well. This time, however, the lesions worsened and came back to stay—for two and a half years!

During that time, Rita Thompson underwent an ordeal few people could endure. The joint pain intensified. And the lesions, even though they appeared to get better, always snapped back more severely than before. After nearly three years, her condition had deteriorated to such an extent that she was hospitalized frequently, and her skin trauma was treated with every conventional modality of healing — topical creams, special wraps, solution soakings, and some fairly radical therapies. For systemic implications, she received oral prescriptions by the dozens. She was given steroids, painkillers and other anti-inflammatories, none of which worked. In fact, she had finally reached a point where nothing worked to alleviate any of her symptoms.

What's more, these were the early days of lupus awareness, so her infirmity went misdiagnosed for nearly a decade. Finally, the condition advanced to such a state that she was able to wear no clothing at all but instead had to be kept in a plastic wrap lubricated with special solutions. Eventually, she was treated by a rheumatologist who prescribed a radically strong steroidal tandem of creams and capsules to be taken in megadoses. This was a sort of shock therapy, as it turned out, that couldn't have been worse.

Those who treat the disease on a regular basis have found to their dismay that lupus erythematosus has one of the strongest bounce-back factors of any disease known to science, and one of the worst things you can do is prescribe a strong regimen and then withdraw it. This was the case with this doctor's regimen, and in fact Rita's condition became even more severe. By now, Rita had lost her hair and her fingernails. To compound her frustration, she was told that there was little chance of either growing back.

One of her attending physicians later confided that, by this time, he had given her no more than two months to live—so grave had her condition become.

Never underestimate the resolve and resourcefulness of a patient with the will to live and a faith in her ability to recover. Rita Thompson soon set out to be an agent in her own cure and, when she had heard of the benefits of Aloe Vera, started using a regimen of products I had formulated, specifically Aloe Vera drinking gel.

To dramatize the significance of the "systemic" aspect of lupus, this gel was the only application of Aloe Vera that Rita was able to use at the time. At first, she took moderate doses. Later, when she realized how quickly and rapidly her condition had begun to improve, she started taking megadoses. Met with both incredulity and scientific curiosity by her attending physicians, Rita was encouraged to quit taking the Aloe gel to see if the skin lesions would recur, but Rita was steadfast in her refusal.

"I know it is the Aloe Vera," she insisted.

But the test, it seemed, would befall her in any case.

One time, quite by accident, Rita Thompson ran out of her supply of Aloe Vera drinking gel, and was told it would be two days until she could get another shipment. Within that two days time, the lupus symptoms returned. Her body started to break out in lesions, and the pain recurred. Once the new supply arrived and Rita was able to resume drinking the gel, her system normalized, and the lesions disappeared within a remarkably brief period.

So dramatic was Rita Thompson's recovery and so strong her intent to give others hope and show them the Aloe pathway to hope and remission, that she penned a short book entitled, *Lupus, Aloe Vera, and Me.* It is recommended reading for anyone who wants to learn about what one person, in the face of all odds, can do to take charge of his or her life, health, and future. Rita Thompson is a remarkable woman, and we are glad we could have some small part in helping her find a new life and a new wellness lifestyle.

We are also happy to say that we have some before and after photos of Rita's condition. All's well that ends well, and this story certainly did.

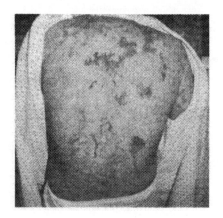 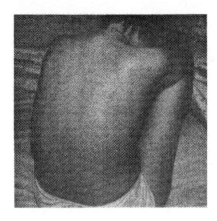

Lupus Erythematosus. Rita Thompson's back late in January 1983. The syndrome in one of its most extreme expressions.

Rita Thompson's back late in January 1984—one year later. With daily intakes of Aloe Vera drinking gel, the remission was complete.

The Rita Thompson Story has a wonderful footnote in that, during an appearance she made to promote the benefits of Aloe Vera and to tell her story, I approached her to congratulate and to tell her how much her story had moved us all. Instead I found her thanking me, and having brought a very special gift for me.

"Bill," she said. "There's something I've been saving for you. Wait just a minute."

Returning moments later, Rita presented me with a rather large apothecary jar filled with dozens of prescriptions and hundreds of pills that had failed to work to treat her condition. The note on the jar stated, "Dispose of these medications as soon as possible. They have all been replaced by Aloe Vera."

The photo, which we include here, is both astounding and sadly poignant. One's first reaction is to be taken aback in horrified amusement at the sheer volume (and cost!) of these prescription drugs Rita was forced to take over the years. Then you're struck by it: Just imagine the years of personal purgatory this woman had to go through and the liberation she must have felt at being freed to live a normal life again.

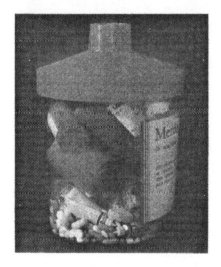

Rita Thompson's apothecary jar. Over the years, Rita reported that she had taken more than 200 different kinds of medication.

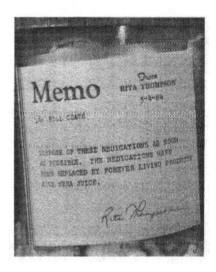

A note from Rita, and the one line that announces the ultimate happy ending.

No question, such syndromes as systemic lupus erythematosus, scleroderma, bilateral scleroderma, and similar autoimmune diseases are actually on the rise. Perhaps it is the age of the supervirus that spawns this kind of outbreak of debilitating and often disfiguring diseases. More than likely, they are springing up because of the pollutants that invade us both from our atmosphere and from the toxins that now come as a part of the package of the high tech, high stress modern lifestyle, much of which is prepackaged and sold to us in foods, cosmetics, and even the water we drink. These kinds of autoimmune diseases are now recorded on the rise because public awareness of them is now at an all time high.

Finally, especially in the last decade, they have come to be diagnosed accurately and treated with intelligent compassion. And many new breakthrough treatments, we feel, are on the way. In the next five to ten years we anticipate seeing these diseases brought to an end.

Meanwhile thanks to Rita Thompson and people like her, lupus and scleroderma support groups have been set up all across the country where women and men can go and receive personal and emotional support for their conditions and learn about some treatments that work. One of them, certainly is the silent healer, Aloe Vera, an old therapeutic friend that we believe still has a significant place in the future.

Diabetes. For the unfortunate few, there are some autoimmune diseases that are 90% hereditary. type 1 diabetes mellitus is one of them. Also known as insulin dependent diabetes, it often comes at an early age and stays with the child through adulthood and what is often a shortened lifespan.

By definition, *diabetes mellitus* is a syndrome characterized by abnormal insulin secretion, excessive blood glucose (sugar) secretion, and resultant biochemical balances in the various governing systems within the body. Although traditional scientific analysis remains mystified by the actual "etiology" or causality of diabetes, it is generally acknowledged that it is the combination of certain hereditary susceptibilities and environmental conditions (almost all of which, it has recently been determined, may be diet-related). To observe that this is a highly complex disease would be to belabor the obvious, and passes as an understatement in any vernacular. Diabetes in its two principal expressions may adversely alter metabolism, blood circulation, and normal cell generation. In its more advanced stages, it can prompt accelerated degeneration of nerve endings, highly impeded wound healing, deterioration of the body's immune system, and opportunistic infections that can lead to death.

Diabetes is commonly sub-classified into *diabetes mellitus type 1* and *diabetes mellitus type 2.*

Diabetes in both its forms affects over 10 million Americans. It is almost always chronic.

Diabetes type 1 is also known as juvenile diabetes due to the fact that it is either congenital to the sufferer or found present very early in life. "Type 1" is what is known as insulin-dependent diabetes in that the sufferer (usually thin) is inflicted with a lack of insulin production and must receive periodic injections. It is a more severe manifestation of the syndrome, and consistently prompts a symptom known as *ketoacidosis,* in which the body's acids and sugars reach relative proportions that are dangerously out of balance. For that reason, it often results in such frequently occurring expressions as impaired sight, even blindness, and early death. Many type 1 diabetics do not live past the age of 35.

By contrast, diabetes type 2 usually develops after age 40, is commonly referred to as non-insulin dependent diabetes and is not generally considered as dangerous, primarily because it is not officially classified as an autoimmune disease. However, that too should be measured in degrees. In fact, there are occasions in which people with Type 2 and people with Type 1 suffer manifestations that differ only in nuance.

In this case, the nuance is the autoimmune dysfunction in Type 1 diabetes that is not (yet) present in the Type 2. We say "not yet," because type 2 diabetes can develop into type 1 if it is not properly treated. And that can have grave consequences indeed.

Once the autoimmune system goes awry, only grave consequences will follow.

Almost all victims of type 1 diabetes will experience an increased risk of glaucoma, cataracts, kidney disorders, impaired circulation and retarded wound healing (sometimes leading to gangrene), heart disease, and various types of vasoconstriction leading to the body's extremities.

Loss of all feeling, failing to heal, gangrene and resultant amputation are all catastrophic results that can and often do result from these syndromes. What's more, recent lab studies showed that excessive tissue degeneration and premature aging are all consistent to the pattern, especially of sufferers of type 1 diabetes.

As is the case with most autoimmune diseases, mounting evidence points to proper diet, nutrition, and appropriate absorption of protein as pivotal in helping to minimize the negative side-effects of diabetes. Certainly no diabetic can expect to smoke or drink without risking disastrous consequences. Heavy intake of fat, chemical preservatives found in processed foods, and high levels of cholesterol also offer serious damage potential to these very susceptible subjects.

Recent studies offer even more dramatic indictments: Medical surveys in the last two decades report findings from Scandinavia as well other parts of Europe indicate that there is a direct corollary between the consumption of sugar (sucrose) and occurrences of diabetes. In every instance these studies report that when a nation's sugar consumption rises, there is a proportionate rise in the rate of diabetes. (Additionally, similar findings also indicated that in every country where the high fat, high-cholesterol American "fast food" franchise diet is introduced there is a proportionate rise in incidence of cancer and heart disease.)

At this point we belabor the obvious. Not only do many autoimmune diseases such as diabetes and lupus point to diet and lifestyle choices as villains, they also strongly indicate they may also act at least in part as deliverers. And we feel it essential to observe our belief that what havoc has been wrought on the system can also be brought into repair within the system while the symptoms themselves are being treated.

At the risk of brooking a misunderstanding, we do not for an instant lay the primary cause of type 1 diabetes at the doorstep of diet and lifestyle. It is invariably hereditary, largely suffered by young girls and women (about 70%), and is an expression of autoimmune disease at its most unforgiving. Having said that, we do know that diet and nutrition have become increasing points of concern among practitioners treating these patients, especially those of nutrients in which the system is deficient.

One of the most profound evidences of diabetic immunodeficiency run amok is in the extensive depletion of zinc from that system. In fact, it has been demonstrated in at least one study that impaired wound healing, one of diabetes' worst symptomatic calling cards, has been the depletion of zinc from the system. Since zinc is essential to protein synthesis that goes into normal healing and is a major constituent in eighteen different enzymatic processes leading to tissue healing, including DNA and RNA synthesis, this seemed like a logical place to start.

One report describes the gross aberrations that accompany zinc deficiency and just how much one mineral can mean to the chemical balance of the body:

> When denied zinc for a long time, the person becomes zinc deficient…Nails assume a spoon-shaped appearance accompanied by fissuring soles. Normal bone metabolism becomes disrupted with growth centers suffering decreased DNA, collagen, and glycoprotein synthesis, arresting development. Generally, clinicians observe gross aberrations including hair loss, growth retardation, enlarged spleen and liver, loss of appetite, eye abnormalities, a wasted appearance, small testes, iron deficiency anemia, and learning difficulties.[10]

In this same report from a research team led by Elliot Engel, Nelson Erlick, and our old friend Robert H. Davis, a study was conducted on a test group of laboratory mice diabetically induced to determine the effect of "Impaired Wound Healing from Zinc Deficiency," and the reverse of this, to determine if, "administering oral zinc sulfate to these diabetic mice reverses their relative zinc depletion, completely restoring wound healing."[11]

Citing a number of previous studies in which both organs and tissues showed depleted zinc to be implicitly related to debilitation in diabetics, the Engel, Erlick, Davis group set up two discrete control group studies.

The first study involved 60 mice broken down into three groups of 20. The control group was allowed normal allotments of zinc. The test group was given zinc-deficient diets, and the second test group was fed zinc supplements sin liquid form.

Then the three groups were submitted to a second test in which the mice were given diabetes-induced treatment and then "wounded" to gauge the relative healing abilities.

Surprising to some advocates of the "zinc" healing school, mice fed up to 100 times the normal levels of zinc showed no greater relative ability to heal than the control groups of mice fed normal levels of zinc. Yet both fared better than test group (2) who had been left zinc deficient. Those showed a severely impaired ability to heal.

So what conclusions can we draw from this? First, it appears that a lack of zinc, characteristic of the diabetic system, does contribute to impaired wound healing. Second, megadoses of zinc don't necessarily improve the ability to heal markedly over standard levels of zinc in the diet, probably because zinc absorption after basic levels is difficult to come by. It is also safe to say that zinc deficiencies were only part of the problem and zinc supplementation only part of the solution. The rest might well be laid at the doorstep of the system's ability to accept certain elements—especially minerals—without the aid of a good conductor medium.

We cite this study for a couple of reasons. First, because it was a logical precursor to the two studies we're about to examine next. Second, and perhaps most important, is the reiteration of the scientific truth that things are never quite what they appear to be. And the greatest role of the researcher is to put *every* hypothesis to the test.

The Next Step: A study headed by Robert Davis, Mark G. Leitner, and Joseph Russo is conducted to determine the role of Aloe Vera as "A Natural Approach for Treating Wounds, Edema, and Pain in Diabetes."

Since diabetes is so broadly degenerative and since there are no consistently effective therapies for its side infections, this study was intended to show Aloe Vera as a potent therapeutic alternative for physicians to use especially when it came to treating the lower extremities. It is commonly known that loss of circulation, feeling and ability to heal in the lower legs and feet are among the most common manifestations in advanced diabetics. So therapists are constantly searching, usually in vain, for viable treatments.

Already having shown Aloe Vera's profound wound healing ability in other tests, including an earlier one involving mustard-induced edema, Dr. Robert Davis was optimistic that a properly modulated Aloe therapy would work in meeting the diabetic challenge.

This 1988 study by the Davis, Leitner group was intended to introduce Aloe Vera as a player and perhaps *the player* in this therapeutic field. Perhaps notably, Aloe Vera does contain some measurable levels of zinc, as well a virtual arsenal of other ingredients.

But the Aloe Vera nutrient complex is so varied and potent, as Dr. Davis and group were careful to point out, that it offers a veritable potpourri of wound-healing potentials, and zinc can only be considered in that context. Vitamin C, Vitamin E, and zinc do work to promote collagen formation, prevent free-radical damage, and promote tissue regeneration. Additionally, lignin, saponins, enzymes, and a complete amino acid complex also help promote wound healing, as well as help potentize the activity of such key minerals as zinc.

In this study, the Davis group established a criterion to test Aloe Vera as an anti-edemic (anti-inflammatory), analgesic (pain reduction) and wound healing agent against opportunistic infections in the presence of diabetes, and to prove that Aloe Vera works effectively even in "an abnormal physiological state."

In this study, mice were divided into five groups, one control group of non-diabetic mice, and one control (placebo) and three test groups of mice subjected to a diabetes induction agent and given time for the diabetes to set in place. After 48 hours had lapsed, wounds were induced on all groups. Afterward, the two test groups were administered decolorized Aloe Vera in varying and incrementally higher dosages—1 milligram per kilogram, 10 mg/kg and 100 mg/kg. In simple terms, they were administered doses that were set at two very high levels, the second one being the highest that their systems could physically support.

And the control group was administered no Aloe Vera. Then the five groups were tested at intervals of four and seven days to determine what effect, if any, the introduction of Aloe Vera had on pain, edema, and the treatment of wounds.

In direct contrast to the zinc/deficiency tests undertaken six years earlier, the Aloe Vera control group studies revealed a strikingly affirmative result for the test groups. Not only did increased doses of Aloe Vera help accelerate healing and aid in the rapid healing of the wounds, the percentage of wound reduction increased in direct proportion to the amount of Aloe Vera administered during treatment. By day seven, the average level of healing had increased to 43% for the 1-mg/kg group and all the way to 56.6% for the 100-mg/kg group. That marked a jump of nearly 30 percentage points for the test group of diabetic mice treated with large doses of Aloe Vera.

Not surprisingly, in the same series of tests, when the mice were tested for analgesic effects and blood edema tests, the Aloe Vera test groups showed equally dramatic positive results in exhibiting lessened inflammation and improved pain response.

This elaborate and painstakingly accurate test has proven to be something of a landmark in diabetic research in that it unerringly showed the broad spectrum potentials Aloe Vera offered in treating many of the troublesome side-effects and opportunistic infections that accompany diabetes. And it did so by showing that

Aloe Vera, when used in heavier doses, actually showed even greater abilities to heal wounds and reduce pain and swelling.

In a follow-up study by Dr. Robert Davis and Nicholas P. March a year later, Aloe Vera was measured again for its anti-inflammatory activity in diabetes. This time, it was tested in combination with *gibberellin*. Gibberellin is a naturally occurring glycoside and growth hormone found in plants, including the complex chemistry of the Aloe plant.

Again the diabetes was adjuvant induced with the diabetic agent, *strepto-zoticin,* on adult male mice in control and test groups. In fact when tested individually and in context with the Aloe over the apportioned number of days, the gibberellin did show almost identical anti-inflammatory results. So the evidence, in this test at least, seemed to point to the fact that the glycoside gibberellin might indeed hold the key to the healing plant's anti-inflammatory powers. At least those were the conclusions of the researchers.

Once more, we have to point to the pieces to support the complete puzzle of Aloe Vera's remarkable chemistry. Assuming the gibberellin is the key to Aloe's remarkable anti-inflammatory capacity, it is still only one element that marks one aspect of this plant's panoply of superior qualities.

Given Aloe's ability to penetrate tissue, heal, relieve pain, increase enzymatic debridement in both degenerative and reparative stages, accelerate healing, reduce inflammation and swelling, salve and repair burns and ulcers, normalize circulation, repair and rebuild tissue, kill viruses, bacteria, fungi, monilia, and hosts of other microbes, we also add the x-factor of its almost mystical ability to hyper-generate into the system.

All things in the realm of scientific discovery come in chain reaction. No doubt these tests by Robert Davis and his research associates had to prompted Dr. Davis' decision to test Aloe Vera for its absorption in later years. And his milestone "Aloe Vera and Aspirin" tests were the result.

To be sure, this and many findings in the field of Aloe Vera and its ability treat autoimmune deficiencies has helped thousands of people being treated for these rare and dread diseases. We have, from personal experience, seen a number of sufferers from diabetes helped both systemically and topically.

By now, there have been so many sufferers of diabetes, particularly Type 1 diabetes, that we have been able to help with regimens using stabilized Aloe Vera. In a way, at least from our level of experience, they are best summarized in our first exposure to this debilitating syndrome and to one of the most dramatic stories of calamity and recovery to which we have ever been exposed.

Brenda's Story. All the laboratory findings, impressive though they may be, can only be given perspective when translated to the human condition.

Brenda's story is perhaps best illustrative of this. Having experienced it early in my career with the healing plant, I was left with the indelible impression that Aloe Vera was the perfect panacea for diabetics. It was a theory that is now being given clinical support two decades later.

I first met Brenda in 1968. Brenda was a young woman in her thirties who had been suffering from type 1 diabetes and was beginning to experience its most savage aspects. In the months before she originally got in touch with me, she had developed a hangnail on one of her toes that had ultimately resulted in the amputation of that toe. This is not necessarily an exceptional occurrence among type 1 diabetics.

Later while Christmas shopping, she developed a blister on her left foot which became so severely infected she had to have a major debridement on her foot. To further aggravate her condition, the foot was not responding to post-surgical treatment. She was in constant pain. Infection was mounting. And her doctor was considering partial amputation as the only remaining option to save part of her foot.

Imagine for a moment the terrifying universe in which many diabetics must live. So susceptible are they to immunological breakdowns and failed functions, that the least injury or illness can pose a serious threat to their health and even their lives. By the same token, some diabetics, forged in the steel of adversity, become gifted with steely resolve and great courage. Brenda was such a person.

Convinced this problem could be solved without surgery, she refused to sign her surgical release papers and instead got in touch with me.

"You don't know me," she said. "But I've seen pictures of work your products have done to heal skin ulcers." Brenda had already used our pharmaceutical cream for pain relief for sore jaws and wanted to know if it might work to help her condition.

I expressed the belief that it would and recommended daily applications of the cream. Brenda followed my recommendation, used the crème in a daily routine, and kept it up for the next fourteen weeks. By that time her condition that had been diagnosed as untreatable by conventional modalities had completely healed, without scarring.

With that, Brenda's first chapter ended happily.

Chapter two began darkly on one chilly mid-autumn evening in 1978. Unfortunately, one of the most severe manifestations of the advanced diabetic syndrome is the loss of sensation in one's extremities. Brenda had long suffered from this and, after falling asleep, her feet extended toward a fire she and her husband had built, awakened to find to her horror that her feet had severely burned. They were tumescent, swollen and actually smoking. Due to what amounts to a total suppression of her PGE 2 prostaglandins, she had a lowered pain-alarm system. She had no sensitivity in her lower extremities. So she wasn't even aware that, even as she slept, her feet were receiving second and third-degree burns. In fact her left foot had burned nearly to the bone. A trauma for anyone, this was a life-threatening occurrence to Brenda.

The immediate challenge, treating the scorched areas, was answered by packing them in Aloe Vera cream. But by now profound fluid loss and side-infections had caused her to run a fever in excess of 104° for the next thirty-five consecutive days! Antibiotics failed to kick the infection, and to compound the dilemma Brenda reacted adversely to them. What's more, in addition to her burn trauma, Brenda developed a stress ulcer. Her hemoglobin count plummeted to a level of six. The situation and her condition were critical.

By this time, however, Brenda, her husband, and their attending physicians had become aware of what Aloe Vera had been able to do for her in the past and not only permitted her to be treated topically but also introduced her to our drinking gel to help alleviate the pain that the stress ulcer had caused. And to some degree, Brenda improved. Nevertheless, the treatments could only take her so far, and it was generally agreed by the physicians treating her that surgery would be required.

Enter a specialist, a podiatric surgeon.

At this point, it is difficult for the average person to fathom the chamber of horrors to which the advanced diabetic is subjected. Given Brenda's history of trauma and severely jeopardized body chemistry, surgery was literally a life-threatening option, and yet the only one she appeared to have. Initial surgery was successful, and a debridement and skin grafts were performed on both feet entailing the partial removal of three and a half toes on each foot. The surgeon then ordered her feet to be elevated and kept soaked in a betadyne solution. After further treatment, Brenda's feet were not responding and in fact were worsening. The condition appeared to be irreversible. By then it was February 14, 1979, and the attending surgeon did not have a pleasant Valentine message to convey.

Seeing no other way, he strongly recommended additional surgery and expressed the belief that complete amputation of the feet, and replacement with artificial limbs would be the only way to save Brenda's legs and life.

Brenda still believed there was another option and took it. Again refusing to sign her surgical release papers, and, over heated protests from the surgeon himself, she insisted on returning home. Reluctantly, she agreed to let them apply pigskin wraps to her feet, and agreed to continue applying them for several days. Pigskin is an acknowledged healant for certain burn conditions, but in this case it proved useless. After several days of applying it, Brenda found her condition worsening, and she returned to the Aloe Vera cream and drinking gel tandem treatments.

Almost immediately the infection diminished. The skin on both feet began to heal and continued to heal markedly. By August 1979, the regular Aloe Vera regimens—crème treatments to her skin and daily intake of the drinking gel—had brought Brenda to a nearly complete recovery. At that point, there were only two small spots that had not quite healed, one the size of a quarter on her left foot, one on her right foot the size of a dime. To dramatically illustrate, we have included some photos of Brenda's condition on these pages.

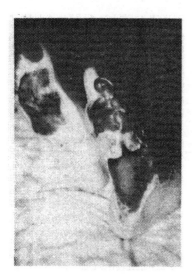

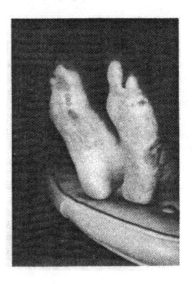

Brenda's burned feet prior to treatment with Aloe Vera with some loss of digits.

Brenda's burned feet six weeks after treatment with Aloe Vera. There is a nearly complete level of healing. with only marginal scarring.

Upon last checking with her in 1984, Brenda was completely healed, walking on her own two feet, and standing very tall indeed.

Since that time, I can say happily that we've seen many diabetics helped both systemically and with topical treatments from Aloe Vera. But Brenda's story will always remain in our mind and in our hearts. It stands as a testament to what one person with the courage of her convictions can accomplish...and to the simple but eloquent powers of a healing plant that never ceases to leave us both grateful and humble.

Summary

We are continually grateful for the progress that has been made in the last ten years especially in the diagnosis, treatment, and amelioration of autoimmune diseases such as the ones we have described in this chapter.

More than that, we are particularly heartened by the research, clinical studies, and new medications that are now pending approval by the FDA and governing health ministries worldwide for the treatment and cure of such perennial maladies as multiple sclerosis, psoriasis, bilateral scleroderma, systemic lupus, and pernicious anemia.

We also recognize the fact that such advances are taken in baby steps, and that final release of such treatments and products to the marketplace may be years in coming.

In the meantime, Aloe Vera remains steadfast in its service of the patients and practitioners to who turn to it as a healthy alternative. It is non-toxic, profoundly non-interruptive of current treatments, and perhaps the best adjunctive therapy God ever created. It counters with no antidote and offers only the true essence of healing: First, it does no harm.

For that, and for all its accomplishments in this constantly evolving field of discovery, we continue to give praise and thanksgiving.

Chapter 6

Memories and Miracles

This chapter, replete with anecdotes, might be a sidebar to the clinician but a Godsend to the average reader. That's because it brings us, at last, in touch with the human element where the poetry of healing truly begins. Touching upon everything from lung tumors to parrots with frostbite, it will bring Aloe Vera into a context of usage that everyone can understand—often as a last best hope for the individual's struggle to regain command of his health, his life and his future.

The past 40 years for us have been those of singular focus: to bring Aloe Vera out of the wasteland of mythology and conjecture and into the Mecca of universal professional use. Still it is the power of personal experience that underscores, at a very human level, just how much miracles help to transform us every day of our lives—how they touch the divine in us and keep us both aware and humble that there are gifts at our disposal of which we are yet unaware. Yes, for the most part, the stories we are about to relate involve Aloe Vera and how it has helped so many people who, in some cases, had lost all hope for recovery. More than that, they are also a celebration of human ingenuity, grit, determination, and faith that we so seldom get to experience and yet so often long to share.

For the most part, what I am about to tell you offers no structured personal chronology. What follows are merely memories that come cascading into my consciousness from time to time, a reflection of miracles held in gratitude's mirror.

Fortunately for me, I was able to be a part of so many of them. In so many other instances, I would get reports either from my fellow professionals or individuals helped by treatments in which Aloe Vera was the principal agent of cure. Knowing of my dedication to Aloe Vera research and development, they would come to me either with personal experience or close encounters that reinforced my belief in the plant and its mission here on earth. Of course, it seldom comes as a surprise that so many seemingly miraculous cures involve the healing plant. Nevertheless, it's always food for the journey.

1962—What started it all.

In 1962, I had just started experimenting with Aloe Vera in my first pharmacy. I had recently developed an Aloe spray that I had adapted from the fresh plant when an attorney friend of mine's wife, Coy McClung phoned me with a request for some sunburn medication for her arm. She told me that the day before she had been out playing a long round of golf in the hot Texas sun.

Coy was in considerable pain when she called asked for a popular sunburn treatment, Decadron, to treat her red scorched arms. Even though Decadron was a popular steroidal anti-inflammatory, it does little to relieve pain. And I personally felt, given the severity of her burn, that it wouldn't be enough to do the job. So, I asked her to do me a favor and try a bottle of Aloe Vera liquid I had just helped formulate.

"I'll refill the prescription," I told her. "But do me a favor. When you receive your Decadron, I'm going to send you a little bottle liquid. If you would, please try this: Put the Decadron on one arm, use a cotton pad and rub this liquid all over the other. Do that for a day or so and get back to me."

Since Coy and her husband were friends and neighbors, she agreed. Although she was skeptical, and I was only mildly convincing, she suspended her disbelief and became the principal in what amounted to my first test case. Of course, I sent her the Aloe liquid without charge, but never actually told her what it was. In fact, I felt it might do her a great deal of good. In truth, I was still experimenting with this unknown quantity and wasn't altogether certain.

When she received the two treatments, she applied the Aloe Vera to her left arm and the Decadron on her right, she admitted that within the first five minutes her left arm started to feel both soothed and improved, while her right arm, where she had applied the Decadron, was still in considerable pain.

About two days later, she came by to show me the conclusive proof of what would soon prove to be Aloe Vera's calling card to the world. Her left arm, where she had continued to spray the Aloe Vera, had tanned and healed without incident. Her right arm, where she had applied the Decadron on a regular basis, still hurt and had thousands of tiny blisters.

At the time, I gave her the Aloe Vera to use, I still knew so little about what it could do, but I decided then that if this little plant could make that kind of impact when tested head-to-head against a known steroidal cream that I would spend the rest of my life finding out just how good it really was.

Now, 40 years later, I realize how momentous that decision was, and I remember the parable of the mustard seed.

An Early Lesson.

Nothing underscores the importance of appropriate treatment more than a crisis that strikes you where you live. In the late 1960s, my oldest daughter Kimberly, then 10 years old, occasionally experienced a kind of severe allergic reaction whose origins we could never quite determine. But we became painfully aware that these seizures were immediately accompanied by a rather pernicious fungus. What we could also determine was the fact that these reactions would occur spontaneously and seemed to increase in both intensity and duration, as did the fungus.

In the beginning, all the remedies the doctors tried to use to combat this pathological one-two punch netted little effect. In fact, nothing we had tried seemed to have much effect, until I started cultivating my soon-to-be lifetime relationship with Aloe Vera. During Kim's allergic seizures, we found that the Aloe Vera was about the only thing that could control it. But not even the Aloe seemed to be able to cure it. Then we experienced a dire emergency with Kim that brought the issue to a head and provided me with a valuable lesson in the process.

At the time, my wife Jewel and I had to go on a brief trip and, as we often did, dropped our two children off to stay with their maternal grandmother down in Quitman, Texas. During the time that we were gone, Kim's hands broke out in a severe infection. The lesions reappeared, and there were streams of red streaks up her arm—an indication that blood poisoning might be setting in.

In truth the lesions appeared to be getting gangrenous, and if they did, the situation for my dear daughter would become dire indeed.

By that time, my wife and I had been contacted, flew in and shot down to Quitman immediately.

As soon as we arrived, I soaked Kim's hands and arms in 100% Aloe Vera gel. Within 30 minutes, she had already shown remarkable improvement. Still concerned, and still not out of the woods as far as I could determine, I took Kim to a physician friend of mine, M.A. Pearson, M.D. Dr. Pearson had worked with our original formula for Aloe Vera and had also had some success in using a steroidal cream called Micolog to treat certain kinds of allergies. So, it was Dr. Pearson's suggestion that we combine the two treatments into an Aloe Vera/Micolog cream to use on Kimberly's hands and arms.

The result we achieved was as groundbreaking as it was heartening to me personally because, for the first time ever, my daughter's condition cleared up and stayed clear. Was she cured? I hesitate to declare it categorically. One can never entirely determine the perverse, persistent nature of some pathologies any more than one can underestimate their propensity to recur. All I know is that neither the allergy nor the fungus returned. And that was cure enough for me.

That personal experience also drove home to me two profound aspects of Aloe Vera.

First, it reaffirmed my previous experience that Aloe Vera was the perfect adjunctive therapy in that it never seemed to antidote any treatment with which it was combined. Second, it not only seemed to complement the other medication, it also almost always enhanced its properties in very synergistic ways. It was a revelation that we would have confirmed for us time and again over the coming years.

The Breath of Life.

With all the recent increase in awareness about Aloe Vera, we often tend to dismiss the courage and pioneering spirit of some of the people we have worked with in the past. I try to transform that tendency to oversight and embrace these memories like diamonds—because they were the first! Such is the case with a distributor on one of my first Aloe companies, a woman named Dot Pierce.

The year was 1969. The city was Baton Rouge, Louisiana. Dot Pierce was the number one distributor in my first cosmetic company. As is often the case with so many early converts to the healing powers of Aloe Vera, Dot had personally experienced a number of instances in which our Aloe products had helped salve and heal all kinds of conditions for her at a topical level. I had also discussed with her the fact that both historical findings and my personal research indicated that the healing plant was equally effective when used internally, especially for challenges to the respiratory system.

It only stood to reason then that when her husband Charlie was admitted to the hospital with a rather large mass on his lung, she would come to me with the fragile hope that Aloe might be able to help improve Charlie's apparently advanced condition. In fact, according to Dot, the mass on Charlie's lung was sizeable, appeared to be dangerous, and that the doctors were all but convinced that, pending further tests and x-rays, they would have to perform surgery to remove the lung.

Having historical and laboratory precedent from which to work, as well as several doctors who had used my Aloe internally for a list of respiratory conditions, I felt confident that it could help. By the same token I knew that in 1969 Charlie

Pierce's doctors were not even going to consider letting our Aloe Vera drinking gel be the treatment of choice, if for no other reason than it was an unknown quantity. (In fact, Dot had requested that they consider this and had been turned down flat.) So we took what, at the time, was the only option opened to us: We smuggled the Aloe drinking gel into Charlie Pierce's hospital room.

At the time, we were also aided by the fact that Charlie was currently suffering from a mild case of pneumonia. So, according to standard medical procedures, the attending physician and surgeon agreed that he could not be operated on until the syndrome cleared up.

Despite the cloak and dagger antics, I knew at the very least that the Aloe wouldn't harm him. Tests we had conducted before had convinced me that it was utterly non-toxic. Dot had complete confidence in that. And so we proceeded.

Virtually working under cover, Dot would sneak her husband Aloe drinking gel into the hospital every day with the encouragement to drink as much as possible. Due to Charlie's accompanying bout of pneumonia, he was able to take in no more than about a pint a day. And yet within a few days, he had not only completely recovered from his pneumonia, the doctors were amazed to discover that the seemingly cancerous mass had been greatly reduced in size. Convinced that their original diagnosis had been a miscalculation of the mass, Charlie's doctors did not operate. Instead, they released Charlie Pierce under the condition that they check him periodically to see if the mass size had increased. Subsequent examinations revealed that this seemingly carcinogenic mass, once having shown up to be considerable in size, had disappeared altogether.

Whether it was fifteen years ago or yesterday, the personal accountings of the curative breakthroughs Aloe has made in so many applications have been no less dramatic and no less frequent in their occurrence. They offer a series of daily miracles no less significant and certainly no less impactful now than ever before. In fact the list continues to be endless, and the rolls of the true believers continues to grow…in legion.

A Fish Story.

It is an unfailing truth that the healing wisdom that comes in Aloe Vera announces itself in direct proportion to the vision of the people who embrace it. And there is always something to be said for the audacity of innocence.

Such was the case with my son Shannon who, at the age of 13, decided that our Aloe Vera gel was just what his tropical fish needed to get rid of their skin rashes.

Tropical fish live in a precarious environment indeed. Their water has to be properly pH balanced, or they'll die. They have to get just the right amount of oxygen, or they'll die. If they don't receive the proper degree of nutrition, they'll die. If their aquarium becomes polluted, they'll die.

In this case, Shannon's tropical fish—all 12 of them—had contracted a skin rash from some fungus that had started to run rampant in the aquarium. Having spent his entire childhood around Aloe Vera and my constant experiments with it, my young son was convinced that this healing plant could do anything, including treat and cure his fungus-plagued fish. So, he plopped eight ounces of Aloe in his 10-gallon aquarium with unshakable conviction.

"If Aloe Vera can get rid of fungus, it can cure my fish," he told me. And without a trace of doubt, he continued to pour the doses of Aloe into the aquarium.

Within a week, the fungus on the scales of all the fish had healed. Their appetites had improved. Not a fish was lost. And Shannon remained convinced that the Aloe had done it. Who was I to argue?

There is a company today that has a usage patent for putting Aloe Vera in fish bowls. I know, because I was hired as an expert in the field by a company that was being sued for an improper application of the patent. Their contention was that this was common usage folk remedy that was recorded in ancient times. On that basis and according to the law of precedent, if something in historical record (such as an excerpt even from one of Pliny's *de Materia Medica*) refers to a product as being in common use, it may fall into public domain and therefore deregister the patent. Unfortunately, despite the intense amount of research involving Aloe Vera and all its many applications, there was not one shred of evidence, even in folklore, of it ever having been used for this purpose. As a result, the company that sponsored my "expert testimony" lost the case. So it occurred to me during the trial that my son, Shannon, was something of a visionary.

Help for the Heismann Hopeful.

Changes in the course of greatness often hinge upon small things. There is no doubt that Earl Campbell, while an All-American tailback at the University of Texas, had suffered a deep thigh bruise during the latter part of the football season during his junior year through the summer and up to the early autumn of his senior year for the Longhorns in 1974.

Due to have another All-American year with one of the college football juggernauts of the 1970s, Campbell was losing hope even of starting the first game, if his deep thigh bruise didn't improve.

Thigh bruises are both debilitating and deep-seeded. And they can be so painful that, given certain degrees of severity, can even prevent the sufferer from any semblance of mobility. So Earl Campbell was not only in danger of missing a few games, he might, were the injury to continue, miss a large portion of what might well be the pivotal year of his entire career.

Fortunately, Earl Campbell's trainer was the redoubtable Frank Medina. As you might have read in our Chapter 3 "Super Stars." Frank Medina was the first trainer in either the collegiate or professional ranks to espouse stabilized Aloe Vera products for broad-spectrum use on athletes in all fields of sports. The fact that he would not hesitate to use it on his star running back, and do so with complete confidence, said everything about Frank Medina and even more about his confidence in the healing plant.

Ordering hot and cold Aloe Vera massages for Earl Campbell's thigh kept up every hour during the day (and keeping it in Aloe Vera liquid wrap at night), Medina saw to it that Earl Campbell not only started the first game of the season but also that he played every game of the season.

Later that year, Earl Campbell not only garnered all NCAA rushing awards and led the University of Texas to a Southwest Conference Championship, he also won the Heismann trophy and went on to an all-pro career with the Houston Oilers.

Having made all these observations, we hasten to note both the character and determination of a remarkable man like Earl Campbell. Renowned not only for his Spartan work ethics and his ability to play when hurt, Earl was also praised as being the paragon of a courageous athlete. For us to place all the credit for his recovery and lengthened career upon his connection with Aloe Vera would be both self-serving and inaccurate.

Nevertheless, one has to weigh the potential consequences had he not had access to it. Reflecting upon the careers of running backs like Dallas Cowboy Emmitt Smith (who did have access to Aloe Vera) and Denver BroncoTerrell Davis (who did not), one can only begin to ponder these simple twists of fate.

Hog Heaven.

There is no accounting for the affection people often show their creature companions or the ends to which they will go to take good care of them.

In 1971, we were in Hawaii at a convention for our first cosmetic company when one of our key distributors who was based in Honolulu came to me in distress about what she could do for her sunburned hog.

Apparently, she had adopted the creature when it had been a mere piglet and had kept it sheltered as a pampered house pet, even though it grew to be several hundred pounds in weight.

Perhaps not surprisingly pigs (and hogs) have very fair complexions and, if not exposed to the elements on a regular basis, can sunburn just as severely as human beings, often with the same results—pain, blistering, peeling, scaling, and subsequent possible skin cancer later on (should they live so long).

Somehow, while the woman was off at our convention, her pet hog had gotten out and was finally found by some neighbors wandering around on the beaches of Oahu. Since pigs are highly intelligent and, especially if brought up around people, can be very docile, she obediently followed the neighbors back home. At the same time, the neighbors took note of her severe redness and the fact that she squealed from the pain of it all the way home and all the time thereafter.

Remembering all that Aloe had done on many instances past, this woman applied what was then our Aloe Moisturizing Lotion all over the sow's sunburn. And, even though this was a diluted solution (no more than 35% Aloe) not only did the creature experience immediate relief, she even came around for more rubdowns.

The end result? The hog healed without peeling…and ended up with some pretty smooth skin in the process.

A Mouthful.

Any one who has ever undergone periodontal surgery will tell you that, in terms of excruciating pain and discomfort, it has few equals. For that reason, when such surgeries are performed, periodontists will only perform them on one quadrant at a time: one upper or lower quadrant on either side, at properly spaced intervals. Given the guidelines of prudent periodontal surgery that is not only customary, it is also entirely prudent.

It is commonly accepted that, were they not to do so—were they actually to perform periodontal surgery on all four gum quadrants at once—the patient might easily find the process of eating so painful that he or she might actually become dehydrated, anemic or even die from an inability to pass food of any kind through the mouth.

That's why it seemed almost foolhardy to some of his co-workers when a young dentist friend of ours, Dr. Lynne Tenny was about to undertake gum surgery on a woman and decided to proceed with a full four-quadrant surgery. Suffering from intermediate periodontal gingivitis, the woman he was working on was a successful career woman and didn't want to lose any more time than was necessary. So she was not only willing to have the four-quadrant surgery, she preferred it. Since Dr. Tenny had used stabilized Aloe Vera a number of times on his patients and had borne witness to its exceptional healing powers, he felt confident in what it could do, but his assistant didn't share his belief.

"If you do a full mouth surgery on this woman, she is going to die of pain," his assistant told him.

Usually after just one quadrant of periodontal surgery, the patient has several days of discomfort and often has to take a series of painkillers such as Vicadin to alleviate the pain. So, at the time, the four-quadrant surgery seemed to be an extreme and perhaps imprudent decision. Dr. Tenny, however, was insistent. "This is a great product," he told her. "I'm going to use it on this lady."

Before and after the surgery, Dr. Tenny swabbed all four quadrants with Aloe liquid and also gave the woman a bottle of special Aloe Vera solution to use as a mouthwash.

After Dr. Tenny's successful surgery, the woman returned home. And on several occasions during the next two days, she would rinse about two ounces of the Aloe Vera solution in her mouth (and swallow it). As a result, her mouth healed without incident, and she was even able to eat some solid food as soon as the second day. What's more, she got through her entire recovery period without having to take any pain medication, not even a single aspirin.

Synchronicity.

Synchronicity, loosely defined, is a "coincidence" that is divinely ordained. In the early 1970s a doctor friend of mine came to me with a unique problem. A patient of his, a woman about 45 years of age, had gotten a case of fever blisters in her mouth that had blossomed into a severe case of ulcers that soon spread all the way down into her throat.

The clinical name for fever blisters is Herpes simplex (1). It is a virus that attacks the mucous membranes. And it is one thing against which Aloe Vera has proven itself effective time and again. Knowing this, and aware of our clinical findings both in the Sims-Zimmermann and Jean Setterstrom tests, this doctor came to me with his report.

"The poor woman has such severe (herpes) ulcers in her throat, she can't eat. In fact, she can't even swallow," the doctor told me, then asked. "What can we do for her?"

I recommended a regimen of pure 100% Aloe Vera gel used as a mouthwash and gargle. The best remedy was for the woman to swish the gel in our mouth for as long as she could and then very slowly swallow the remainder—and to do so as often as possible. That way she would not only get the topical benefit of the gel directly on the ulcers but also the systemic benefit by absorbing the Aloe into her system where, frankly, the Herpes simplex virus does its worst work.

Later the doctor reported to me that after following this regimen for just 30 minutes, the woman was able to eat soft food again. And he informed me of something else.

"Apparently, this woman knows you, Bill. It seems she was a classmate of yours in Greenville High School."

There are no accidents.

A Wonder Down Under.

It was 1983, and I was down in Sydney Australia giving a speech on Aloe Vera to a group of highly motivated distributors. In fact, it was almost like the miracle of healing in the old time tent revival. The only difference happened to be that I was the speaker at the Sydney Opera House. Not only is the Sydney Opera House a bastion of artistic dignity, it is also the cultural linchpin of the island continent of Australia and its architectural signature to the civilized world. So I suppose the sudden appearance of the woman I was about to meet caught me a bit by surprise.

Before my lecture to this already supercharged assembly, a lady in her 60s came out of the wings, introduced herself to me, and asked if she could give her testimony before the crowd. I agreed to have her on, but when she did appear, she surprised me as well as the entire gathering with her story.

"Eighteen months before I came to talk to you tonight, I was confined to a wheelchair, because I had arthritis in every joint of my body. I couldn't walk. I could barely move. I even had to have corrective surgery..."

At that point, the woman pointed out some scars on one wrist and one knee where her joints had to be replaced—so painful and crippling had her condition become. Even then, she declared, she had still found little relief and was now saddled with the prospect of decreased mobility.

Then, upon the advice of a healing professional she started taking oral doses of Aloe Vera drinking gel which she would combine with several tablets a day of bee propolis. (Bee propolis, besides being credited with certain anti-bacterial qualities, has now been found to be an anti-inflammatory agent as well.)

After several months of drinking the Aloe Vera juice and taking the bee propolis, the woman was not only able to come to this meeting she was also able to walk up the sixty famous steps required to enter the Sydney Opera House.

"And I did it," the woman proudly proclaimed, "without experiencing a single moment's pain."

Interestingly, I was there on a promotional junket to sell the concept of Aloe Vera to a group of distributors for a private label marketer of my products. After that very touching and poignant moment, there was not much selling left for me to do.

Malaysian Miracles.

Some of our most dramatic stories of cures and treatments involving Aloe Vera have occurred in places like Malaysia, Korea, Taiwan and mainland China. But it has always seemed to have been Malaysia where some of our most dramatic encounters have taken place.

A mysterious country, as steeped in the poetry of tradition as it is in the ever present dragon of poverty, it has some of the best and worst of what Asia represents. Certainly among its best attributes are the people.

Firestorm. In the spring of 1983, I received a letter from Malaysia. It was urgent in tone and desperate in nature, and came from the parents of a 10 year-old girl whose severely burned legs and body had been completely been healed by stabilized Aloe Vera gelly.

Apparently while working on a rubber plantation, the young girl's father received a panic call from his wife, telling him that their 10-year-old daughter had brushed near a flame and had caught her dress on fire. While, desperately trying to put it out by any means necessary, the little girl had suffered first, second and third degree burns over 50% of her body. Her father rushed home to tend her but immediately saw that the severity of the burns would require immediate medical attention.

In trying to tend the girl, her parents felt hopeless and alone. Because their daughter was crying out loud with pain and they were at least 30 kilometers away from the nearest physician, the young couple quickly set about to find one before the situation became even more critical.

During their journey to the doctor, they stopped off at a local service station to get some gas and ask directions.

Meanwhile, the little girl was sobbing non-stop from the pain and infection and, since there was no doctor within 30 kilometers of their plantation, she'd received no relief whatsoever.

As it happened, one of the salesmen representing an Aloe Vera company to which we were providing product happened to be at the service station, and happened to have a large sample bottle of Aloe Vera gelly with him. So, with the father's permission, he was able to apply it to the little girl's burns. Almost immediately, they reported to me that the girl stopped crying and declared at the same time that she no longer felt any pain.

These sales people of course left the bottle with the young man and his daughter, and were delighted when he got in touch with them a few days later to report what had happened. The doctor he did find, it seemed, was conversant with the virtues of the healing plant and had noted that the girl had "received the best possible treatment she could have for her burns."

He gave the girl a tetanus shot for any possible tetanus infection, but also informed the girl's father. "You're using the best possible product in the world on your child. Just keep it up."

Afterward, the young girls grateful parents sent me the photos along with the complete details of her remarkable recovery. I've included them here as a graphic example of Aloe's special healing power.

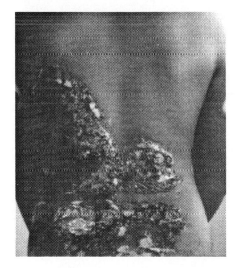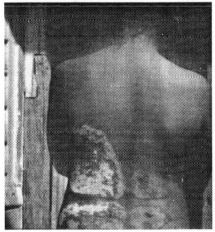

A ten-year-old Malaysian girl's back prior to treatment with stabilized Aloe Vera gelly. Evidence of first, second and third degree burns.

A ten-year-old Malaysian girl's back 90 days after to treatment with stabilized Aloe Vera gelly. Note the healing with minimal trace of scarring.

The Danny Chow Story.

Although I didn't originally go to Malaysia in 1985, I was offered a free trip and accommodations plus a hefty fee if I would look into helping treat a very distraught young man named Danny Chow.

In a letter from an associate in the Kiwanis Club in Ipo, Malaysia, I received news that Danny had been severely injured in an auto accident and, unless something were done and quickly, the doctors were going to have to amputate both his legs.

Apparently his legs, already badly injured from the wreck, had also developed massive ulcers that had now formed and would not heal. A distributor for a family of products manufactured under my formula had actually collected a considerable sum of money to send Danny to U.S. so that I could examine him and recommend treatment.

I told them, I would be willing to do so, but I could advise them to do the same thing in Malaysia that I could do here. So, I very specifically set up a program of treatment for Danny as follows:

First, I recommended that his attending physicians take 100% stabilized Aloe Vera gel, saturate a clean wash rag with the liquid and allow it to run down the legs twice a day for 30 minutes at a time. Between the soakings, I recommended that they apply a generous portion of Aloe Vera lotion every three to four hours.

They followed my directives and treated the boy accordingly. And though I didn't hear from them immediately, I received news that Danny Chow's legs had been saved and that he did recover from the incident.

Two months later, I was back in Malaysia on a lecture tour and was informed by that same distributor that Danny wanted to meet me personally. We went to Danny Chow's house later in the evening and found the young man sitting on floor with his feet in a pan of Aloe Vera gel. After he had finished soaking his feet and legs, he showed us what the Aloe gel had been able to accomplish: Danny's legs, once so entirely ulcerous that the doctors had considered amputation as the only viable alternative, had completely healed except for one small area about the size of a quarter.

Delighted for the young man, I asked him what he was going to do for a career in the future. His answer was as ironic as it was unequivocal.

"Why, I'm going to sell Aloe Vera products," he said, with a broad grin. And so he did.

The Plane Dealer.

Sometimes, small stories make for the most eloquent expressions of Aloe Vera's amazing healing powers. On one such occasion in the early 1990s, I was on a flight from Miami to Atlanta when I noticed an elderly couple across the aisle undergoing some difficulty. The 80-something husband was trying to console his wife, who apparently was suffering from osteoarthritis and was in such pain that she was on the verge of tears, so much so that even the act of consolation, a slight pressing of the hand caused her to scream outloud.

For a moment, I wondered whether or not to invade their private agonies. But when you've been given the secrets to healing that I've been blessed to receive, you contract a certain missionary zeal that overwhelms any personal sense of reserve. So I introduced myself and mentioned that I might have a product that might help her.

"My mother had the same condition," I noted and presented the pair with a small bottle of Aloe Vera liniment. "Now, I'm not saying this will cure your condition. But I feel pretty optimistic about the fact that it can relieve you of your pain."

I handed them the liniment and then fell back into my book, trying not to become too overbearing in the process. Still, I spied them out of the corner of my eye and noticed that the woman began applying the liniment every two or three minutes, and seemed to be doing so more vigorously each time.

We landed about 20 minutes later, and when I went to the baggage carousel to pick up my two-suiter, the woman came up to me.

"Where can I buy some more of this?" she asked.

To that I answered, "I know just the place…"

Lupus and the Lady in the Lobby.

Some of our most poignant experiences with Aloe Vera come when we least expect them. Not long ago in our offices and factory I was doing some research in the lab when one of the girls in our office came to me and announced that there was a woman in the lobby who wanted to meet me.

"I think you'll want to see her," she nodded, in a way that precluded denial.

Still in my lab coat, I stepped outside to find an attractively dressed woman in her forties waiting for me with tears in her eyes.

I invited her into my office, and as she took a seat on my couch she began to reveal a story that moved me as well.

"I had contracted Lupus (erythematosus) in my nose nearly two years ago, and it had developed to such a stage that I was now beginning to look grossly malformed. After several months, the doctors had tried every modality they could think of, and nothing had worked. I had just about given up hope, and then I finally went to a chiropractor, Everett Combs, who knew something about Aloe Vera."

The woman remembered that she went to a doctor who had read some of our material, had become familiar with the Rita Thompson story, and had also used our Aloe Vera products from time to time. Sympathetic to the severity of the woman's condition, he ordered some of our topical Aloe Vera cream and had the woman apply that, while she began daily to drink several ounces of our Aloe drinking gel.

In a short time the lupus cleared up and, after a few weeks, seemed to have disappeared entirely."

"I don't know how I can ever thank you enough," the woman told me.

"Thank God. He's the one who made the plant," I told her. It was a reaction I gave that was as spontaneous as it was surprising to me. It's just that I've always felt that way and always will.

A Frostbitten Parrot Speaks Out.

One of the advantages of having a bird with a vocabulary perhaps rests with the fact that it can let you know how it is feeling—even if you might not always want to hear what it has to say. So it was with a working associate of mine, Marty Young, and his large golden macaw named Nugget.

Nugget's story is quite a unique one, and it's a testimony to both the bird and his new owner that it turned out as well as it did.

To begin with, Marty didn't originally own Nugget. He actually bought the large beautiful golden breasted, teal blue bird from a family in Waco Texas, and had done so shortly after an untoward winter freeze.

Except for the infamous blizzards of its notorious Panhandle, massive freezes across the state of Texas are something of a rarity. But early December of 1983 proved to be a violent and punitive exception. For three solid weeks of that month, the temperatures hovered just above zero degrees Fahrenheit and were accompanied by wind-chill factors that sent the real temperature well into Arctic lows. Crops in the fertile Rio Grande Valley were laid waste. Cattle in west Texas, despite ranchers' attempts to herd them into barns, froze to death in the fields. And we were all headed toward an economic disaster as well as a danger to plant and animal life, alike.

Bad weather for anyone under any circumstances, this could prove to be an especially difficult if you're a Gold Macaw who is used to the tropical climes of the Matto Grosso in Brazil.

Most domesticated avians such as macaws, parrots, cockatiels and other exotic birds are used to thriving in warm, balmy Amazonian climates and feeding on the rich fruits, berries, and nuts of the rainforests. They do not adapt well to arctic temperatures and, even when exposed for relatively short periods, are in peril of not surviving them at all.

Apparently, the day before the big freeze of 1983 hit the state of Texas, Nugget had literally flown the coop, got out of his owner's house and vanished from sight. Braving the wilds through the Nordic chill in search of him for days on end, the family finally gave up. Deducing that Nugget had probably frozen to death, they gave up the quest, lamenting but accepting the fact that he had fallen victim the devastations of a terminally cold winter.

But one can never underestimate the intelligence of birds that can talk as well as any creature's instincts for survival. Somehow, Nugget had found his way to partial shelter from the devastations of the freeze. And thanks to one of the family's cousins who would not give up on the lovable bird, he was finally found and brought home nearly two weeks later.

To everyone's surprise Nugget seemed to be in satisfactory (if not perfect) shape, particularly in view of his recent purgatorial experience. Naturally concerned, Nugget's family took him to a local vet who examined the bird and assured them that he was all right.

"There's nothing wrong with him," the vet said, giving his rather sunny if ill-advised diagnosis.

Despite the fact that the macaw's feet, normally ash grey and quite soft had now become black and stiff, the family took the vet's professional opinion as gospel and brought the bird home.

About a week later, the family sold Nugget to Marty Young. A well-known Dallas documentary film producer, Marty had long held a fascination for tropical birds and took an instant liking to Nugget. The price was right. The family seemed intent on seeing to it that the bird got a good home. And Marty took Nugget, aviary and all, back to his Dallas film studio.

Before selling the bird to Marty, the family had told him about his traumatic incident but assured him that Nugget had gotten a clean bill of health from their local vet.

But after Marty got his newfound tropical companion back home, he couldn't help but notice that something literally didn't smell right. Nugget was favoring one foot, held it up almost perennially and would seem to go nearly berserk whenever anyone would approach him "to perch."

Normally tropical birds like parrots and cockatoos are quite amenable to perching on a human's fingers, hand or wrist. It's the way they affiliate. And most domesticated birds are quite used to it. But in this case, Nugget was not only resistant to that kind of contact, he was paranoid about it.

Now, convinced that Nugget was not in good shape at all, Marty took him to a local vet who specialized in treating tropical birds.

"Good grief, this poor fellow's got a terrible case of frostbite," the vet declared. Immediately, he treated the bird with a clear betadyne solution, rinsed his feet and toes several times, and then came to Marty with a rather fatalistic prognosis. "He's going to lose two toes on his right foot and probably three, which means he'll lose his foot. If that happens (and I think it will), I suggest we put the poor creature out of his misery and put him down."

Marty thanked the vet but declined the 'ultimate solution' he suggested. The vet acquiesced to Marty's love of the bird and prescribed Nugget some antibiotics to help cut down on the infection. When he did, Marty implied that he had one alternative left that he'd like to pursue.

As it turned out, he had worked with me on a number of film and video projects about Aloe Vera and had a very good idea about what the healing plant could do. So he called me up with his and Nugget's life-and-death dilemma, and asked me what I thought we could do. After listening to his problem, I suggested that he first wash Nugget's toes as thoroughly as possible with stabilized Aloe Vera liquid and then follow that with Aloe Vera gelly—and do it as often as possible. (I knew the liquid would get rid of the dead tissue and clear up the infection and that the gelly was the perfect medium to apply Aloe's various healing powers and to help rebuild the tissue on the toes.)

Marty didn't have much trouble washing Nugget's toes in the Aloe liquid; in fact, the big bird seemed to enjoy it. Applying the gelly was a bit more of a challenge.

Macaws are good-natured birds as a rule, but they're also the largest members of the parrot family and have beaks that can snap a pencil in half with a single bite. Nugget was in a very tender state of mind and had little inclination to let his toes be touched.

But the bond between man and his creature companions is often a rare and wondrous thing to behold. By now, Marty and Nugget had established a level of trust that broke through the pain and resistance. And despite Nugget's rather vocal complaints and occasional feints toward combat, he started letting Marty apply the Aloe Vera gelly.

After about four days, Nugget stopped resisting the application at all and in fact started sticking his toes up at Marty to be treated.

In two weeks time, Nugget's toes had, for all intents and purposes, healed. Within five weeks, Nugget's toes had healed without a trace of frostbite and without the loss of a single toe or claw. Except for the occasional dose of antibiotics to cut down side-infections, the Aloe Vera was the only treatment used.

Since Marty Young was also a part-time photographer, he took some before and after photos of Nugget's feet and toes. They, of course, show the results better than we could hope to describe them.

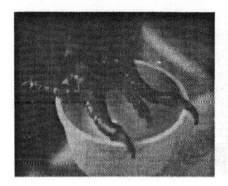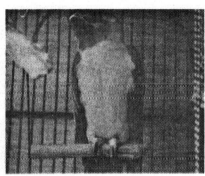

The Golden Macaw: Nugget's frostbit-ten feet and toes shortly after Marty got him from the family. Note the hard, black, distended toes.

Nugget about six weeks after his treat-ment with Aloe Vera Gelly. Note the return of color and health to the toes.

As a happy footnote to the story, I paid Marty a visit about three weeks after he had completed treatment on Nugget's feet and toes. Marty was putting in a new computer program, and Nugget was off in one corner, whittling away at what remained of a stump of wood, grasping it with his very healthy toes and claws.

"You've got to admit one thing about old Nugget," Marty acknowledged, looking up from his screen. "The bird's a survivor. "

"Sure is," I agreed.

"Sure is," Nugget repeated.

I could have sworn he understood me. It only seemed appropriate that he did.

Of Small Dogs and Snakebites

This story happened to my co-author, Robert Ahola, and is one of the most dramatic life and death episodes I've ever heard of. Robert and I have been friends for nearly 25 years and have co-authored a number of books on Aloe Vera. So he has, by osmosis if nothing else, come to know as much about the healing plant as any lay person in the world. Over the years, he has networked his knowledge of Aloe Vera to people he thought might benefit from it, and actually routed a number people to me who were in need of product advice and counseling.

Not surprisingly, he has amassed a library of experiences on his own, many of them involving our creature companions.

One of them involved a type 1 diabetic queen cat named Dede to whom he fed Aloe Vera and watched thrive to the ripe old age of 17. Another involved a wounded oriole that he nursed with Aloe for two days, until she finally bit him on the finger and flew away. (Some display of gratitude!)

But the most dramatic story Robert told me was about his (then) girlfriend's prize Havanese Bijon Frises, George and Gracie. "Bijons" as they are called are great dogs—small dogs in the poodle family with a large dog sense of self. At a fighting trim 10 pounds, George, being the male, was the larger of the two dogs and the most adventuresome.

On Mother's Day in 1999, he was out roaming the grounds at Robert's cliffside home in Malibu, California when he was bitten on the right front paw by a very young rattlesnake, no more than fifteen inches in length.

"That day brought home a couple of issues to me," Robert recalls. "The first one was that I still had a lot to learn about snakes. The second was that I still had a great deal to learn about Aloe Vera."

Robert remembered thinking at the time that, since it was a young rattlesnake, its venom might not be as potent. Then he checked up on it and found that just the opposite was true—that young rattlers have the most potent venom and the least self-control about using it. Unlike older rattlesnakes that learn how much venom to use with each strike, young rattlers tend to empty their entire sack into the object of their rage. And even though this was a defensive strike, young George had received quite a wallop.

Since it was late in the day on a Sunday, all the local vets were closed except for an emergency facility in Westwood about 15 miles away through heavy beach traffic. So any antidote would be at least an hour through heavy weekend beach traffic. That was virtually a lifetime when you had a small dog getting delirious from his reaction to the snakebite.

Remembering the incident with the Mexican rancher's prize bull that we discussed years before, Robert wasted no time. He cut a medium-sized leaf of Aloe from a plant he had on his upstairs balcony, split the leaf and wrapped it in a poultice around George's paw, holding in place as his girlfriend Yolanda manneuvered through stop and go beach traffic.

"I remember noticing at the time," Robert told me, "that the Aloe Vera leaf had almost flattened out in my hand. All the gel seemed to have evaporated. And

I silently questioned my own choice of the leaf: Had I gotten one that was a 'dink'?

"Then I realized that the leaf had actually been unloading all its healing potential into the dog's paw.

"As it turned out, it took us nearly an hour and a half through snarled, Sunday, Mother's Day beach traffic to finally get to the emergency veterinary clinic. And that can be a dog's lifetime in a dire situation like that.

"Ordinarily, a snakebite will manifest by imploding into the system. Swelling, distension of skin and high fever will be the immediate result. But none of this happened with George. In fact, about five minutes before we arrived at the vet's, George's paw had unloaded blood, puss, venom and everything else—about a pint of it in fact—all over my trousers and onto the floor of the SUV. Seeing this, I actually let out a shout for joy.

"'Oh great!' I said. 'The Aloe's done it! It's done it!'

"'Done what?!'" Yolanda asked, with a mixture of surprise and concern.

"I started to answer but didn't need to. Because by the time we reached the front door of the clinic, George was standing in my lap, perched with his front paws resting on the dashboard, barking and wondering when we could get out of the car."

The vet decided to administer the antivenom anyway, as a precaution, but noted, given George's size and the severity of the bite, that she was surprised the dog had made it at all.

"We lose a lot of little guys that way," she noted. "But not this time."

"It was the Aloe Vera," Robert told her.

"I'm sure it helped," she nodded, patronizing his conviction with faint regard.

Robert thought to pursue the issue, but experience had taught him by now. The greatest healing is always done in silence.

The Grass is Always Greener.

In the 1960s, billionaire H.L. Hunt was not only noted for being one of the richest men in the world, he was also renowned for his devotion to Aloe Vera and all he believed it could accomplish. It might also be said of him that he was a classic example of the fact that all the money in the world does not always provide the appropriate leverage for success if you're misguided in your efforts. Because, try though he may, he could never figure the plant out.

Even though he set up a state-of-the-art facility devoted to the research and manufacture of Aloe Vera, even though he hired what he felt were the best research scientists and plant processors, he still wound up with a product he could never quite bring successfully to market without some unfortunate repercussions.

Still, I never once doubted that the man's heart was in the right place. And, because of my success with formulating Aloe Vera, we would often communicate either directly or through one of his staff.

One time, his plant manager in Dallas called me with a request from Mr. Hunt that could only be termed unique.

"Bill," he told me, " I have an agronomist, Dr. Rowe, and his associate with me from Mississippi. And they're very much in need of a sterile safe Aloe Vera product. If I sent them over, would you be able to sell them some of your stabilized Aloe Vera gel?"

"No problem," I agreed to the request. And in a while, the two doctors Mr. Hunt had told me about pulled up to my plant in their truck and requested two large barrels of Aloe Vera juice. When I asked them what they were going to do with it, they showed me some photos of tomatoes that appeared to be about the size of cantaloupes. In fact, they apparently had to build special (bird) cages so they could carry them around for display.

What Dr. Rowe and his associates were doing was growing tomatoes hydroponically with a special growth enhancement medium consisting of a specially treated dirt medium, parchment, bat guano, seeds, and Aloe Vera that they would lay on in the dark of night.

In a rather unique multi-tiered growth process, Dr. Rowe and his associate would take parchment, put dirt on put some bat guano(an excellent fertilizer) on top of that, pack more dirt on top of that, plop in their seeds, and pour Aloe Vera juice on top of the layers of parchment, dirt, bat guano, dirt, parchment and seeds—somehow remarkably performed in the dark. In this process, the Aloe Vera would run slowly through the dirt, parchment, bat guano and tomato seeds and perform the unique task of killing the troublesome little virus that is germane to all tomato seeds, thereby performing the function of an antiviral agent and growth medium all at the same time.

When I asked them how they came to discover that Aloe was such a tremendous plant food, they recounted the story of their first encounter with Aloe Vera. Apparently the two men were traveling through a plantation area of southern Mississippi when they came across a pasture and noted that one section of it contained grass that was much greener, fuller, and taller than any other. When they inquired at the plantation, they learned that the people had been processing Aloe Vera and had used that patch of ground to dump the Aloe rinds.

"That's when we decided to use this on our tomato crops," Dr. Rowe confided.

I couldn't say I was surprised, but I was delighted. So were they.

Hair Raising Tales.

Some of my best stories about Aloe Vera surround its ability as a systemic replenishment following critical treatment. I recall a couple of instances in particular.

One night in the early 1980s, I was a giving a lecture to a group of key distributors in Shreveport, Louisiana. At the break, a young man about 40 years old came up to the podium and introduced himself.

"Mr. Coats, you didn't know me," he said. "but I just wanted to thank you for putting out such a remarkable product. And I'd like to tell you why." Almost tearfully, the man related his experiences from about two years before when he had suffered a case of severe throat cancer.

At the time, the young man's doctors were insistent that to save his life, they would have to administer heavy doses of chemotherapy and alternate that with extensive radiation. Radiation and "chemo", provided the host is young enough, work well enough for certain types of cancer. But invariably the radiation will cause massive scarring of tissue. And the chemo brings on such vicious side effects as nausea, vomiting, and an inevitable loss of hair.

Terrified but willing to explore the alternatives, the young man took the recommendation from a friend and put two ounces of Aloe Vera gelly in a glass with two ounces of our Aloe Vera drink (to coat his throat) and took them together liberally every four hours prior to his radiation treatments and regularly during his doses of chemotherapy.

(After the treatment, he would drink four ounces a day of our Aloe Vera drink and treat the outside of the throat topically with Aloe Vera gelly.)

After considerable applications of these two types of "radical" treatment, the young man proudly proclaimed that he suffered no scarring from the radiation treatments, and no side-effects from the chemotherapy. He even kept his hair.

Amazed that the young man not only appeared to be clear of the cancer, the doctors were equally astounded that he had survived his ordeal without apparent side-effects and actually looked better than when he'd started the treatment.

On a similar occasion while I was lecturing in Dallas in 1990, one of the distributors from a major network marketing company came up while signing books and said, "Bill, about six months ago I was diagnosed with internal cancer. And I was told I would have to have chemo to save my life.

At the time, I was warned by my physician about the side-effects I could expect from extended doses of chemotherapy.

"So remembering what I'd read in one of your earlier books about Aloe Vera and its positive effects as an adjunct in easing the effects of radical therapies. And a few days later, I started drinking about 12 ounces of Aloe Vera a day to prepare for it. I would take it prior to chemo and then take again for a period of time in anticipation of further chemotherapy.

"After I finished the regimen of chemo a few weeks later, the physician treating me asked me to come by for a final check-up. Expecting to hear the usual horror stories about how serious the side-effects had been, he was flabbergasted to learn that I had actually experienced none whatsoever.

In fact, I told him that I was already feeling better than I was before I developed cancer and that I credited the Aloe Vera for much of it. He nodded indulgently at me. But I'm pretty sure he didn't believe me."

The Mysterious Plague of Mr. Barefoot.

Our final story is one I'm repeating without apology. Because of the profound impact it has made on the lives of so many, and because it is the summary story of how Aloe Vera can make a change in anyone's life, I emphasize it yet again.

It involves a truck driver named W.R. Barefoot. As the principal in an independent trucking business out of Johnson, Kansas, Mr. Barefoot had been a trucker all his life. After operating his business for years without incident, W.R. Barefoot eventually contracted what we still refer to as "the disease with no name." We call it that because he was examined by physicians in legion, and no one was ever able to make a successful diagnosis.

It began with discomforting and prolonged pain in his knees and legs that presented all the symptoms of being rheumatoid arthritis. In fact that was what one physician had diagnosed, and for some time, he took various standard prescriptions for that kind of ailment. Over time, nothing had worked. The condition worsened and finally took a sudden sinister twist. Whether it was a complex reaction to his medication or an extension of the condition itself, W.R. Barefoot soon began to experience unsightly blemishes that would pop up anytime he bumped anything, even casually. Those blemishes would soon turn into painful oozing sores.

This pervasive and debilitating condition actually went on for years, until it had reached a point where any cutaneous contact in Mr. Barefoot's extremities would draw blood, infection, and suppuration of tissue.

At one point late in 1977, the condition had degenerated to such a degree that many doctors believed the man's life was in danger. And at least one doctor had recommended amputation of both legs as perhaps he only way the man's life could be saved.

Late in the autumn of 1978, another pair of physicians diagnosed the condition as vasculitis (or angitis), which was an irritation of the blood vessels. But that only seemed to address part of the complex package of pathologies that W.R. Barefoot was forced to endure on a daily basis. By that time his physical condition had degenerated to such an extent that he was hemorrhaging and in grave danger of losing his life.

Able to determine that his red blood cells were reproducing too slowly, this team of physicians drained his blood one pint at a time. They in turn replaced that with blood reinforced with new red cells reinjected into his circulatory system. And temporarily at least that stemmed the hemorrhaging. He was then flown to a special immunological center in Denver Colorado where he was examined by a team of specialists from all parts of the world. Although this noted team of immunologists commonly agreed that the condition was not vasculitis, they were able to agree about little else. In fact none of them, many of whom were noted diagnosticians, had ever encountered a disease quite like it. So all attempts to treat the syndrome ended up being the medical equivalent of the Tower of Babel.

In fact, they virtually sent the man home to die with the request that if he did find anything, to be sure and let them know.

Left with a diagnostic stalemate and little hope of recovery, the beleaguered trucker finally received a glimmer of hope. He met a distributor who had worked with our stabilized Aloe Vera, she shared with Mr. Barefoot numerous accounts of how it had helped so many other people with syndromes that had also seemingly been impossible to treat. He was also informed that our Aloe had no relative toxicity. So he could take as much as he needed, and he could do so without the need of a doctor's prescription.

By that time, it was the week before Thanksgiving in 1978. Desperate to try anything, W.R. Barefoot began drinking moderate doses of our Aloe Vera drinking gel (no more than four ounces a day) and continued that regimen religiously. Within six weeks, all his lesions had either healed or were in advanced stages of repair, and only traces of the once pervasive mystery disease were evident.

By the following May, Mr. Barefoot was sufficiently convinced that he was healed to call his doctors and inform them that he was completely recovered and that the Aloe Vera had done it.

The doctors were incredulous and immediately informed the man that he had experienced what is referred to in medical terms as a "spontaneous remission." At the time, medical professionals were still in the Dark Ages as far was their Aloe awareness was concerned. So the reaction, though lamentable, was understandable.

W.R. didn't need convincing, but the team of physicians did. And so they asked him what might seem to be the unspeakable:

First, his principal consulting physician, in Denver, Colorado made a special request of him (and of me).

"Mr. Barefoot, I want to see you and the product and the man who makes it in Denver as soon as possible. Can you do that?"

We both agreed that we would, and the next day, I met W.R. in his doctor's office. After reviewing the data I brought him and after talking with both of us, the physician remained unconvinced. And to this, Mr. Barefoot himself threw down the challenge.

"Doctor, what do we have to do to show you this works?" he asked.

To that the doctor gave a bone-chilling reply. "I want you to stop taking the product."

At that, Mr. Barefoot could only respond with what amounted to a spontaneous expression of disbelief. "Doctor," he reminded him. "Not long ago just two floors up from here, you were one hour away from taking off both my legs. Do you realize what you're asking me?"

"I know it's a great deal," the doctor acknowledged. "But we have three other people with this same [incurable] condition. And if you would try this for us, you might be able to save some lives."

"Okay, I'll do it," Mr. Barefoot agreed, with one condition. "If you will promise me that when I start bleeding, the first thing I do is get back on this gel."

As a testament to his courage, to his sense of humanity, and to assuage the professional skepticism of his doctors, Mr. Barefoot agreed to quit drinking the Aloe Vera gel for a designated period of time. And, as he knew they would, his rapacious symptoms returned within in a matter of days. Unfortunately, they did so at the worst possible time, because W.R. Barefoot was back on the road and making a run in his truck. Fortunately, the trucker had enough presence of mind to take a couple of bottles of Aloe Vera gel and began swigging it at least to keep him balanced enough to get him back onto a plane and back to the clinic in Denver where he could be examined.

After examining him and noting how profoundly his symptoms had returned and listening to his accounts of how—yet again—only the Aloe Vera had worked to assuage them even slightly, his doctors told him to go back on the gel. With almost light speed swiftness, he went back into remission. All his symptoms disappeared. Mr. Barefoot was once again on the mend. And in the meantime, he had helped some other victims of this vicious syndrome find relief and renewed hope.

In retrospect, there is little doubt that that this vicious syndrome W.R. Barefoot experienced was some sort of autoimmune disease. It is certainly one we hope does not begin to reappear at any time anywhere else in the world. But if it does, we have remedy that will treat it successfully both topically and systemically.

And that is a combination Aloe offers that no other single modality can hope to match.

I'm happy to say that W.R. Barefoot never had a recurrence of this mysterious and rapacious syndrome. He remained a devoted and consistent patron of stabilized Aloe Vera for the rest of his life. It was a full life; one that ended 22 years later, in the year 2000, with Mr. Barefoot dying in his sleep after a heart attack— a kind and gentle end for a courageous man.

Summary.

Chapters such as this are mutable. When we first began to address this subject, I wondered if we would have enough stories to make a full chapter. Once we got underway, we had to make choices about which ones to leave out.

There are so many personal accounts of the marvelous achievements of Aloe Vera, we realize in the end that we could probably make a sizable edition of those alone. Perhaps we'll do that one someday. Meanwhile, personal experiences involving the healing plant punctuate every week of our lives, and they bring to life in a very personal way all the many miracles we experience every day. Some of them are announced with fanfare. Others come in the Silence, allowing the natural process of healing to take place without so much as a whisper of recognition.

Chapter 7

AIDS, Cancer
and the Aloe Answer

This chapter gets to the heart of some of the most profound and controversial advances in Aloe Vera research and therapy in the last 10 years. Some of them bring new hope. Others revisit old debates. All are essential to understanding the expanded role the healing plant now faces in the changing arena of world health. Whatever you find on these pages will stir you to question and to rethink some long held positions about dread diseases and just how we go about treating them. At best, it is in itself a handbook for hope. At its worst, it is food for much consideration, research and examination. In either case, the reader will emerge from this chapter better informed and more willing to consider intelligent alternative therapies for these two pandemics.

Cancer. AIDS. Mention either, and you bring terror into a room. Consider them together and you cite two of the global community's most shattering health concerns. In terms of etiology (or cause), expression and contagion, they have little in common. But when you consider them in terms of long-range impact and the prospect of individual mortal combat, they are twin horsemen of the Apocalypse. Left untreated, they are certain death sentences. In terms of causality, they are both very often diseases of lifestyle.

Propensities toward cancer can have genetic bases. AIDS almost always presents itself as a situational disease. AIDS is a contagious pandemic. Cancer is seldom contagious and can only be spread in the rarest of circumstances. AIDS is often viewed as achieving epidemic critical mass in developing countries. And sexual transmission is often misperceived as the primary cause. Cancer is very often perceived as being the scourge of more advanced societies, the cellular hazard of a complex lifestyle. This can also be a misperception.

Cancer Update. Recent Developments.

Our literature—both patient applications and personal anecdotes—is peppered with accounts of Aloe Vera's ability to treat various kinds of cancer from basal cell carcinoma to lung tumors. What we long for, and what cries out for attention, is the validation that can only come from laboratories and clinical research. So we offer some of them here. We do so while fully aware of the fact that cancer as a disease is a quagmire. So much of it relies upon prevention. And cures, if they come at all, are protracted and often fraught with complications. They are also immeasurable in so many ways. So many times, we have seen Aloe Vera applied in cases that were written off as hopeless. So, rather than the treatment of choice, it was a treatment of last resort. Because of that, even its most exceptional results have been clouded with the doubt of "spontaneous remission" and the deadly tag of "anecdote."

So, we yearn for further vindication; the kind that can only be achieved with clinical findings and scientific research surrounding the healing plant.

With that in mind, we begin with a categorical imperative: Despite the billions of dollars spent on cancer research, treatment and cure, there are just as many new cases of cancer that develop in America now as there were recorded in the early 1970s. The good news is the fact that there are fewer fatalities per capita. So in real terms, though we are finding ways to prevent fatalities from the disease, we have yet to achieve success in our attempts to prevent the disease.

Of course, we're not saying cancer is entirely preventable. There are genetic dispositions toward the contracting of certain kinds of cancer that cannot be denied. It can also not be denied that certain types of cancer such as lung cancer, throat cancer, skin cancer, even many kinds of breast and stomach cancer can be prevented by conscious lifestyle modifications and attention to healthier pathways of living.

The question however remains: What does one do when the reaper strikes, when the dark Narcissus comes to announce the end of normalcy in one's life? That's the way cancer so often affects us when quite possibly it shouldn't. Now we have become sufficiently educated enough to know, when we hear the "C" word, to discreetly inquire, "What kind?"

If it's a skin cancer, it is usually treatable if caught early enough. If it is pervasive or "metastasized," it may carry a death sentence. But today's cancers, though far more universal, are also considered treatable. And sometimes the best way to talk about it is to demystify it.

Technically there are about 170 different kinds of cancer that fit into two major categories: carcinoma and sarcoma. Carcinoma is by far the more prevalent of the two representations and covers the skin, the epithelial cells and the body cavity. Sarcoma involves the connective tissue—vessels, blood, bone and glands. although carcinoma is often thought to be, by force of presentation alone, the more prominent of the two, sarcomas, once they take hold, are almost always an indicator of probable terminality.

In a strict sense, a cancer is any unusual, advanced or extraordinary growth of tissue on the body's surface. That includes the systemic functions of the body where abnormal cell proliferation is less visible but nonetheless perilous.

Technically, this applies to about anything. Any polyp on any organ or mucous membrane is, by definition, cancerous. Any sore that won't heal, any ulcer that persists, or any wound that won't close is experiencing abnormal cell response and may be cancerous. Any skin tumor that forms is, by definition, cancerous. Although we have the choice of examination and through that examination the ability to reveal it as either benign and therefore harmless, or malignant and potentially deadly, we must invariably treat both as the threats they mean to be.

If a cancerous tumor is benign, it is experiencing abnormal cell growth that is not spreading to other tissue or hop-scotching into other cells and organs of the body. Since the body possesses tremendous wisdom to heal itself, especially at the cellular level, one may look forward to a number of occasions when small "cancerous" growth such as polyps, warts, and moles may erase themselves and fall back into the parade of normal cell reprocessing.

Encouraging though that may seem, in the majority of cases the tumor almost always has to be removed before it can become malignant. If a tumor is malignant, it has the potential of spreading into other tissue, overproducing itself, finding toxic pathways through the neural and circulatory system, running rampant through the body at large and eventually bringing death to the host.

That is when we have to address the immune system and the cell production that goes on inside it, and that's where Aloe Vera may prove to play its most important role.

Malignant cancers, whether carcinoma or sarcoma, have a way of multiplying cells in ways that are both rampant and destructive. They form abnormal growths either in the form of tumors or of sores that will not heal (either in the normal course of time or at all). Especially in certain types of cancer, all forms of drugs (or chemo) therapy have been tried. Surgery is often the only alternative, and even that must be both invasive and largely destructive even of healthy tissue (just in case). When this occurs, it is an admission on the part of the physician that both the innate and adaptive immune systems have failed.

There is, however, one last alternative to radical surgery that might come in the form of a sympathetic immune system created by such a synergistic therapy as Aloe Vera.

Although we will shortly reveal a series of laboratory tests that show Aloe's ability to reduce tumor growth, lower carcinogenic activity and promote wound healing, we also acknowledge the reluctance on the part of most clinicians to offer explanations as to how it works.

We will play the fool here and offer our attempt to explain the mystery in as simple terms as possible. Since all disease occurs at the cellular level, it stands to reason that all healing also begins at that level.

Cancer's signature is abnormal accelerated cell production. In its way it gets into a negative "punch up" with the body's adaptive immune system B-cells (or lymphocytes) that try to overcome it in various ways to create a growth system of their own. In this way, they themselves virtually become converted into villains and form tumors and wounds that won't heal. Otherwise, the cancer antigen (such as that which exists in leukemia) just shadow-boxes the host, encouraging the white blood cells to keep reproducing in their own geometric proportions so that they devour the red blood cells and eventually destroy the organism with their own over-expressed need to fulfill their function.

For all these and other forms of cancer, we introduce the Aloe Vera orchestra and its own symphony of immune system symbiosis. Whatever Aloe Vera's "mysterious chemistry" may reveal, it has shown this much: It assumes the rhythm of healing tissue at whatever level it requires. If the body's cells are reproducing at unhealthy and pernicious rates, the cancer finds its counterpace and produces itself. If, as we soon shall see, the antigen is an insidious imposter (such as occurs in HIV) then Aloe Vera can provide that cellular cavalry to reinforce the T-cells under siege.

To give example to the healing plant's remarkable effects against cancerous growth conditions both in and out of the labs, we cite four distinct cases, each pointing to an aspect of Aloe that has been possibly taken for granted before.

The first test has to do with a clinical study reported in 1981 on the "Effects of Aloe Extracts on Human Normal and Tumor Cells In Vitro," another catchy title that nonetheless caused justified reverberations through research communities around the world.

In this test, a group of research scientists from the University of Texas Health Science Center tested extracts from three different varieties of Aloe Vera (Aloe Chinensis, Aloe Barbadensis, and Aloe saponaria are all variations of the "true aloe").

Following the guidelines set for the test, fresh clean leaves were cut from the sample plants, homogenized in a Lourder blender and tested against a "commercial preparation" of Aloe Vera. All the preparations were then tested against cells of two kinds of carcinoma—human fetal lung and human cervical carcinoma—in a special medium of bovine serum and antibiotics.

The tests, although complicated in a number of ways, did point to one set of conclusions: that the substances in Aloe fractions did diminish the lectin-like free-radical activities in the cells and disrupt the growth particularly of the human (cancer) cells.

For a number of reasons, the reverberations surrounding this experiment came more in retrospect than occurred at the time the tests were conducted. In the first place, in vitro testing was not viewed to be as valid as live patient tests. Second, there was not the awareness for criteria of testing Aloe Vera that exists today. In truth, the three types of Aloe that were tested are variations of Aloe Vera given regional labels that reflect the part of the world from which they come. Third, there was no data to substantiate either the quality or efficacy of the commercial preparation of Aloe Vera used for the test.

The history of Aloe is rife with such inconsistencies, and yet there is also a constancy of curative potential that pierces all the veils of conjecture. Through all the issues of types of plant, commercial origin of extracts and whether or not the extract comes from the gel, the rind, or the blended whole leaf—whether or not it is extracted, concentrated, freeze-dried, or air-dried—it is the bottom line that matters.

It works. It becomes the pivotal point of cure. It exists as the unequivocal winner in comparison tests of all kinds. Surrendering all conjecture about it, it proves itself to be the overall superior adjunctive therapy, perhaps of all time.

And yet questions remain.

One of the greatest concerns about Aloe Vera has been the possible existence of carcinogens inside the plant itself—particularly in what is known as the anthraquinones. In truth when tested for this possibility, the anthraquinones, aloin, aloe emodin and emodin have all shown certain immunosuppressive qualities. In fact, the Japanese Health Ministry has, beyond a very slight percentage of presence (below 50 parts per million), outlawed aloin from any products brought into that country.

Two tests in particular—one in Taiwan in 1992 and one in Dallas, Texas in 2000—found certain anthraquinones to be both toxic and immunosuppressive. And yet in both instances, there was an upside to the findings.

In the 1992 test at the National Taiwan University College of Medicine, a team of six Chinese scientists used a control group in vitro study to show that the anthraquinone emodin, measured on its own, displayed distinct immunosuppressive characteristics. By the same token, they determined that it was the perfect x-factor to be introduced during organ transplantation to prevent the rejection of tissue. They also deemed it to be potentially helpful in the regulation of certain types of autoimmune diseases where immuno-suppression may be occasionally necessary.

Of course, the control group study was made on emodin as a separate chemical element and not as a specific component in the intricate chemistry of Aloe Vera.

Tests such as these emphasize some exceptional aspects of biochemical research and some flaws as well. One is the natural inclination to try and isolate ingredients to determine their role in the process of disease and cure. This often nullifies its contribution in the complex chemistry of a plant like Aloe Vera and unnecessarily villainizes an element that might not be culpable, especially when it works in concert. Having made note of this (more than once in this book), we also acknowledge that there are so many ways elements—flora, fungi, bacteria, anthraquinones, amino acids, even vitamins and minerals—are flip-flopped back and forth into the roles of heroes and villains. In truth, with intelligent application, they may be put to maximum positive use. In the case of such anthraquinones as emodin, this is potentially the case.

Such became the case again in the year 2000 when my good friend Dr. Ivan Danhof conducted an extensive series of tests to determine whether or not anthraquinones (such as those found in Aloe Vera) were genotoxic or carcinogenic especially as they affect the process of digestion. Since aloin and Aloe emodin in particular were often extracted from Aloe Vera for individual use as potent laxatives, the question raised was a pertinent one.

(In fact, for centuries Aloe Vera was singularly perceived as a strong purgative agent, often a last resort to remove the blockages caused by constipation.)

In a private paper entitled "Are Aloe Anthraquinones Genotoxic or Carcinogenic?" Dr. Danhof reported his findings that resulted from a 10-patient animal subject crossover study. Working under the supportive hypothesis that orally ingested anthraquinones were "partially absorbed by the small intestine with the material subsequently secreted into the colon, as well as partially passed unchanged into the colon," he ran a 10 patient two way, crossover study.[22] In his study, he determined that anthraquinones, specifically Aloe-emodin-9-anthrone, did cause Melanosis coli, ordinarily considered a precursor to tumor initiating cancers of the colon.

At the same time, he was careful to accompany his findings with the appropriate caution that, even though his findings did indicate the carcinogenic intention of the Aloe-emodin that, as a short term laxative (its original intent), it would work satisfactorily with little danger that it would cause cancer.

Later in the same year (2000), Dr. Danhof ran a series of tests to determine "The Antitumor Effects of Aloe Vera." Factoring data that measured pleural tumors in a small test group of rats, Dr. Danhof determined that the combination of vitamin C and Aloe Vera gel (ours) did in fact reduce the chemically induced tumors in the rats.

In another test, testing the anthraquinone emodin for its ability to reduce tumor growth in breast cancers, Dr. Danhof was able to determine that this anthraquinone tested on its own was in fact able to suppress the malignant transformation of a cancerous growth medium artificially introduced into human breast tissue. So, it might be surmised from these tests that the anthraquinone tested (emodin in this case) might be carcinogenic in its effect within the digestive system and yet fulfill an equally important role as an anticarcinogen when introduced to other tissue in the body, such as the mammary glands or reproductive system.

Granted, these tests run by Dr. Danhof were conducted against very small samples. So further testing would be needed before any solid conclusions could hope to be reached. And each of these tests points to the perilous game of Russian roulette we often play with our curative agents.

As it was pointed out a number of times in Chapter 1 and other chapters in this book, we now must face the prospect of Salmonella bacteria being used as a possible agent in the cure for cancer and scorpion bites as possible treatments for arthritis. A "snake oil" from the deadly bushmaster snake is one of the homeopath's tried and true treatments for what are called rabies miasms in our canine companions. And people now routinely inject modified forms of deadly botulism (as Botox™) into their skin to improve their complexions, get rid of wrinkles, and to mitigate the effect of migraine headaches.

In this world of cause and effect, we have to acknowledge the possibility of anything working in the divine tapestry of disease and cure. And yet we cannot help but wonder about the Law of Cause and Effect itself. Is there not, in some of these instances of usage, an equal and opposite reaction to the some of the radical therapies being used to address the maladies that now come into our lives in so many different ways?

Such possibly drastic treatments as hormone replacement therapy are already coming under hard scrutiny for their possible toxic implications. And stem-cell research, valid though it seems, carries a kind of moral baggage that might well tie up its unrestricted usage for years.

So, we'll beat the drum yet again for the original "genius" that resides in Nature's original formulations—in the myriad plants themselves. "Genius" like another root word, "enthusiasm" can be literally translated to mean (en Theus or en Deus) "filled with God." As herbalists, naturopaths, and ancient pharmacologists have been insisting for years, sometimes its best to work with what we have already been given in the plant and to improve upon recreating its best possible presentation.

Still, we acknowledge the noble attempts to isolate the key ingredient in Aloe Vera, and point to the fact that some very pivotal findings have been achieved in Aloe Vera research in the last 15 years. And yet the questions persist: Is Aloe Vera more effective when left intact to do its work? Or does the "silver bullet" truly exist? And has it been found already?

Nothing underscores that debate more intensely than our next section on Aloe Vera and AIDS—the millennium's critical mass. And even though it may not arrive at the unequivocal conclusions we would all like, it does raise the issue that for any one disease, there are a number of viable treatments. That is exactly how it should be.

Aloe Vera and Chemotherapy

By now we know that chemotherapy refers to a general category of drug treatment therapy, invariably a highly potent one, administered to severely ill patients who cannot successfully stave off the disease in any other way. True to the allopathic tradition of treatment, the patient is set upon a treatment regimen of massive doses of this chemical drug therapy in hopes that it will find new ways of combining with the adaptive immune system to form new fighters to help it destroy, drive off, or at least amend the invading organism.

Chemotherapy is often ageist in its choices of how well it works. And it is a rule of thumb among practitioners that the younger the patient the better chance they have that the "chemo" will work. (This is especially true if the patient is under 30 years of age.)

There is little question that this has a great deal to do with the fact that the adaptive immune system is more inclined to be potent and therefore able to recombine with therapies and nutrients introduced to it. Later in life, the system loses its reserve and its flexibility so that by the time the subject is in his or her eighties there has occurred such erosion of immune system stamina that the "chemo" becomes nearly as debilitating as the disease itself.

Although chemotherapy occasionally works well, it extracts a heavy toll at any age in terms of what it does to the host body. First, the physical side-effects in most cases are severe: frequent nausea, vomiting, inevitable loss of hair, possible alteration of personal appearance, swelling of body areas, and premature aging are commonly accepted side-effects that go along with this kind of treatment. It is almost traditional for cancer patients to embrace "chemo" as their first option to cure a carcinomic tumor. And such treatments are very often combined with radiation.

What's more, chemotherapy radically depletes the system of its much needed nutrition, nutrients that are needed to keep the body healthy and balanced so that its other systems may function properly. This is one area that doctors and other helping professionals often overlook. Especially when undergoing this kind of treatment, we recommend that patients should take large well-balanced doses of nutritional supplements and eat as many fresh whole foods as possible. This is easier said than done, because nausea is one of the most frequently occurring side-effects of any kind of chemotherapy, and it's often difficult for the subject to hold down food of any kind.

It is here where stabilized Aloe Vera has performed in one of its most effective roles as the consummate adjunct to chemotherapy. In the first place, Aloe Vera appears to be an ideal systemic balancer. It has, in our clinical experience, never risen up to antidote a single medication, and it's compatible with almost all broad-spectrum antibiotics, steroids, and even the most radical treatments introduced to the body.

We have instances in legion, including scores of physician's reports, in which Aloe Vera juice taken internally helped alleviate not one but all of the side-effects of chemo and radiation. In almost every case we have ever come across, the patients experienced little or none of the negative spinoffs from chemo. Explicitly, the patient experiences little or no nausea, vertigo, severe loss of energy, or chemical "seepage" that is so often characteristic of patients with chemo.

Many prep sheets that oncologists commonly provide for their patients going on chemo contain a macabre laundry list of traumatic side effects that the patient can expect during his or her regimen of "chemo." Principle among them is the hideous assurance that the patient can and probably will lose all his or her hair, accompanied by the sincere belief that, in most cases, it does all grow back.

Perhaps one of the best tangible measurements of Aloe Vera's subtle but brilliant contribution to the system lies in the fact that, in many instances, patients who took regular orally administered doses of Aloe in combination with the chemo experienced no hair loss. Neither did they experience nausea, malformation of tissue nor excessive fatigue.

And if didn't presage a jaunty return to life as normal, it most assuredly softened the blow and (who is to say until appropriate testing is done) quite probably aided in speeding the recovery.

In our Chapter 6, "Memories and Miracles," we cited three instances in which Aloe Vera was used as an adjunct to chemo and radiation and virtually eliminated the side effects so common to those treatments. What's more the patients who endured the treatments showed every sign of recovering more quickly and having higher levels of energy and physical presence after treatment. In one case (that of Charlie Pierce) we noted, after the patient ingested massive doses of Aloe Vera juice, that the large mass on the man's lung disappeared entirely. It was praised by Charlie Pierce's doctors as a medical miracle and written off as a probable spontaneous remission.

That's why they call it "the silent healer."

Aloe Vera and AIDS. The Millennium's Critical Mass.

It is an appalling consideration, but undeniable: AIDS recently celebrated its twentieth birthday. And it was noted with the casual acceptance of marking the anniversary of a head of state, the funeral of an international figure, or the marriage of a celebrity couple.

Somehow, on a global scale, we have come to learn to live with AIDS and HIV as part of the peril of life on a busy planet. Even though it is still a global pandemic, it is now too often viewed as someone else's problem. Even though it is now estimated to have killed more than 22 million people worldwide since 1982, we somehow view it with less grave concern because, in the U.S. at least, it is not quite the death sentence that it once was. In fact, it was recently removed by the Centers for Disease Control from the list of the 15 deadliest diseases in the United States.

Today, AIDS and HIV have spawned fewer targets for termination in G 7 countries, because education about the diseases is higher and treatments are in place to forestall their deadly effects, sometimes indefinitely.

That is due in part to a more sensible approach to treatment alternatives, intelligent drug "cocktails," and modified lifestyles geared toward rebuilding the immune system rather than wholesale blanket chemotherapy that can be blamed in part for tearing it down.

AIDS (no longer referred to by its full name, Acquired Immune Deficiency Syndrome) may not induce the panic it once did in the decades of the 1980s and '90s. But to most of the developing world, it is still the ultimate terminal virus, the undefeated unencumbered non-stop pandemic "Pale Horse" of the Apocalypse, waiting in their next blood transfusion, the next shared needle, the next monkey bite or the next blood-borne encounter of any kind.

At this moment, it has sidled its way out of our consciousness. After all, we are told, more than 85% of all outbreaks of HIV in the world take place below the equator, the majority of those on the continent of Africa. So...it is something removed, a thing a part. "And besides…" we ask ourselves. "When is the last time any of us ran into anyone who was HIV positive?"

Still, there are 40,000 new cases of HIV reported in this country every year (compared to over five million cases globally). And though its occurrences have risen among women, especially in the southern United States, and though it is now the number one cause of death among African-American men between the ages of 25 and 44, we tend to stratify its susceptibilities, and now make it a social phenomenon of the lower classes. Much of this has to do with that fact that HIV is being found to be related to intravenous drug use and sex-for-drug trafficking that still plagues the poor in ghetto areas.

Now, we're being told that HIV might not have been as much of a lifestyle disease as it was a response to the environment, and that "sex" did not play quite as much of a role in its transference and spread as was once believed. Although HIV is still viewed as a sexually transmitted disease, new evidence indicates that much heightened susceptibility to AIDS and its precursor HIV was much more often acquired through poor immune system response to conditions—to sexual transmission of course, but also to direct blood transfer as can be found in transfusions, shared needles, the passage of fluids through sex, and bites from infected HIV infected animals (such as monkeys).

Today famous celebrities such as basketball legend Magic Johnson and boxer Tommy Morrison go about their days in relative normalcy promote the belief that HIV can be put under control. They do this while proclaiming the benefits of lifestyle moderation, nutrients, and therapies and supplements that most of them are reluctant to discuss publicly.

Still, we overlook one inescapable truth: To date there is still no announced cure for it. Nothing to date—no treatment, antibiotic, medication panacea, or surgical procedure—has worked to take it out.

Despite all our research thrust against it in the last 20 years, it still attacks the innate human immune system and devours its T-cells with rapacious persistence, leaving the body's' defenses so ravaged that other opportunistic diseases can come in almost at will and finish the job. So what begins as HIV ends up as an opportunistic disease that rides in on the wake of HIV and inhabits the host body with such universally known maladies as seemingly infinite kinds of cancer, lymphomas, and a panoply of skin diseases and respiratory complications that would make the pathologists "Who's Who" of the microbial killer elite.

This is of course an oversimplification of what may be the most misunderstood disease in scientific history. In fact, AIDS is not the virus itself, but the syndrome that represents the ultimate expression of the virus. The original virus from which AIDS emanates is HIV (or Human Immunodeficiency Virus).

In fact, HIV is not so much an invader who like, Attila the Hun, rapes, pillages and plunders as much as it is the consummate trickster, the super-saboteur very low-profile antigen who hides, disguises and insidiously sets its agenda, gaining its initiatives cleverly. Step-by-step it completely eludes the police patrols of the Innate Immune System and Adaptive Immune System until it finally acquires its legion. Then, and only then, does it strike, surprising the T-cell and B-cell defenders so completely that they do not have time to fortify against it and put it down.

Whenever T-cells, and even more so B-cells, expend themselves they need time to redevelop, to reform and grow new "helper" cells to enroll in the disease-fighting corps. What the HIV virus does so well, once it has infiltrated and multiplied, is wage a war of attrition against the body's innate immune system, literally wearing it down so that no T-cells or helper B-cells are left to do battle. This takes time, of course, and patience is HIV's strong suit. Once it is entrenched, seemingly nothing can prevail against it, time is literally on its side.

Initially, to be sure, when the body first encounters HIV, the immune system mounts a vigorous attack against it. Macrophages and the lymphocyte T-cells come at the new invader, guns blazing and actually are convinced they have overcome it. That's exactly what the HIV does best: It plays possum for while. It keeps a low profile, deceiving the host into thinking it is harmless. And then it waits for its window of opportunity to open wide.

Interestingly enough, it is HIV's low-profile personality that renders it so pervasive and so hard to combat, because despite its continued presence it manages to confuse the body's immune systems into accepting it as a normal "good guy" and letting it stay on.

The important issue to understand here is that T-cells only proliferate if they have a job to do—if they have an antigen to arrest and destroy. If not, then they no longer feel needed, and like the worker bee with nothing left to do, they simply die off. And only a certain number stay in reserve.

Since T-cells and B-cells, must have time to recreate themselves, but at this stage this sudden antigen Armada is something for which they are not in the least prepared. By this time in the HIV's recognizable stage, the antigen presence is so overwhelming the T-cells and other helper cells lose all their rank and file, and their numbers fall drastically—literally being destroyed more quickly than they can reproduce.

AZT. The Rest of the Story.

First of all, we need to be very specific about one thing: AZT is a kind of chemotherapy. Technically, any form of drug therapy that has a pharmaceutical base maybe referred to as chemotherapy. But usually the chemo label is reserved for highly invasive regimens of use that come with measurable and occasionally drastic side effects. That certainly applies to AZT.

AZT (technical name, *Amyozicolictryptomiacin*) is initially less traumatic than most other kinds of chemotherapy in that its side-effects and overt discomforts are, on the surface at least, less severe. In view of the debilitating side-effects that AZT can manifest later on, however, those initial good impressions have not only proved misleading but, to many people's way of thinking, fatally so.

In other ways, AZT is typical of other types of chemotherapy in that, in the beginning, it does appear to do a good job of bonding with the Adaptive Immune System and forming a viable wall of defense against the insidious low-profile HIV antigen. If it doesn't succeed in putting it in remission, at worst it has enjoyed the reputation of forestalling the onslaught of HIV and of slowing its rate of growth. On the surface, these initial evaluations of AZT help explain its adoption originally as the "treatment of choice" for suffering AIDS patients.

Even now, even though it has fallen from grace as the treatment of choice, it is still kept in the loop of elaborate drug cocktails that are so frequently prescribed to patients suffering from HIV.

Taking a historical perspective, we feel obliged to note that when AZT was first introduced to the market, the medical community, then in a panic to find something that would work to forestall onslaught of this dreaded pandemic, sponsored a series of control group tests involving 281 patients in 12 different hospitals. (As in all control group studies, the test groups were given the actual medication, and the control groups were given a sugar pill placebo.) It is important to emphasize here that though the average test time—four and a half months—was unusually short for any kind of conclusive testing much less a landmark decision such as the FDA was about to make, it was somehow deemed sufficiently conclusive to generate licensing and release into treatment.

At the time, pharmaceutical companies and research scientists, pressured by government agencies and desperate to find something—anything!—that would make a difference, somehow determined that AZT just might be the magic bullet needed to stem the stampeding epidemic and accompanying panic that AIDS had spawned in the early 1980s. So all tests were put on a fast track and the usual time parameters that the FDA usually insisted upon for review and discussion were suspended. And almost all the weight of expectation was placed upon this one control group sample.

Despite the fact that the patients on AZT exhibited serious depressions in blood hemoglobin (45% as opposed to 14% in the control group) and reductions in granulocyte count (47% in the test group versus 10% in the control group) the outlook for AZT was deemed promising. And even though the quantities in the drug that had netted the positive results had to be drastically reduced for fear that they might overdose the patients with high accompanying toxicity, AZT was declared the only viable panacea for the deadly new HIV virus.

This declaration was based on the fact that, during that 4 1/2 month period, there were 19 deaths from opportunistic diseases in the placebo-control group as opposed to only one death in the AZT test group. It is ironic that the most effective duration for AZT as an isolated therapy has been found to be about 4 1/2 months. But the FDA, already under tremendous political pressure to get something out there, declared the AZT retrovirus the clear winner among all current drugs then under consideration and allowed it to be released to the market (along with an accompanying fine print warning list of potential side effects that nearly took a full page).

At this point, who is to say that AZT was not the right drug for the time? Nothing else had even come close to working and, despite the severely measurable side effects, this retrovirus did make some positive initial impact. Doses were adjusted to more manageable levels, and virtually hundreds of thousands of patients were to be treated with the drug over the next ten years. At worst, it bought many of them some time, and time gives wings to hope.

Nevertheless, the controversy over AZT's benefits versus its side-effects rages to this moment. Corroborative of its somewhat questionable beginnings, recent findings indicate that AZT is very often counterproductive in the long run. Especially in the latter stages of HIV and fully developed AIDS, it seems the AZT therapy may actually hasten the depletion of the Innate Immune System's T-cells and helper cells and accelerate the demise of the host body. This makes sense, since even in early findings, it showed itself to be immunosuppressive and actually strip mine nutrients from the system. Even recent tests showing its debilitating impact on muscle tissue and systemic recovery have been dismissed as inconclusive and "lacking sufficient data." So, the beat goes on. And AZT is often left in the mix of therapies, even though its impact may be deleterious.

One of the most frightening aspects of AZT lies in the politics surrounding its continued use in other areas. Since it's still cheap to manufacture. And since acceptance standards in developing nations are somewhat lax, AZT is more than occasionally used as a primary, if not exclusive, therapy in many nations of Africa, Asia and South America.

We also note that in Africa, Asia and other parts of the world, the mortality rate from AIDS is much higher than it is now in the U.S. and parts of the developing world. And though we do not in the least intimate that there is a direct corollary between the mortality rate in Botswana and the exclusive use of AZT as a primary treatment, we also note that in many nations where occurrences of the disease remain epidemic, there is poor sanitation, poor access to pure water, and geometrically matching incidences of poor nutrition, health education, and general hygiene.

Today, in the developed world, the drug persists, as part of, if not the main player in, a number of drug cocktails. Part of the reason it holds on despite the controversy surrounding it lies in its proven strength in two areas: 1) It has shown to reduce the impact of what is known as *AIDS related dementia* (or people losing mental capacity due to the severity of the disease; 2) it has proven effective in preventing expectant mothers infected with HIV from passing the disease to their unborn children.

In a way, it only stands to reason, since as we understand it the immune system is under such pernicious and irrepressible invasion. Yet thus far, at least, standard therapies for it have all but ignored the key element responsible for its protection—making certain it has a chance to be properly built-up in the first place. And even though AZT and other drugs in the cocktails now used to treat HIV pass the brain-blood barrier to get into the system, all of them possess a few qualities in common. They often bring on anemia. They're generally regarded as accelerating the effects of any drugs that may be harmful to the kidneys. And they are without exception viewed to offer "diminished benefits over time." That is euphemism for creating what is known as a "Bell Curve" effect.

The Bell Curve (named after Dr. Bell) is a phenomenon indicative of many drugs and therapies in applied use. That has to do with the fact that a medicine, when introduced to the body, induces a short-term positive effective. So, often because the human system is adjusting to the new chemistry thrown its way, the healing process appears to accelerate. The immune systems go churning into action trying to take measure of the new biochemical "guests" as friends or foes, and assimilate them accordingly. And for a time the patient seems to show marked improvement. Then, often in geometric progressions, the body in question reverts to its former syndrome often finding it susceptible to even more rapid deterioration.

Some longstanding clinical findings have indicated that susceptibility to HIV varies greatly, and that if the immune system is built up strongly enough in the first place it stands a far better chance of resisting HIV. The questions, however, remain: Can one ever truly build a resistance to HIV? And, once HIV has set in, is there something out there that can arrest it without radical side effects?

The answer to both questions is a conditional yes.

Prostaglandins, Aloe, Acemannan, and HIV.

When discussing the immune system there exists the temptation to draw too many players into the game and, though they're important, to add too many "tech" names to what is already a highly complex mural of invaders and defenders, good guys and bad guys. Nevertheless we need to add *prostaglandins* into the mix. We covered some of the importance of prostaglandins in our Chapter 5, "Autoimmune Diseases and the Aloe Vera Orchestra." But we will devote a little more attention to them here.

We do so because they are frequently mislabeled and almost always misunderstood.

There is now profound evidence to indicate that prostaglandins live in every cell of the body. They are in essence hormones but ones of such intense personality and force that their impact cannot be denied. As recently as 20 years ago, very little was known about prostaglandins. But since that time volumes of scientific papers have been released about them and their impact on the human immune system.

And yet knowledge about them and the full spectrum of their activity, even among clinicians and M.D.s practicing at this very moment is frighteningly sparse.

Even today, if canvassed about the significance of prostaglandins in the human body, we estimate that half the health professionals surveyed would view their formation in the human system as pathogenic in origin and often detrimental to the host. Nothing in the necessary context of understanding prostaglandins could be further from the truth.

Based upon our awareness of prostaglandins we now know that there are three major types of—PGE-1, PGE-2, and PGE-3.

As we noted earlier, PGE-2 prostaglandins make up what we have come to understand is the body's alarm system, and for this reason are more than occasionally maligned as bad guys. Some practitioners even believe, because of the reputation of PGE-2 prostaglandins, that *all* prostaglandins are bad. This is a common oversimplification. What the PGE-2 prostaglandins actually do among other things are to manifest symptoms whenever something is wrong with the body.

Example: Whenever you have measles you break out in spots, bumps and lesions. These are the PGE-2 prostaglandins at work, letting you know something is in fact wrong with the body. They also express themselves in the form of fever (another manifestation of measles).

Example 2: Whenever you have a cold or the flu, you may have a runny nose, aching joints, headaches, and mild nausea. These symptoms are the PGE-2 prostaglandins at work.

Herpes blisters are PGE-2 prostaglandins at work. Turf burn lesions, pain and draining wounds are PGE-2 prostaglandins at work, all letting you know something is not right with your body. And if it seems as if these PGE-2 prostaglandins are nothing but trouble, the real trouble comes when they're not working at all—as is often the case with type 1 diabetics. When many insulin dependent and advanced diabetics lose feeling in their extremities, when they can't sense something as simple as pain, their PGE-2 prostaglandins have not been allowed to kick-in. The same, by the way, applies to the early stages of HIV (often for years, until it is found). PGE-2 prostaglandins have not kicked in to alert the body's immune system that something indeed is wrong until it's truly damaged.

As we know by now, PGE-1 and PGE-3 prostaglandins are considered primary passages to the immune system in that they work through omega-chain fatty acids to actually help reconstitute much of the body's immuno-defenses. The challenge with both PGE 1 and PGE 3 prostaglandins is that once they are depleted from the human system there are very few ways they can be brought back into play. It is when the body's immuno-defenses are strong that the T-cells can send out their macrophage policemen to do their jobs properly.

In a narrow context, PGE-3 prostaglandins are responsible for the build-up of the body's cardiovascular immune defenses, and PGE-1 prostaglandins are largely responsible for the immuno-efficiency of everything else.

Genetics play an important role here, because our primary immune system defenses are inherited. They are provided us at infancy through mother's milk and the simple passage of genes. That is very often why predispositions to every kind of disease from diabetes to cancer and heart disease tend to run in families. And generally speaking, healthy immune systems start out at full potency with the infant and the very young child and are gradually eroded over the years. Ultimately through wear and tear, substance abuse, environmental contaminants, fighting diseases, stress, and the onslaught of old age the immune system wears out entirely.

By recent evaluations, most men and women between the ages of 21 and 31 have 85% of their immune systems operational and fully ready to meet environmental challenges. The majority of people over 80 have less than 25% of their immune systems intact. So illness, old age and death come to us as inevitable players in the process. That's not something that's likely to change. But what may have changed considerably is both the character of the process and its inevitable waltz with time.

Until recently, there was little that was thought capable of rebuilding the immune system. In the last couple of decades, it has been found that certain elements in nature and in our natural diet can in effect help rebuild the immune system, and that diets consisting of live enzymes from fresh whole foods and juices can keep it from getting torn down.

Now it is understood that PGE-3 prostaglandins and cardiovascular immunity may be aided greatly and rebuilt to a large extent by the intake of Omega-3 fatty acids (known as EPA or eicosopentanoic acid) that come from deep water salt-water fish such as cod, halibut, herring, mackerel, salmon and tuna. (Yes, when our parents forced us to take those awful tablespoons of cod liver oil, they were definitely onto something.) The best source of those are fish oil capsules or gel caps available in most nutrition stores, whole food stores, and pharmacies

PGE-1 prostaglandins are a far more difficult to come by, and it seems that a limited number of foods offer the Omega-1 and Omega 6 fatty acids (such as GLA or gamma-linolenic acid and CIS-linoleic acid) to rebuild them. Evening primrose oil, and borage (from gooseberries and blackcurrants) seem to be the most potent candidates. But due to the nature of the foods, they must always be supplied in gel-cap form, and the formulations are relatively expensive.

It is also now understood that good nutrition, a diet replete with fresh foods, fruits and vegetables with phytochemical content, and the proper daily intake of antioxidants (either through diet or supplementation), can go a long way toward fortifying the immune system and keeping it from tearing down. "Live enzymes," such as those that come from fresh fruits and vegetables and from "juicing" become increasingly important for their roles in disease-prevention, anti-aging, and as bulwarks against free radicals.

Although theories hold strongly supporting these purported omega chain fatty acid contributors, entire new roles of candidates have been enlisted as major immune system enhancers.

Everything from shark cartilage and Reishi mushrooms to pygeum from tree bark and grape seeds (considered the ultimate antioxidant), have been proposed as new protagonists in the immune system's fight against opportunistic diseases such as cancer, various kinds of cardiovascular conditions and a broad range of other pathologies. Many of them such as shark cartilage in cancer treatment have already been discredited. Others may offer some curative potential but they seem to come and go in the flow of events and then go out of style like last year's fashions. Many of them that may be viable fall out of favor due to a lack of data, and frankly the criticisms of many of them are justified.

New candidates have also arrived that may be contributory to the rebuilding of PGE-1 outside the intake of GLA and other Omega-1 fatty acids. Those come in the form of bovine organotherapy derived from the glands of healthy free-range cattle. What they are beginning to discover in initial tests is that certain maladies such as those of the heart, kidney, liver, stomach and spleen can be treated by enzymatic therapy provided from freeze-dried desiccated organs of free-range cattle. The therapy, though still experimental, does show some promise.

Asian studies in Reishi mushroom therapy for both cancer and heart disease have been profoundly successful. All these natural products have received high praise in their abilities as immune system helpers, and just as many detractors who denounce them as being useless and exploitive.

One new set of "players" in the realm of anti-aging and systemic have been with us for a long time, but have only in the last ten years been banded together in a group identity. They're called HGHs or Human Growth Hormones. And there is a movement in many wellness circles to bring Human Growth Hormones into play as a part of everyone's daily regimen of supplements.

More popularly referred to as HGHs, these growth hormones are primarily formed out of precursor amino acids such as arginine, ornithine, L-glutamine, melatonin, glutathione, glucosamine sulfate and GABA. Thus far, these HGHs have shown a remarkable ability to forestall the effects of aging, refortify immune system responses, help build muscle mass, and reduce weight gain through unnecessary water retention.

There is, however, a mixed blessing that comes with them, and there are still conflicting reports as to whether HGHs, though they may be effective in other areas, truly make a positive impact on the aging process.

In truth it is not length of life but quality of life in our winter years that make the real difference. And HGHs may or may not carry part of the answer. But some recent field tests have shown that they are delivered with greater effect into the human system if they are combined with stabilized Aloe Vera.

No less significant, and perhaps more prolific than any, have been studies involving Aloe Vera particularly as pertains to its ability to aid the immune system and trigger its effectiveness.

We have already cited a number of studies in previous chapters that have documented Aloe Vera's contribution to the immune system, especially in regard to its role in the delicate balance of autoimmune diseases.

Now we invite you to examine how it has helped to effect advances in AIDS research in the last twenty years, and how profoundly it may affect it in the future. Some of these studies are most impressive. And though some are more completely rendered than others, all offer a great deal of hope to the legions who suffer from this syndrome for which they have yet to announce a cure or even an effective vaccine.

The Terry Pulse Studies.

Terry Pulse was an M.D. and internist in Grand Prairie, Texas who later in his career came to specialize in the treatment of HIV patients, and whose reputation as being something of a risk-taker and a bit of a sensationalist both aided and hindered his attempts to make breakthroughs in AIDS research and related palliative therapy.

Willing to take chances in treating his HIV positive patients, and having patients willing to try new modalities in their attempts literally to gain a new lease on life, Dr. Pulse began early in 1989 to initiate a series of what were then considered radical treatments.

The first one was significant because it involved a combination of megadoses of omega-chain fatty acids (GLA oil in the form of evening primrose oil and EPA oils), a potent whey based nutritional drink, and eight to twelve ounces of stabilized Aloe Vera every single day (a whole leaf formula developed by Coats Aloe and Associates).

All of the subjects were allowed to continue their AZT and other prescribed therapies. And though they varied as to degree and type, there were no interruptions of normally scheduled treatments.

(In retrospect, we feel it necessary to emphasize that the treatments were not truly radical in the sense that Dr. Pulse didn't attempt any therapy that was in any way harmful to his patients. All of the ingredients used in the test were in fact nutritional, were GRAS qualified, and as such created no side-effects. Nor, in fact, did Dr. Pulse ever act outside acceptable parameters established by FDA guidelines. In fact, he even submitted his testing criteria along with the constituents to be used in the study to the FDA for approval but was told by FDA officials that, since the products were nutritional supplements and beverages given GRAS approval, that they were actually categorized as "food" and as such did not require FDA approval. We bring this up here, because this fact seemed to elude critics who attempted to pillory Dr. Pulse later in the study.)

With a specific test design in mind, Terry Pulse set a group of 30 volunteer HIV positive patients ranging in degrees of severity on the Modified Walter Reed Scale and subdivided them into three groups.*

---

* The Walter Reed U.S. Government Hospital originally established a means of rating HIV- positive patients on a scale of HIV 1 through HIV 15. Ratings of HIV 1 through 7 referred to patients who were adjudged to be in what are controllable stages of the syndrome, or ARC (AIDS related complex). In this stage, physical symptoms are not yet manifest, and opportunistic disease have not yet had time to develop and work the full extent of their mayhem. In the stages of HIV 8 through 15, the patients are now experiencing the full expression of the syndrome, including radically lowered T-cell counts and hosts of opportunistic diseases many of which have advanced to life-threatening stages. Invariably, death for these subjects is only a matter of time.

The participants in Group I were HIV 0+ to 1.9 (or the early stages of HIV). Group II were HIV 2.0 to 5.9 (in the ARC, or AIDS Related Complex range). Group III were HIV 6.0 to 14 (or fully manifested AIDS). Taking volunteers evenly divided into the three groups Dr. Pulse planned to have patients tested at 30, 60, and 90-day intervals with final measurements and ratings scheduled for the 180-day termination of the study. What Terry Pulse found after just a few days was a remarkable degree of turnaround. And out of the three groups into which he subdivided his study, he found the following in just 90 days time:

5 patients from initial Group III improved to Group I
10 patients from initial Group III improved to Group II.
10 patients from initial Group II improved to Group I
1 patient from initial Group I improved to score 0-negative (indicating no presence of HIV)

Upon full 90 day examination of the three distinct test groups, Terry Pulse also noted another significant set of developments involving the presence of the AIDS virus in his current list of patients.

On a 90-day measurement of P-24 core antigen levels, 5 patients have tested 0, indicating an absence of HIV viral activity in the body. And on the Karnofsky Quality of Life Scale, wherein a score of 100 indicates normal activity, 11 patients are now rated at the 100 level.[12]

After just 90 days of full day-to-day involvement in this study, Dr. Pulse dramatically announced his findings. "In 30 cases, all have shown significant improvement. I've seen T-4 cells double and triple. And many patients are now able to function and lead normal lives."

Having revealed these findings to two nationally acclaimed physicians, Dr. John Boyer and Dr. Howard Pyfer, Dr. Pulse then solicited their review and oversight of the study. Dr. Boyer, an M.D. and former Chief Medical advisor for the President's Council on Physical Fitness, and Dr. Pyfer owner and operator of a highly regarded wellness clinic in Bellevue, Washington also found the quick turnaround in the HIV positive patients to be highly promising. They also viewed them to have profound potentials for being landmark, "provided a full evaluation of the patients in this test group is allowed to run its course."

Encouraged by professional evaluations that coincided with his own, Terry Pulse became convinced that the good news should be shared with the world while the study was in progress. That, in the highly political world of critical clinical research, is never a good idea.

In the complex world of HIV, 90 days is simply too short a time to declare any study of this kind either bona fide or successful. In the first place, it was neither a control group nor a double-blind study and therefore would not have passed muster by any system of acceptable measurement. Second and most important, it was declared a success prematurely and long before final evaluations could be made. Caricatured in past as being something of publicity hound, Dr. Pulse nonetheless allowed himself to be pressured into releasing his initial findings early. He announced the results of his studies as "works-in-progress" to both press and public, and found himself perhaps justifiably in a welter of controversy. Elements of the test were denounced as incomplete. And reporters, sensing a profit agenda in the early release of findings, quickly used their "bully pulpit" to viciously denounce both Dr. Pulse and the company sponsoring the study as sensationalist and unprofessional.

In subsequent months, the pattern of the tests became corrupted for a couple of very significant reasons. First, due to pressure by one faction of the product's sponsors, the Aloe Vera was removed as part of the regimen of healing from the group tested, so on that basis alone the study had to be declared incomplete. Second, because of the overexposure in regional newspapers and television, some of the test subjects dropped out of the test, while a few others began to relapse.

Apropos to the relapses was the third aspect of this now altered study—the fact that with the Aloe Vera entirely removed from the treatment regime, some of the other patients in the group started experiencing less than satisfactory results. And from the time-frame of the Aloe's removal, the test came completely unraveled.

Needless to say, any time you interrupt the pattern of any clinical study, you invalidate any conclusions that might be extracted from it.

As it turned out, much of the study was altered due to the conduct of the participants themselves. Of the thirty participants in the study, three dropped out, one was removed because he had violated the guidelines of the test, and two others exhibited no measurable improvement.

Of the 24 remaining volunteer test subjects reviewed within the initial [Aloe Vera] frame of reference, all showed levels of improvement that ranged from moderate to remarkable. Five of the subjects went from levels of ARC ranging from HIV 7 to HIV 2 to HIV 0 Positive. Three others went to HIV 0 negative; in other words, there were no longer any traces of HIV that registered. Even those with HIV ranges of plus 8 and higher saw their levels drop as many as six and seven points on the Modified Walter Reed Scale. One patient who was judged HIV 14, riddled with tumors from opportunistic lymphatic cancer and written off by two oncologists as terminal, was able to reverse his condition and was measured at the end of the 90-day period as HIV 1 with a rapidly rising T-cell count. Especially during the initial 90-day period during which all modalities of treatment were conscientiously adhered to, test subjects saw their T-cell counts increase, some by five times the previous level, and all saw improvements in their condition.

All in all, this initial mixed element Pulse study fell into disarray. Yet despite the misperceptions of its intent and purpose, three major conclusions could be drawn from the initial findings that bring the findings out of hypothesis and into the realm of the axiomatic.

The first and most significant conclusion indicated that the omega-chain fatty acids, although they exhibited profound impact in helping to build up the immune system initially and make it more resistant to disease, including the AIDS virus, might do little to actually reverse the effects of HIV once it was entrenched in the human system. Second, the question had to have been raised: If, once the stabilized Aloe Vera drinking gel was removed as a constituent in the treatment regimen the therapy started to unravel, then wouldn't the Aloe Vera merit a study in itself?

A third aspect of this study tended to go little acknowledged, though it is consistent of Aloe Vera in all of its uses as an adjunctive treatment in every pathology against which it is tested. And that aspect is this: There are no instances in which it appears to antidote or countervalue existing modalities of treatment. And in this study as in others, neither the whole Aloe Vera juice nor the omega chain fatty acids either exhibited any antidoting effect on the AZT or be negatively affected by it.

Having recognized the light that failed in what amounted his second study, Dr. Pulse saw the merit in the possibility of testing Aloe Vera exclusively as a means of treatment, and proceeded late in 1990 with another study, this one using only stabilized Aloe Vera drinking gel in megadoses (of 10 to 14 ounces a day) as a sole treatment modality.** Thirty new HIV positive volunteer patients agreed to participate in the study. As in the study before it, all HIV patients were allowed to continue their AZT or other standard medications in conjunction with the stabilized Aloe Vera. This time, the test, though checked after four months was permitted to continue over the course of the next year. Similar in

---

**Dr. Pulse had conducted an earlier pilot study in 1986 with Dr. H.R. McDaniel using a commercial form of Acemannan. We will review this study and the conclusions stemming from it in our next section on doctors McAnally and McDaniel.

character to the first test, the patient sample experienced three drop outs (one for personal reasons and two who were dismissed for failing to adhere to the criteria of the test). Of the remaining twenty five, all but one experienced moderate to highly remarkable improvement in their test results. After nearly a year's time, six were determined to be HIV 0-positive, one was determined to have gone HIV 0-negative (with no remaining traces of the HIV) and one patient was virtually brought back from a condition of terminal with pronounced tumors to a level of HIV-0 positive in a five-month period of time. All the patients experienced a dramatic rise in their T-cell count accompanied by either a diminishment or a complete elimination of opportunistic diseases.

This time, the patients tested continued into a total test period of 18 months, and though two more participants dropped out of the test, it was largely completed intact. Dr. Pulse allowed the remaining 23 patients to continue on the Aloe Vera gel as a part of their treatment regime.

Once more, due to the fact that there was no control group study as such and no double-blind study, these Terry Pulse tests were deemed inconclusive.

In defense of his testing methods and in the name of humanity, Dr. Pulse refused to issue placebos to people already dying of this dreaded disease. However, what may have been an act of noble intent in fact proved detrimental to the long-term credibility of the cause, because none of the Pulse findings could gain lasting credibility either among his peers or among the scientific community at large. This highly dramatic set of findings by this somewhat controversial doctor was literally given a death blow when Dr. Pulse died suddenly in Europe in 1993. This unfortunate occasion saw the loss of one of the most valiant crusaders against the AIDS scourge, and one of Aloe's most ardent spokesmen.

The McDaniels/McAnalley Studies.

All this might have been dismissed as merely fascinating and perhaps (that old jargonistic scientific disclaimer) "meriting further study," had it not been for a series of equally dramatic and infinitely more verifiable studies sponsored by Carrington Laboratories of Irving, Texas. These involve the work of two men: Drs. B.H. McAnalley and H.R. McDaniel.. From 1985 on, Dr. McAnalley and later Dr. McDaniel can be credited for two major breakthroughs. The first is McAnalley's successful isolation of the Acemannan molecule as what is possibly the active ingredient in the Aloe Vera complex. Second is the successful determination of the immuno-stimulating capacities of Acemannan in high concentrations (both as a part of the Aloe complex and as an individual ingredient) in treating a number of conditions: herpes simplex, measles, cancer, FLV (Feline Leukemia Virus) and AIDS. So, like Aloe Vera, its disease-fighting capacities as affects the immune system are broad-spectrum indeed.

Acemannan is a *mannan* or a *mannose monosaccharide* derivative molecule found in the Aloe polysaccharide complex. The acemannan molecule was isolated and successfully identified by Dr. McAnalley as carrying the bulk of the immunomodulatory potential of the Aloe Vera complex. (In all fairness, however, there is so much more to the entire polysaccharide complex and to Aloe Vera itself than can be embraced by any one ingredient. Nonetheless, as the following disclosures may confirm, if Aloe Vera has a "singing sword" at least as far as its disease-fighting and its contributions to the body's immune system are concerned, it appears that Acemannan is a viable candidate for that honor.

Initially, Dr. McAnalley's attention was drawn to the potentials of Aloe, and later of Acemannan, through a group of informal and admittedly anecdotal reportings from eight AIDS patients who seemingly did not know one another and had only the common ground of their consumption of a then popular Aloe Vera drink to serve as their touching point.

However discrete their origins and intentions, these eight AIDS patients offered comparable levels of improvement in such areas as elimination of fever, lessening of fatigue and opportunistic infections. In every case these patients, all of whom had advanced to HIV-positive (plus 5 or higher) had previously been unable either to work or attend school yet, after three to four months of drinking the Aloe drink, were able to return to normal activity.

It was at this point that Dr. McAnalley, a research scientist, turned to Dr. H.R. McDaniel, a respected physician to evaluate the reports from these patients, who in turn dismissed them out of hand as being fanciful and unfounded.

By his own admission, H.R. McDaniel was skeptical when first approached by his colleague, Dr. McAnalley. Even after being exposed to the data surrounding Aloe Vera and the Acemannan molecule, he admits he still found them to be of questionable merit.

"I took a look at the data Dr. McAnalley had been compiling since 1985, including the responses he'd been getting from HIV positive patients, and I still refused to be convinced." Dr. McDaniel remembers, with amusement. "Then, after observing the results and consistency of testing for several months, I finally allowed ego to prevail over 'logic,' and I had to become a part of this exciting new research."

In 1985 under the aegis of Carrington Laboratories, Dr. McDaniel joined Dr. McAnalley in setting up a full time virology lab largely devoted to the research and development of Acemannan as the isolated ingredient in the Aloe Vera complex that most strongly carried its healing potential. Acemannan was originally isolated and used in experimental wound therapy treatment by Dr. McAnalley, McDaniel and a group of associates in 1985, and found at that time to be highly effective in the production of macrophage (phagocyte) cells to aid in tissue rebuilding.

As we have established by now, it is the macrophage cells that go about the business of policing for trouble spots in the human system and fixing them, through the release of cytokine SWAT-teams that bond with the T-cells and act as triggering agents or "whistle blowers" to help them locate, isolate, and destroy the invader antigens and convert the new cells into good citizens.

Shortly afterward, Dr. McDaniel set up a series of three pilot studies, the first in 1985 under the full guidance and oversight of an FDA consultant. Following the filing of a treatment protocol with the FDA, 14 AIDS patients were given regular daily oral doses of Acemannan. In setting the protocol and monitoring the study, Dr. McDaniel was able to observe significant symptomatic improvement in all but the most advanced AIDS patients. "Using a combination of clinical and laboratory criteria, at 90 days therapy a 71% improvement in the group was documented."

A second pilot group of AIDS patients involved Dr. McDaniel's participation with Dr. Terry Pulse and constituted Terry Pulse's first exposure either to Aloe Vera or to any constituent of Aloe Vera, in this case the commercially prepared Acemannan product.

We note here that Dr. Pulse was one of the first and most adventuresome practitioners on a national level to pursue AIDS treatments on an experimental basis with his patients. Dr. Pulse's fatalistic but accurate appraisal was that these people had been given a terminal prognosis anyway, and was willing to pursue "any means necessary" to help his wards. Apparently his patients agreed, because the rolls of volunteers for these studies were very quickly filled.

In this 1986 study, 15 AIDS patients were treated with oral Acemannan, and at the time Dr. Pulse had neither bias nor exposure to the test results achieved by Drs. McDaniel and McAnalley in the first pilot study. In the clinical and laboratory parameters that Dr. Pulse established he noted a broad base of 69% improvement in all the patients after 90 days of the Acemannan therapy. And in the 29 patients in the two initial pilot studies, helper B-Cell levels previously decimated by the HIV virus rose from low to normal levels and some to triple the pre-treatment levels. Core antigen levels for the virus dropped or became negative, patients gained weight, saw their infections subside and skin test reactions become positive. Finally, 75% of the group tested returned either to their work or schooling.†

---

† Patients in the 1986 Pulse/McDaniel study were offered continued supplies of oral Acemannan and were provided free annual examinations and evaluations. Of that group, three patients continued using the product indefinitely. As of the late 1990s, those three (all having met the Centers for Disease Control standards for AIDS), experienced neither hospitalizations nor serious opportunistic infections. All three are still living functional lives.

In a third pilot study again in 1986, Dr. Terry Watson joined Dr. McDaniel to participate in the treatment and examination of 26 symptomatic HIV-1 patients (that is a large group of nascent ARC patients). Part of the purpose of this study was to establish a pre-treatment prediction of how patients would respond and compare actual results to the criteria and predictions from the first two pilot studies. After a similar period of study, an 87% accuracy rate emerged for predicting who would and who would not respond to treatment. And the large sample of patients indicated (now characteristic) increases in levels of CD-4 lymphocytes, reduction in P24 core antigen levels and an overall improvement in weight gain and energy levels. These clinical findings, like the others before them, were reported to the FDA, which put the orally administered Acemannan capsules on hold in October 1986—a standard practice by the FDA.

Prohibited, for the time being, from conducting further clinical studies on active patient groups until scrupulous FDA efficacy testing requirements could be undertaken, Dr. McDaniel continued to research the apparent myriad advantages Acemannan exhibited in treatment, therapy, and positive suppression of the HIV antigen group.

In a further study in 1987, Dr. McDaniel and some associates, working against the hypothesis that Acemannan would in fact have some immuno-enhancing capabilities, ran a study using virally affected sheep red blood cells to determine just how effective this molecule would be in increasing the release of interferons from lymphocytes; in other words, they tested for the possibility that Acemannan might in fact be helpful in treating viral infections. Positive results from this study led to further *in vitro* studies by McAnalley, McDaniel, Carpenter, and associates which showed that Acemannan did in fact exhibit strong anti-viral capabilities against *Herpes simplex, measles, rhino-tracheitis, Newcastle virus*—and against *HIV*. To be sure, in vitro studies (either in test-tube, beaker or petri dish samples) are impressive, but it is *in vivo*, or in live subject tests where the true tale of HIV can be best measured, and it is in actual patient application that some of the best results can be found for the healing plant and derivatives from it.

By now, the research that the McAnalley and McDaniel team was doing was making giant strides, and Acemannan was being examined as a viable adjunct in the struggle against AIDS.

Since 1994, Dr. McDaniel has continued in his studies and relentless pursuit of Acemannan technology. Even today, he continues to be in wonder at the infinite potential this very intelligent molecule seems to exhibit not only against HIV, but also against a host of viral and bacterial infections ranging from Feline Leukemia Virus, to ulcerative colitis and Crohn's Disease.

According to Dr. McDaniel, he has in his findings noted what it is about the Acemannan molecule that makes it unique.

When the immune system is under attack, it sends out these macrophage policemen to find the antigen attackers—to find the 'damaged me' part of the system, seek out the foreign elements and bond to them. The amazing thing that Acemannan (and in fact the whole Aloe Vera complex) does is, when it senses these foreign bodies, it triggers the macrophages to spasm and multiply in geometric progressions, sending a cascade of cellular defense to bond with the T-cells and take out these foreign antigen invaders.

Working well in the facilitation of the immune system's white cell (lymphocytes), Acemannan, Dr. McDaniel has found, also does an excellent job of allowing the CD-4 lymphocytes to normalize. These cells are extremely important in the fighting of HIV, yet Dr. McDaniel has noted frequently in the past that Acemannan works extremely well in helping the immune system fight a number of other opportunistic diseases, including various types of cancer, tumors, ulcerative colitis, Crohn's disease (an autoimmune dysfunction), and the Coacci virus (also a very low profile antigen and very hard to detect, Dr. McDaniel observes). The undeniable significance of this lies in the fact that both Aloe Vera and Acemannan show highly positive anti-viral effects in the combating of a vast array of the opportunistic diseases that accompany HIV, and in raising the profile level of antigens so the macrophage policemen can spot them and arrest them.

Impressed by the work of Drs. McDaniel and McAnalley, doctors Debra Womble and Harold Helderman of the University of Texas Southwestern Medical Center conducted their own tests in 1987, using Acemannan against a number of viruses, including HIV. In this study, they found it to be effective in conjunction with AZT and its legacy drug, ACY, in arresting HIV while at the same time cutting down on the deleterious effects of AZT in lowering the effectiveness and numbers of the macrophage cells.

In their conclusions, Womble and Helderman observed the following:

> In summary, Acemannan, the active substance derived from the Aloe Vera plant...has been shown to be an immuno-enhancing agent in vitro with respect to allergenic responsiveness in the mixed lymphocyte culture, perhaps by virtue of its enhancement of monocyte function in its capacity to compete with T-lymphocyte for antigenic recognition. This drug holds important promise as a clinically useful anti-viral agent.[13]

This study, though corroborative of the many McAnalley /McDaniel studies, was only a precursor to a series of studies in 1990 and 1991. We refer to three in particular.

The first is a study conducted by a team of scientists from Texas A&M's College of Veterinary Medicine in 1991 that of a complex carbohydrate compound (gel) taken from Aloe Vera, *Aloe barbadensis,* in this case and measured the effectiveness of Aloe Vera and Acemannan as an adjunctive therapy in combination with AZT and ACY to block the spread of both HIV and HSV (herpes simplex virus). Using the Aloe-Acemannan juice compound in combination with reduced doses of AZT, the Kemp group found that the same effective results could be achieved with a volunteer group of patients with daily dosage of AZT being reduced from 500 milligrams to only 50 milligrams per day, as opposed to an accompanying ratio of 16 ounces a day of the Acemannan/Aloe juice. In other words, the Aloe Acemannan/Acemannan compound in combination with AZT could match and exceed AZT's performance with patients without either the high cost of AZT or the enervative side-effects. What this report also indicated was that in vitro lab tests, the Acemannan compound interfered with HIV's ability to reproduce in infected cells. So, on its own, the Acemannan compound had in effect accomplished what AZT had not been able to do—to stop HIV's growth on the spot.

The fact that Aloe Vera and Acemannan as therapies in and of themselves were not examined by the same group is indicative of the mentality that prevails when trying a new type of therapy: That mentality dictates something to the effect that you combine the new modality with a known quantity such as AZT and allow it to perform as an adjunct. Although that does something to soften the pathway toward acceptability of that new therapy of treatment, it does little to justify it as a stand-alone treatment. In this case, though the Texas A&M study was a step in the right direction, the Aloe Vera/Acemannan compound was viewed narrowly and safely as benefiting the patients most because of its relative lack of toxicity and its dramatically lessened cost—both factors worthy of consideration but hardly "the magic bullet" for which the scientific community still searched.

In a similar study in 1991, Dr. McDaniel too had determined that "an ideal 100% inhibition or protection from infection and/or cytopathic (cell killing) effect of the AIDS virus was achieved at a ratio of 15 parts Aloe Vera juice in the form of Acemannan to 0.0001 part AZT." This means that AZT in a greatly reduced blend (literally a infinitesimal dosage ratio of AZT to Acemannan) was able to totally inhibit HIV-1 viruses in vitro in the laboratory.

In tests after series of tests, Dr. McDaniel continued to find the Acemannan juice compound "reflected the release by the macrophage system of increased immune system chemicals such as interferon and Interleukin-1, 'tumor necrosis factor' and other components that 'seek-and-destroy' negative particles, including viruses and bacteria..."

More significant is the fact that in H.R. McDaniel's pilot studies with stabilized Aloe Vera juice alone, he and his research team were able to report that its use—without any combination whatsoever with AZT—exhibited profoundly effective immune-stimulatory capacities against numerous opportunistic infections that routinely attack AIDS patients, both relieving symptoms and stopping the progress of those infections "without any toxic side-effects whatsoever."

There is no question that, over the years, Drs McDaniel, McAnalley and their staff made remarkable strides in developing Aloe Vera and acemannan as viable candidates for AIDS research and treatment. At the very least, they have graduated the Acemannan product to a Phase III category just short of full FDA approval for unrestricted use. Certainly, in view of recent universal findings that have dislodged AZT as a principal viable therapy, this and the advent of Aloe Vera could not have come at a better time to help the millions whose lives now rock perilously between life and inevitable death.

Acemannan and Aloe Vera:
Concentration versus Broad Spectrum Healing Potentials.

We have to begin this segment by qualifying everything we are about to say in that we are firm believers in the "both/and" rather than the "either/or" philosophies. We believe there are positive uses for most treatments developed within the great universal canopy of healing.

Having made note of that, the revelations we have just disclosed about Acemannan are bittersweet for a couple of reasons. The first is institutional and unfortunately somewhat political. Despite all the work that McAnalley, McDaniel and their research associates have done over the years, Acemannan is still not approved for human use. And although it is approved for use in veterinary therapy, it has a very narrow range of acceptance, primarily because there has been little PR done to introduced its profound broad spectrum benefits, but also partly because, due to its concentrated presentation, it must also be sold as a drug. It is even more unfortunate that AZT is now being used in veterinary medicine (and we feel unwisely so) in far greater profusion for treatment of dogs and cats with conditions against which both drugs might be applied.

Another issue, we find both heartening and challenging lies in the fact that pure Aloe Vera and whole leaf extracts from the plant work to serve the same ends as Acemannan and perhaps broaden the potential for curative benefit.

Primarily the issue of developing Acemannan in the laboratories is a simple process of using an alcohol filtering process to isolate and extract the mannose polysaccharide (or mannan) from the rest of the Aloe polysaccharide complex and concentrating its potentials. What is separated away may also be concentrated and utilized for the qualities that complex contains, and both may be applied to specified uses.

The questions one has to raise are the following: Does the separation actually broaden the spectrum of Aloe Vera's potentials to treat, heal and cure? Or does it lessen it? And doesn't isolation and concentration of ingredients bring in the shadow of potential side-effects where none have existed before?

We answer these questions in part by making a comparison between Aloe Vera and its Acemannan derivative.

First, Acemannan has shown tremendous power to fight infection, lessen pain, reduce inflammation, forestall side-effects, and rebuild immunity.

So does Aloe Vera to virtually the same degree when applied to the same criteria of testing.

What Aloe Vera and commercially processed whole leaf extractions from the plant can do that Acemannan cannot is also to penetrate tissue, reduce itching, bring in far superior antiseptic capabilities, act as an effective fungicide, and perform as a nutritive delivery system that is superior to any known to science.

The other issue is that Aloe Vera is a food, has GRAS status, and is therefore not restricted for use. Acemannan, by nature of its extraction as a concentrate, must be sold by prescription, and is in fact only available for use as a pharmaceutical prescription drug in veterinary practice.

The question we must raise again is, when the solution in its simplest form is at hand, why complicate the issue? Pure Aloe Vera has so many of the answers, and one of them is its ability to act as a combinant with other forms of nutrition and deliver it at the cellular level into the immune system which is so much in need of it.

Immune System Fortifiers. The Case for Nutrition.

No question, research and development in the immunomodulatory and disease-fighting abilities of Aloe Vera continue at an increasing rate.

Especially those ongoing studies by Dr. McDaniel and others devoted to AIDS research hold great promise for the future. Dr. McDaniel is to be congratulated for his tireless work and research in this field. His ongoing studies on behalf of Acemannan and Aloe continue to impress scientific bodies and win converts.

In our opinion, one of the primary areas of focus needs to be the ability of Aloe Vera to deal as a preventive measure with the pandemic of HIV. We have already examined the importance of rebuilding the immune system, and focused upon adjuncts that appear to help accomplish this. Aloe Vera, with all its variant capabilities and its seemingly infinite potential for combination would certainly be principal among them. And, as the world of science and medicine are turning more and more toward prevention and environmental medicine as a means of proactive health, there has arisen a need to reappraise Aloe Vera's role as a preventive health measure, including its prophylactic capabilities against such insidious destroyers of human health as HIV, HSV (herpes simplex virus) and the entire rogue's gallery of autoimmune diseases.

Has Aloe, in fact, proven itself effective as a preventive agent against HIV? At least one practitioner thinks so. And not surprisingly his underlying reasons for doing so address nutrition and its role in both the recovery from and immunity to HIV.

It has been observed that HIV is most pronouncedly on the rise in nations of the developing world. In parts of South America, Asia, and especially the tribal communities of central Africa susceptibility due to malnutrition and unsanitary living conditions is still extremely high. Many research scientists and practitioners are finding that susceptibility to HIV, though it is still viewed as a lifestyle disease, is much less an issue of sexual transmission than it is one brought about by other factors.

That was at least part of the opinion of our departed colleague Dr. Robert Davis. After much research into the causes of HIV and AIDS, he concluded that HIV had actually not been created *de novo* over twenty years ago. Nor had it been, as some conspiracy theorists contend, created in a laboratory at Bellevue in New York and secretly released in Africa as a means of destabilizing the Third World.

Characteristic of his penchant for tireless research, Dr. Davis was able to determine that accounts of HIV and AIDS-related syndromes had appeared in Africa as long ago as 1872. He also revealed reports that indicated that HIV, the presumed precursor to the AIDS retrovirus, had actually been around for decades (and possibly centuries) but had existed in a benign form that only recently mutated into the scourge it has become.

This, in the age of the supervirus, is characteristic of so many modern mutations such as tuberculosis, small pox, Salmonella and the Staph aureus flesh-eater, that subtherapeutic levels of antibiotics, various types of chemo and steroids might have also made some nurturing impact contributory the rise of this syndrome.

But one thing that can be derived from the findings of Dr. Davis and so many others lies in the fact that, on their own, pure drug therapies applied to HIV and fully developed AIDS don't work. They can forestall the fatal effects of it; they cannot eliminate them.

Dr. Davis was also able to corroborate, as so many others have, that most prime candidates for HIV are those whose immune systems are suppressed to begin with. In fact, there is so much data to indicate that people whose immune systems are strong enough can experience direct prolonged exposure to HIV and not contract the virus.

What's more, further support has been given to Dr. Davis' theories and those of others that nutrition is most probably the missing factor in both prevention and cure of HIV and AIDS.

In tests of AIDS patients, deficiencies of vitamin C, vitamin E, pyridoxine (B-1), vitamin A, and folic acid have been noted, as have deficiencies of zinc. Anabolic hormone replacement (and Human Growth Hormones) have now been recommended for patients with fully developed AIDS. Given the fact that AZT, or any chemo, virtually strip-mines nutrients from the already immunodepressed human system, replenishment of the vitamins and minerals we previously mentioned is now deemed of critical importance if the patient is to enjoy any true potential for recovery.

But there's the rub here—because proper replenishment requires proper absorption. HIV positive patients, especially those in secondary stages of AIDS, exhibit high levels of malabsorption, diarrhea, and intestinal infections. So they're not only malnourished, they 're unlikely to absorb the nutrition presented to them *unless* it is delivered at the cellular level.

Enter Aloe Vera with its incredible abilities a) as a proven nutrient delivery system and b) with its ability to penetrate at the cellular level. What better answer to the current Caucus race of problem-solution that still surrounds the AIDS pandemic.

In his book, *ALOE VERA/ A Scientific Approach,* Dr. Davis proposed this kind of Aloe Vera/nutritional supplement tandem as an adjunct for the drug cocktails now available to treat HIV—and possibly as an alternative to them. Given Dr. Davis' fearless penchant for testing Aloe Vera in every imaginable kind of clinical setting, he would have doubtless pursued his intended test just to prove the effectiveness of this kind of nutritional team against HIV. Unfortunately, he was taken from us just prior to our undertaking this book.

So, like so many before it, this torch too is being passed to a new generation. And, as necessity is the mother of invention, it is certain to be picked up.

Chapter 8

More Than Skin Deep

This chapter will engage us in the myths and realities of Aloe Vera's role in the personal care industry. By the same token, it has continued to make such dramatic contributions in areas such as plastic surgery, esthetics and cosmetology that it has come to be viewed as indispensable by many authorities in skin care technology. But understanding both the impact and exploitation of Aloe is a matter of education. So we dedicate the following pages to establishing a set of guidelines for use of Aloe Vera in personal care, and to set the record straight about what works and what doesn't.

Let us begin this chapter by offering a truism. People will do almost anything to improve their personal appearance—to stay slim, to look more youthful, to be able to present themselves as more attractive to the world at large. For millennia, it has been the obsession of the upper classes in every society known to humankind, not merely as an expression of vain self-possession but more definitively as a declaration of their enlightenment—that they see their own perfected image as a representation of a higher self. It is no different today. In fact, it is more so. And yet at the same time we make that observation, we also note that today such fixations upon appearance come from a practical basis.

Studies now show that people respond, and do so viscerally, to the dynamics of another's physical presentation. In this age of youth worship, flat abs and smooth complexions, society now very often ties one's personal appearance to his or her sense of inner worth, success potential, economic status and even spiritual development. We have already noted new healthocracy class distinctions being formed around personal fitness versus the blue-collar stigma of "the obese" lower middle classes. Fat is not only out, it has also quite universally become a condemnation to a kind of body-dynamic caste system.

185

Now, it begins to go even a step further as expressed in the narcissism of the "wrinkle-free" market cap affluent baby boomers of the 1990s and early 2000s.

In certain parts of the urban U.S. (especially in the Sun Belt) there has come to be a virtual cottage industry in tummy tucks, liposuction, plastic surgery, face-lifts, dermabrasion and what is euphemistically referred to as cosmetic surgery. People are willing to pay the price, almost any price, to look better, to feel better, and to offer a better physical front to a highly judgmental universe.

It is inevitable that this universal fixation would filter down to a general public who are looking for something, *anything,* that will help them keep up "appearances." Naturally (and we use the word advisedly) they want to obtain the same results as the glitterati without paying the same heavy toll for their restructured good looks. That means they're constantly searching for key ingredients, one-word answers that will help them regain their lost beauty, slim them down, bring them more energy and tone up their face and body. So, they too are in constant search for, if only peripherally aware of, such elements as vitamin E, collagen, placenta, hormones, essential fatty acids, eucalyptus, and (of course) aloe vera. We use the small "a" and "v" in this point of reference, because there is precious little mass market "aloe vera" products have in common with the real thing.

Aloe Vera and the Myth of the Magic Complexion.

Nowhere has Aloe Vera been sabotaged by its own popularity more thoroughly than in the arena of skin care, or what is now placed in the mass market grapeshot category of "personal care." By our last count there were hundreds of personal care products that not only contained but also featured "Aloe Vera" as a key ingredient.

These days, every imaginable cosmetic hitchhiker—from sun tan lotion to facial massages, from shampoos to shaving creams—make specific mention that their product contains "Aloe Vera" or even "Pure Aloe Vera" (as if they would be selling impure Aloe). At the same time, they imply that this is the x-factor that sets their product apart. By and large the actual Aloe content in many of these products is negligible, offers little more than marquee power, and is typical of the shadowy ethics of many popular manufacturers whose only motive is profit and whose actual knowledge of the benefits of Aloe Vera is superficial at best.

It would perhaps be unfair to characterize the vast majority of them as impostors. We do not wish to judge the motives of others in this highly competitive field. And yet were we not to hold them accountable, we would not be vigilant in our quest for making the best of the Silent Healer.

In fact the new American healthocracy is no longer easily gulled. They're at least reasonably educated about healthy personal care products and intent upon learning even more about them. They're not fooled by bargain basement prices. They can spot a craze when they come across one, and they're willing to ask the hard questions that will help them weed out the imitators and embrace the products that come with true intrinsic value.

Unfortunately, that still leaves us with the mass of the public (about 61%) who may fall prey to the perils of pop marketing.

Perhaps we should be more philosophical about this long-term exploitive trend. Even if the general public is getting "junk aloe" in a cheap drugstore product, it might be reasoned, at least they won't be getting hurt; no harm no foul. Well, that's not exactly the way the real scenario unfolds.

In truth, Aloe Vera has made greater strides in the fields of plastic surgery, cosmetology, advanced skin treatments, and personal care products in the last twenty years than all the years before it in history. We have the data to show for it, and we will present them in some detail in the rest of this chapter.

We also offer a system for determining a truly effective Aloe Vera product used for personal care and one that is merely capitalizing on the name. In a way, making that determination is just a matter of common sense.

First we can establish that, in personal care, most cosmetic products have a water base. No harm in that. But not much benefit either. These basic $H2O$ formulations may feature specially filtered purified water, an ionized water base, osmotically extracted water, Hansa water, or even micro-cluster water. But it's still just water and as such offers little therapeutic value other than the fact that at least the manufacturers aren't using tap water.

Aloe Vera extracted from the whole leaf, properly stabilized and formulated, possesses not only considerable therapeutic potential but also a live enzymatic potency that, when it comes to treating the human skin and hair, creates a synergy all its own

By now we understand that pharmaceutical grade Aloe—stabilized formulations of Aloe Vera juice (or gel), lotion, jelly or crème—it is recommended as a rule of thumb that you use no less than 70% stabilized Aloe Vera, although occasionally when placed against such conditions as *Herpes zoster* (shingles) and *Candida albicans* (the cause of everything from yeast infections to chronic fatigue syndrome), a 50% concentration is sufficient to be 100% effective.

In many formulations designated for personal care, as little as 25% stabilized Aloe Vera may be used in the foundation and still be deemed effective. But let us be mindful of something here. In order to be truly effective as a cosmetic compound, whether it's a facial masque or a body lotion, it should have a foundation whose principal ingredient is stabilized Aloe Vera. We believe it works best at levels of at least 35%, and we often recommend pharmaceutical grade Aloe Vera at full strength to be pressed into service for all facial treatments in which some extensive therapy may be required.

Aloe Vera actually thickens the cellular walls of the skin, strengthens them and brings its own special kind of native chemical synergy that promotes rejuvenation and overall skin health. We shall soon see this in a number of tests and laboratory studies, and offer it now as reassurance as well as a challenge.

Understandably, such profound impact, properly formulated, will come at some additional cost, and yet it is a cost that women especially are willing to undertake if it means they will enjoy better nutrition for their skin, enhanced skin health and an improved appearance.

We pay homage to women here, not to sound sexist but to cite the statistics. Despite a larger percentage of the male population of the United States over the age of 40 now more actively involved in pursuing the secrets of skin health, facials, and even face lifts as aspects of longevity, women still comprise about 84% of the total "cosmetic skin care" market. That's a $168 billion dollar industry in personal care, largely dominated by one gender. That's not a surprise. What is surprising is the fact that in this new millennium personal care consumers—both women and men—are more aware, are better educated about what truly matters when it comes to their personal appearance. And they have a greater understanding of the fact that skin health is more than skin deep. It's also the by-product of a healthy diet and a more sensible lifestyle.

New Paradigms for Personal Care.

We note with some pride and no small amount of admiration that the personal care industry is one that is constantly striving to enhance both its standards for efficacy and through them its credibility in the consumer marketplace. As such, there has risen from it a new kind of higher consciousness, especially in the last 20 years

When we first wrote about personal care in our first two editions of *the Silent Healer*, we were facing a different set of concerns than we are today. In the late 1970s, what were then referred to as cosmetic companies were to a large degree putting out products that were *comedogenic*. In other words, they tended to cause acne. In 1979 in fact, a dermatologist and occasional working associate of ours, Dr. Robert Fulton exposed many ingredients, specifically *isopropyl myristate* (a petroleum based extender), as being largely contributory to the formation of acne and acne related skin problems. Since such ingredients are base carrying agents and in that role are used very much in the way one would use flour to bake bread, this revelation justifiably brought on quite a few shockwaves and caused quite a few "cosmetic" companies to rethink the way they formulated their products.

It is not always easy to identify these tipping points that bring about major milestones in any one area. But in retrospect, Dr. Fulton's discoveries and reports to the CFTA (Cosmetic Toiletries and Fragrance Association) may well have created the paradigm shift in consciousness that the industry needed. And in the wake of them even many mainstream personal care giants came to realize that beauty truly was more than skin deep and that skin health rather than the artifice of personal appearance was truly the Holy Grail upon which their clients had set their quest.

Today, practically no one uses isopropyl myristate for care of the human skin. But today, there are still more culprits that hide in the corners of the personal care industry and hope to escape detection.

In the year 2003, we have a suspected villain thought to be of similar lineage now being used almost universally as a fundamental ingredient in shampoos and hair conditioners, and that is *sodium lauryl sulfate*. Although there is still more research to be done on this, early research indicates that sodium lauryl sulfate blocks the sebaceous glands surrounding the hair follicles. That in turn clogs the pores and prevents the growth of healthy new hair. Although this might not present as much of a problem to women, it is a major concern particularly among middle-aged men or any man who might be experiencing the challenges of *alopecia* or what we refer to as premature balding.

There are even some reports, though presently deemed spurious, that sodium lauryl sulfate and its chemical chain cousin, *sodium laureth sulfate* may both be carcinogenic; that is how far the paranoia in personal care has extended. In a way that's a good thing, because it indicates that the CTFA and the FDA—even though they may occasionally be at odds about the findings—are more vigilant than ever in their pursuit of the highest possible standards for what is now becoming a health issue marketplace.

(Of course, most of the ingredients in question are put into play for one reason: They're cheap. In large quantities they provide gargantuan savings to the manufacturer. Until recently, they were perceived as benign. That has changed over the years, as have perceptions of what truly comprise cost-effective ingredients. With the exception of low-end drug store cosmetic lines, users in the general public both expect and demand that the products offered them have "skin health" as their primary *raison d'etre*).

Underscoring the "health aspects" of personal care even further is the recent debate over the use of antibacterial soaps, scrubs and cleansers, one that has placed the CTFA, the SDA (Soap and Detergent Association) and the AMA at loggerheads. This once again brings us to the fascinating potential for fusion between the environmental sciences and traditional medicine in that environmental medicine emphasizes the perils in our environment as well as helping us find both systemic and topical remedies for dealing with them. Traditional medicine protects old criteria for health measurement and yet provides an invaluable service in that it challenges the newer standards of scientific measurement to prove themselves.

In this instance, the AMA has expressed the research-based concern that new antimicrobial soaps, cleansers, and scrubs—though they work in the short term—might ultimately be helping to spawn new strains of super bacteria resistant to any form of cleanser or anti-bacterial soaps. Some scientists, including many doctors and CTFA members, take an opposing point of view, declaring these antimicrobial cleansers and complexion soaps to be not only helpful but also essential in the war against these new bacterial terrorists—the super-microbes. These super-germs, they claim, have quite possibly mutated to resistant strains due to flagrant use of antibiotics, both by prescription and through sub-therapeutic levels fed to cattle and livestock.

According to its critics as well as some doctors who have quit the AMA, physicians have for years been dispensing broad-spectrum antibiotics "like candy," while they have now chosen to fight home hygiene as a genuine cause for concern in the war against the super-germ.

Although this new spate of name-calling seems to have extended itself well into the wasteland of the counterproductive, we offer a simple solution to most of the issues presented here: stabilized Aloe Vera.

In the first place, since stabilized Aloe Vera has already proven to be bactericidal, bacteriostatic, virucidal, fungicidal, antipruritic and antiseptic, it presents itself as the perfect ingredient to be put into any cosmetic cleanser, scrub or antimicrobial soap. Quite the opposite of sodium lauryl sulfate, isopropyl myristate, sterol stearate, squaline or any other cosmetic extender, Aloe Vera is innately hypoallergenic and has proven itself for pharmaceutical use as a probable "treatment of choice" for seemingly every cutaneous condition known to modern medicine.

Since Aloe Vera has been traditionally recognized for its effectiveness against burns of all kinds—sunburn, radiation burns, turf burns, scrapes, lesions, and injuries—it stands to reason that it would become an immediate focus of interest for its use in personal care. Since Aloe Vera has proven effective in study after study involving its use in wound-healing, enzymatic debridement, and helping accelerate cell growth in the rebuilding of tissue, it soon becomes a primary candidate for all the multifarious uses demanded of properly structured skin-care programs.

We like to refer to it as "skin health" or "prescriptive skin care," and yet the personal care industry is prohibited in both its advertising and its product claims from referring to "health" as an aspect of what they do. For them to make such references pushes them perilously toward pharmaceutical classifications that make much higher demands upon the formulation and purveyance of their products. These are standards that few "cosmetic" companies can adhere to without incurring production costs that few of them could tolerate. And yet it has been our eternal contention that for any personal care products to truly stand out they should adhere to the highest ethical pharmaceutical standards.

Today, there are some highly efficacious personal care lines now offered both through the network market and esthetics clinics that provide truly exceptional formulations for skin and hair. Not surprisingly, they come with a high price tag, and frankly much of it is justified. Some estheticians are virtually "designing' personal formulations for their clientele that include a precise study of their pH balance, their personal body chemistry and skin types that are now often broken down into complex sub-categories.

There has come into existence a cottage industry in which entire personal care programs are structured around an individual's needs and, in certain cases, done so under the supervision of a plastic surgeon, dermatologist or other qualified health professional. Of course, these are ideal circumstances made available either to the highly affluent or to individuals in the fields of fashion and entertainment whose professional leverage is almost entirely tied to their personal appearance.

In most cases, these are regimes that the average person cannot usually afford, and yet they may be indicative of a trend. As is so often the case in the fields of luxury automotives, technology, and even health and nutrition, what begins as a luxury for the privileged few eventually comes to be priced for the mass-market.

This may soon be the case in the world of personal care. And when it is, Aloe Vera is certain to be a major contributor. In fact, if the average consumer were to put to intelligent use the pharmaceutical grade Aloe Vera products available to them today, we could guide them through a program for prescriptive skin care that would benefit people with even the most moderate budgets.

First, it requires a willingness to enhance our awareness of what it takes to be skin savvy not only about what goes onto the largest organ of our body but also about what goes into our systems as well. So the term, inner beauty, may mean more than just personal kindness, spiritual development and a pleasant disposition (although those too make their contribution to the end result). There may also be some nutritional and environmental factors to be considered here as well as an awareness of what works to make for healthy human skin.

The Care and Feeding of the Outer Self.

A new rule of health applies that is as timeless as it is considered revelation. A blossoming complexion and thick head of radiant hair are symptomatic of a healthy human system as much as they are integral to it.

Granted, the skin is the largest organ of the human body. And we are, like most protoplasmic mammalian life forms, about 78% water. So, constant hydration and proper pH balance are essential to healthy skin. That means keeping the system well fed with healthy liquids and the skin's *epidermis*, or outer layer, hydrated as well. That's easier said than done, because an erosion of the skin's surface is as inevitable as aging and just as insidious.

When you get a cut, a burn or an abrasion, you tend to see to it immediately. You tend it, mend it, and make sure that it gets plenty of exposure to fresh air and (one would hope) such healants as Aloe Vera. Exposure to the sun, wind, tanning beds, dry climates and what has now become a very toxic general environment brings just as much insult to the skin but does so over a protracted period of time. So, we tend not to notice the infinitesimal cuts that come to us in myriad ways, until much later in life when all of the damage is done, much of it irreparable.

Due to the politics of gender commodity, women tend to address the issue of skin health much earlier in life than men. In fact, it is often true that a man's only encounter with skin care in his earlier years might be when he shaves and puts on a sunblock. But that too is beginning to change.

There exists a small but growing percentage of men who are now using such regimes of the feminine domain as facial masks, scrubs, toners and creams on a regular basis. Granted this demographic almost exclusively comes in the 40plus range of men and the now notoriously youth-obsessed generation of baby boomers. In fact, there are even some purveyors of personal care who have come out with entire men's (or at least unisex) lines that take into consideration the unique pH balance and special stringent needs of a man's complexion. So, the ranks of men in search of a more youthful appearance are marching in platoons if not regiments toward a generational explosion of considerable proportions. And virtually, if not literally personal care for the individual woman and man is being programmed on an individual basis rather than blanketed, as had been the case as recently as the early 1990s.

This dovetails into predictions we originally made over two decades ago and still validates the need for prescriptive skin care and at least a working knowledge, made as concise as possible, of what goes into the complex chemistry of the human skin.

Skin Layers and Skin Types. What you need to know.

Basically, there are three layers of the human skin: *the epidermis, the dermis and the hypodermis. The epidermis,* the outer layer, is the one we see with the naked eye. Despite the illusion of constancy it presents, it is incessantly in a state of upheaval in that it is always dying, sloughing, and replenishing itself on a daily basis. Bathing, shaving, wind, sun, the abrasions of some clothing, even hugging and kissing, cause the epidermis to go through a daily revolution in cellular impact, cells that are being incessantly and unselfishly supplied from the dermis. When we're young the epidermis tends to slough dead cells easily and bring on healthy replacements form the dermis. When we get older, however, this process needs all the help it can get.

The dermis or middle layer is what is known as the *true skin* and provides the real strength and durability of the cutaneous complex. The dermis contains the blood supply and elastic network of cells through which the blood vessels, nerves, and sweat and oil glands are distributed. As such, it is the nutritional cell bank for the epidermis. When the two are in balance (as they are in a person's youth), the dermis easily supplies new oxygen-rich, blood rich cells to the epidermis. When we get older, the epidermis loses its ability to replace skin as quickly. So the more we need a topical agent to slough dead skin so that the dermis may continue rebuild tissue efficiently. When there is too much sloughing of cells from the epidermis, the dermis can no longer supply blood in a normal fashion, and problems start to arise; some of them pathological (such as is the case with eczema, seborrhea and psoriasis). So it is mandatory that we not only gently and consistently care for the epidermis but also that we supply nutrients to the dermis.

The *hypodermis* is the third layer of the skin housed just beneath the dermis and as the protective casing for bone and muscle tissue. In combination with the dermis, it contains two-thirds of the body's blood supply as well as housing the sweat glands, hair follicles, nerves, blood vessels and other tissue. It is not only a nutritive supply bank for the other two layers of skin, it also specifically insulates the underlying muscles and bones.

In this subtle waltz of interrelation, the dermis acts as the critical connective tissue between the hypodermis and the epidermis. So dermal pliability is crucial to the system as a whole. So creating the proper balance of moisture and nutritional supply to the dermis is the critical issue here.

Just as the human body it houses, the skin is born to die. The way it dies is through exposure to various levels of abuse and a loss of moisture, flexibility and nutritional balance that comes with constant exposure to the environment and aging.

The most perfect expression of the human skin is through the complexion of an infant. Fresh from the amniotic fluids of the mother's womb, it is a marvel of vitality and free access to nutrition from a fully charged immune system. Through the early years, despite struggles between parent and child over nutrition and diet, the skin remains relatively healthy; at least until teenage. During adolescence, the introduction of sex hormones and the violent shifts in chemistry that accompany them frequently causes the skin to overcharge the sebaceous (or oil) glands, which in turn bring on frequent bouts of acne (as *acne vulgaris)* or other problematic skin conditions so endemic to the teenager.

As the glandular changeover completes itself, the individual begins to regain biochemical balance just in time for aging to set in. This starts to take place from between 25 to 35 years of age, and then the challenge of maintaining skin health truly begins.

Having just read this, don't be misled into thinking that we don't have to worry about our skin health until sometime after our 30th year. Maintaining skin health should be a priority from cradle to tomb, and heaven help the woman (or man) who does little or nothing to look after their skin until they're forty-something and then tries to make up for lost time by resorting to some "miracle" treatment.

In the first place, such treatments don't exist. In the second, in terms of appearance and resilience, our skin tends to be less forgiving than the body at large. And even Aloe Vera, as effective as it may be in appropriately applied regimes, cannot entirely turn the course of a personal appearance gone to wreckage. With the help of Aloe and some other effective developments in skin health and biochemistry, the skin may repair and restore itself in large measure. But once the appearance of youth is lost, it can seldom be regained without a great deal of effort. So, we cannot emphasize strongly enough that everyone should give constant, intelligent attention to their skin, hair, and personal appearance; and do so on a consistent basis over the span of their lives.

"Intelligent" is the operative word here, because in order to be intelligently applied, personal care requires a certain degree of education.

Fundamentally there are four basic types of skin and two potential problems associated with them.

1). *Dry skin* usually lacks sufficient moisture and oil. It often feels arid and taut, and is occasionally characterized by the frequency with which it flakes or chaps.

2).*Normal skin* is considered ideal in the average adult in terms of its balance of dryness, moisture and oil. The texture of normal skin appears to be smooth and slightly moist.

3). *Oily skin* is usually excessively oily and characterized by large pores. It is often oily skin that is the seedbed for acne.

4). *Combination skin* comes in two presentations: a) normal to dry and b) normal to oily. In both cases, though the general facial area will appear normal, the "T" zone of the eyes, nose and mouth will exhibit a tendency to be either oily or dry, creating an environment of its own.

Out of these four basic skin types two problematic sub-types arise: *acne or problem skin* and *sensitive skin*.

As we pointed out earlier, *acne (problem) skin* begins in adolescence and may continue well into adulthood. It is more inclined to occur in oily skin but may also appear as an extension of any skin type. Acne is usually due to overactive oil glands that may be prompted by heredity, poor diet, an unhealthy response to environment (such as cheap cosmetics), or a combination of the three.

When it appears, acne manifests itself in four commonly recognized forms: *1) Blackheads.* The early signs of acne, blackheads occur when pores become clogged with residue and oil. These are not critical as such but, if left untended, form the seedbed for other complications. *2) Whiteheads* are clogged pores covered by a thin layer of skin, and are the first warning signs of acne that is about to spread. *3) Pimples* are blocked pores that have become inflamed and may become infected. Left untreated these will definitely compound and lead to unsightly blemishes such as cysts and nodules. *4) Cysts and nodules* are severe forms of pimples that swell, blister, and become infected. These are the final stages of acne that has either been left untreated or has been treated unsuccessfully. In these forms, *acne vulgaris* can leave disfiguring scars and craters in the skin that can only be remedied later in life, possibly with certain kinds of dermabrasion and plastic surgery. And that is not an option people like to be left with.

Sensitive skin is also present in all skin types but is slightly more prevalent in dry or combination normal to dry skin types. Sensitive skin is also possibly hereditary in that it is more acutely sensitive to weather, harsh chemical detergents, or other environmental influences that might not otherwise effect normal skin types. The impact of sensitive skin can never be underestimated because it is often reflective of the biochemical conflict between toxins and nutrients that is going on in the system as a whole. And because that struggle is ongoing throughout a person's lifetime, skin sensitivity can occur at any time as the individual grows older.

Excessive dryness, liver spots, cracks, wrinkles, mottling, drooping skin, rashes, lesions, flaking, scabs, seborrhea, eczema, keratosis, and skin allergies of all kind often can and will occur as a person grows older, partly because of an individual's constant exposure to the environment, partly because the immune system is slowing down, and partly because they've just gotten the wrong roll of the genetic dice.

No matter what type of skin an individual possesses, he or she is going to be primarily influenced by *four factors: heredity, age, nutrition, and the environment.* And it is here that we must give the Environment a capital "E," because now more than ever it has become the potential scourge of personal health.

It is perhaps symptomatic of the complex society in which we live that we now take environmental peril in stride, like the constant stalker of our well-being, always hovering on the fringes of our consciousness, a present but never quite a serious threat.

We prevail upon you to think again. And if our pleading will not encourage you to take our relationship with the environment more seriously perhaps a few statistics might help you better understand the daily proximity of the danger:

- In the year 2000 alone, more than 1.9 billion tons of chemicals were dumped into our nation's water systems.
- In that same year, environmental reports estimated that 160 million tons of air pollution were released into the atmosphere in this country alone.
- That includes indoor air pollutants such as radon, asbestos, formaldehyde, tobacco smoke, carbon monoxide and chemical solvents.
- In the year 2002, the EPA determined that 44% of U.S. coastal waters are not fit to support either aquatic or human life.
- The EPA has also determined that as many as 38% of all Americans are living in areas where their tap water may not be fit to drink.
- Environmental medicine has now become one the fastest growing fields of alternative health practice.

In truth, more people than ever before are now reporting health concerns directly tied to their exposure to a toxic environment. Combine that with a less than prudent fast-food, high cholesterol, acrylomide-laden carcinogenic diet and the pressures of a very quick paced, low touch/high tech pattern of behavior and we have the makings of a lifestyle that is starvation to a healthy system and an outer casing that reflects the inner creature. All the more reason why diligence is required, and discipline about your skin is essential to survival.

Nutrition. Proper facial care has to begin with nutritional intake and continue with topical attention as a matter of daily existence. Beyond the vitamin C, the vitamin E, Beta-carotene and other antioxidants, nutrients such as folic acid, choline-rich lecithin, and Omega-chain essential fatty acids are of paramount importance not only as free-radical fighters but also as elements known to enhance the immune system. Such HGH precursors as L-Glutamine, Lysine, Arginine-Ornithine (recommended to be taken in tandem) and GABA are also showing themselves to be increasingly important to the development of healthy hair and skin. Coenzyme Q 10 and glutathione are also considered by many practitioners of environmental medicine to be essential to systemic defense against the daily toxins in our lives. In addition, proper systemic cleansing is also viewed as essential to forming a clean house for nutrients to do their best work.

Of course, when you add Aloe Vera gel (or juice) to this formidable family of nutrients, you get a systemic double hit, because Aloe Vera not only contains its own synergistic nutritional complex, it also converts into the consummate delivery system for all the other nutrients with which it interacts.

What proper nutritional supplementation and especially a diet replete with fresh fruits and vegetables do is help promote a slightly alkaline pH balance in the body's chemistry.* To be healthy, a human system should be slightly to the alkaline side (7.5 or higher on a scale of 15). This in turn helps promote a skin pH that is slightly acid in its presentation (6.5 or slightly lower on a scale of 15). The highly acid human system is an indication of the presence of extreme levels of toxicity. The highly alkaline human skin is one that is much more susceptible to hypersensitivity, allergies and infection.

This brief encapsulation of our body's delicate chemistry should underscore the necessity of beginning your healthy personal care regimen with appropriately formulated nutritional supplements and a balanced, fresh whole food diet. Then follow it with an intelligent prescriptive skin care and a regimen dictated by stabilized Aloe Vera products.

The Aloe Advantage.

So much new information has been provided us as regards the contributions Aloe Vera has made particularly in terms of its treatment of the human skin and

---

*We cannot stress enough the importance of a daily diet of fresh fruits and vegetables—preferably organic and ideally raw or lightly blanched—to help effect the proper alkaline pH balance within the human system. There are also now tongue and saliva litmus test kits available in health food stores that will help you determine your systemic pH. Unfortunately, most people are pH balanced to acid levels, and no supplementation on its own, not even when used with Aloe Vera, can tip one's pH balance to the alkaline side. Though not as much of a challenge in youth, high acid pH balances in later years can prompt such conditions as gout, rheumatoid arthritis and all sorts of skin allergies, as well as gradual but relentless erosions of the immune system.

its impact on the system that we are almost at a loss to choose which factors are the most important. What we can do here is to take careful note of some of the more notable breakthroughs that have taken place in recent years.

As we have already reported many times in this chronicle and will show again shortly, properly stabilized Aloe Vera products do a number of things to promote a healthy skin.

1). Taken internally Aloe Vera helps bring a natural pH balance to the human system. Applied externally, Aloe Vera provides natural pH balance to the skin. Its predilection to naturally tune into the skin's chemistry renders it ideal in the cleansing of skin, removal of bacteria and fungi, and the supplying of appropriate nourishment.

2). Properly formulated Aloe Vera products have deep penetrating power. Through the presence of lignin and Aloe polysaccharides found in Aloe Vera gel have now proven to posses an ability to penetrate tissue that is truly unique. This carries Aloe's natural synergy of nutrients down into the dermal and hypodermal layers of the skin.

3). The proteolytic enzymatic activity in the Aloe Vera nutrient matrix is important in helping to slough off dead cells from the epidermis and create a natural base from which to bring up healthy new tissue.

4). Since Aloe Vera is a storehouse of synergistic nutrition, and since it helps synergize other nutrients introduced to the skin, it is a perfect adjunct to use with other skin care regimes beneficial to the user.

5). Part of the Aloe Vera synergistic blend is a complete body of amino acids, including all the essential amin0s. Since "aminos" are the building blocks of new cell formation, and particularly since they are interactive with the plant's highly active complex of enzymes, Aloe Vera is proving to be one of the best natural complements to the needs of the skin and hair.

6). Because of its proven effective abilities as an antiseptic, astringent, and cleanser Stabilized Aloe Vera gel (or juice) applied directly to the skin is the perfect natural moisturizer that cleans and allows moisture to form a healthy platform for the skin. What's more the Aloe Vera does so without clogging the pores.

7). Because it is formulated according to pharmaceutical standards, truly stabilized Aloe Vera creates little or no opportunity for side effects or allergic reactions to take place. This is due to two factors. First, Aloe Vera is a wonder of toxicology in that is known to have no measurable toxicity, and that puts it in a category of one where known healants are concerned. Second, for an Aloe Vera product to meet necessary pharmaceutical standards (which is the only determination under which it should be allowed to be used), it is subjected to guidelines established by the FDA rather than those recommended by the CTFA. Without belaboring the issue as to exact microorganisms per gram, we simply acknowledge that CTFA general guidelines for purity of raw materials (for example) are recommended. They're not required, and they're not enforced. In our opinion, basic materials that do not adhere to the highest standards are nothing more than culture media for impure microorganisms to form. Frankly, in order for a "personal care" product of any kind to be deemed entirely pure, all materials should be blended in an aseptic environment with optimum standards for purity applied at all times. As we live in an imperfect world where even striving for perfection is fraught with obstacles, we advocate vigilance in our own sense of responsibility to the markets of the world that place their trust in us.

Prescriptive Skin Care—Why Everybody Needs it.

Prescriptive Skin Care is a term we coined early in our development of Aloe Vera products for the personal care industry. Now, we're happy to say that it has been adopted by a number of other groups in the industry. Since we'd rather have progress than copyright for that kind of philosophy, we welcome the imitators. I also merely note, with some small measure of pride, that it did begin here, and as such it will always have its philosophical home. I can't take credit for all of it, of course. We came upon the system through our work with some of the best dermatologists, estheticians and plastic surgeries in the county. So, as is the case with many great movements, it came as a matter of common accord and pragmatic singularity of purpose—to find a system that works and works well for everyone.

For a system to work well under any circumstance, we believe it has to adhere to a discipline. For that reason, neither stabilized Aloe Vera products nor any other regime will work unless they are applied on a regular basis with daily disciplines and an intelligent sense of limitation.

Ordinarily, we do not preach limitation in any aspect of life, but there are areas in which appropriate prudence is not only recommended but also essential. As we will soon show there are some instances in which you can get too much of a good thing. And some women, in pursuit of perfect beauty and the ultimate physical expression of self go way over-the-top in their application of health and beauty aids.

It is here that we preach that part of applying any discipline comes with the understanding that moderation, along with patience, is often required. No skin care regimen, not even Aloe Vera based products, can repair overnight what the caprices of Mother Nature and the ravages of Father Time have taken years to undo. With that in mind, we recommend this program with the caveat that it be applied with appropriate care and moderation; and with at least the occasional supervision of a true personal care professional.

Step One: Cleansing. Cleansing in both the morning and evening is essential for the success of this program. It is the only way to removed make-up, dead skin, and residue from living in a less than perfect environment. For that, Aloe Vera gel or an appropriately formulated Aloe cleansing lotion are recommended. They're safe for all skin types and bring needed moisture and nutrients to the skin. With this kind of cleanse, scrub lightly or heavily as needed to aid in the sloughing of dead cells and to allow new cells to rise to the surface of the skin. Afterward, remove the cleansing lotion with a *clean* washcloth and warm water.

Step Two: Toning. Toning is a traditional step that is often overlooked. We view it as essential because it helps remove whatever residue may have been left on the skin after the first step. This is best accomplished by using a freshener or astringent to tone the skin, eliminate residue, and prepare the skin for proper moisturizing. And it is here that special attention should also be given to the eyes, nose and throat,—the sensitive T-zone—of the face. This is especially an area of concern for combination skins where oils tend to accumulate. In this case, Aloe Vera in combination with a light astringent helps to synergize the activity. In fact, Aloe Vera liquid (gel), acting on its own provides excellent toning properties.

Step Three. Stimulation. Some of the best forms of stimulation for the complexion come from specially formulated facial masques. (One with Aloe Vera gel and a facial masque powder would be ideal.) Aloe Vera gel or liquid, properly formulated and pH balanced, helps clarify skin tissue and promotes increased blood circulation and nourishment to the cells of the skin. This in turn helps to prompt increased cell production from the dermis and serves as a vital finale to the cleansing process.

Step Four: Pure Aloe Vera Liquid. Some people with sensitive skin will get enough exposure to Aloe Vera in the previous three steps and may eliminate this one. So proceed advisedly here. People with normal skin, however, will find Aloe's ability to penetrate, soften and stimulate the skin to be extremely beneficial. It also deep cleans and aids in sloughing of dead skin and rebuilding of new skin cells from the dermis, as well as fighting fungus and bacteria that often prey upon skin during this sensitive period of transition.

Step Five: Moisturizing. Whatever the individual's skin type, it will need moisture. Moisturizers in a base of Aloe Vera liquid will keep the skin soft, pliable, nutrient rich and as a wrinkle reduction agent. Moisturizers also help facilitate an appropriate gradual blending of make-up and other cosmetics in that a good moisturizer will help stabilize them to last all day.

Step Six: Sunscreen. Sunscreen might be thought of as the hidden Derringer of skin care, because it can either protect or endanger, depending upon the type it is and how it is applied. Essentially there are two types of sunscreen. One very popular version is the UVA and UVB type of sunscreen. This is the darling of the cosmetic (personal care!) companies, because it is superficially more attractive, occasionally filled with fragrance, and now often included with a self-tanning formulation of some kind. It comes in seemingly infinite number of presentations and commercial preparations that carry both advantages and perils of their own.

The second type of sunscreen is a melanin UVL browser that creates a particle size coating that can't be absorbed into the skin. It is a titanium-zinc oxide application that absolutely limits harmful exposure to the sun. Unfortunately, its presentations are often industrial grade and limited in the ways they can be used. They're not very popular; they're merely effective and carry few allergens. There are however a few good manufacturers of this type of sunscreen. And we strongly recommended that you cultivate a relationship with one of them. The use of reflective agents is one of the fastest growing areas of the skin care field today. (The aloin in Aloe Vera is a partial barrier in itself.)

The challenge with the first type of sunscreen lies in the fact that, second only to fragrance, UVA-UVB based sunscreens are the number two external causes of allergic skin reactions.

Despite the purported perils, we need to establish the fact that sunscreen, particularly in today's ozone-depleted global climate, is an essential element of truly conscientious skin care. And there are some very good reasons for it.

The human body, as it turns out, has not one but two discrete immune systems: one for the internal system and one for the body's largest organ, the skin. And though they may be interdependent in some instances, they often function with their own individualized consciousness, especially as it regards their defense.

Notwithstanding heavy burn trauma from fires, acid or chemical damage, the skin's primary immune defenses are established as natural blocks to the sun. Once a child has passed infancy, the skin nicely and naturally secretes a healthy supply of melanin to screen itself against the assaults of the sun. Barring exceptional abuse or overexposure, this melanin connection usually works adequately up to a certain age—usually the early 20s—in the individual's life. From that point on, much like the general immune system, the skin begins to lose its ability to block out the sun. And the older the individual gets, the less innate melanin sunblock his or her skin is able to generate. So, with constant unshielded exposure to the sun's ultraviolet rays after a certain age (usually in a person's 30s) skin cancer becomes an impending challenge and, if the skin remains unprotected, a virtual inevitability.

Unfortunately, the incessant savaging of our ozone by our own pollutants has so depleted the normal screening we enjoyed just 30 years ago that even 20 minutes of unprotected exposure to the sun can net negative consequences for an older adult. Even if someone works indoors most of the time and experiences even light from the window, this to can project complications such as liver spots, Keratosis, and incipient basal cell carcinoma.

More than just the unhappy by-products of aging, these are now possible health risks and must be fended off at all costs. So the addition of sunscreen has become not only a necessary part of any appropriate skin care regime, it is essential to the life of the skin and (often) the individual who wears it.

Step Seven: Protection. This final step is one that is often overlooked and yet cannot be underestimated. Once the skin has been scrubbed clean, toned, rejuvenated, and refreshed, it requires protection. This is a matter of conscientiously applying the first five steps plus an application of foundation and make-up formulated for the individual skin type. (Obviously make-up and foundation is not an issue that most men will face. Nevertheless, diligent care and feeding of the male skin, especially after the age of 35, becomes increasingly important with each passing year.)

Thus far, all emphasis has been placed on the face when some attention needs to be placed on the body. Certainly the rest of the body needs its own levels of cleansing, scrubbing, toning, moisturizing and even exfoliation. And there are some very good products (many of them with foundations in Aloe) that can accomplish this. But there is one aspect of body care that is important to note: The body's own response to both the hazards and the variances of the environment often causes it to assume a different pH balance from that of the face. And because it does, many products such as lotions and creams for the body are not necessarily good for use in facial care. That's why there are special formulations for both face and body. And, yes, they are more than just cosmetic in nature. It is not that they will bring harm if applied. But, all things considered, one fares better when trusting the intention of the manufacturer.

Proof Positive.
The Aloe Vera Skin Savant.

Categorical declarations are often both self-serving and perilous. And yet proof abounds that Aloe Vera and stabilized Aloe Vera liquids, gels, gellies, lotions and creams have become the clear-cut first best treatment for skin challenges ranging from wounds to mild forms of acne. Certainly it has become of crucial importance in the influence it has brought to bear in such areas as cosmetic surgery, plastic surgery, and various aspects of esthetics and dermatology.

One has to be mindful, especially in the advanced stages of many of these treatments, that the potential for infection becomes an omnipresent issue, as does the rebuilding of tissue and the abilities of the wounds made by the surgeries to heal. In such areas there is a delicate balance to be struck between the necessary precautions of medicine and the progressive (and occasionally imprudent) needs of clients to recover quickly and to a point of optimum personal appearance.

Antimicrobial Studies. Wound Healing and Cell Growth.

It often emphasized yet little understood that every aspect of healing and repair to the human skin makes an impact down through the chain of study, treatment and final phase markets. From in vitro laboratory findings to surgery, from surgery to patient application, from patient application to esthetic and cosmetic treatment, one step invariably precedes the other, each one looking to the one before it for both reference and validation.

That's why it's important to note the work and study of such pivotal figures in dermatology, plastic surgery and skin health as Dr. John Heggers. A Ph.D. and Professor of Microbiology and Plastic Surgery at the Medical Branch of the University of Texas at Galveston, Dr. Heggers has become notable for his studies in the various aspects of burn studies and wound healing.

We have already covered some of Dr. Hegger's work involving Aloe Vera in our chapter on "Major Milestones", and yet there is one more study we would like to give some coverage, even though it does not directly involve Aloe Vera.

Obviously, so much of plastic surgery involves repair to damaged tissue that has resulted from some extrinsic trauma such as burns, disfigurement from accidents, blows or abuse, and congenital deformities (from "port wine stain" to structural malformations). In view of many of these challenges, there is a potential for post-operative infection that not only comes from the atmosphere but also one that comes from microbes commonly found on and around the individual human skin surface itself.

In a definitive paper completed in 1993 and entitled "Antimicrobial Therapy for the Plastic Surgeon," Dr. Heggers explored the potentials for antimicrobial drugs being administered prior to surgeries as a preventive (or prophylactic) measure.

Although this might seem to be a simple, direct, and logical procedure, it often becomes complex, because each drug administered has to take into account several factors: 1) the patient's own skin type; 2) their medical history and predisposition to infection; 3) the environment surrounding the surgery, such as the hospital and its characteristic cross-infections; and 4) the percentage of application between topical and systemic use of the drugs.

In a highly complex study involving an examination of basic topical antimicrobials ranging from *sodium hypochlorite, providone-iodine* and *silver sulfadiazine* to more advanced topical antimicrobials such as *Mupirocin,* Dr. Heggers and his staff measured them in the context of what they could do in terms of preoperative, perioperative, and post operative usage, as well as being used individually and in combination.

Although he confirmed that the use of topical antimicrobials did indeed reduce the occurrence of "invasive wound" infections, Dr. Heggers also acknowledged that oral doses of (systemic) broad-spectrum antimicrobials were also needed. In the first part of the test he introduced a group of what are referred to as "cell wall" inhibitors such as *cephalosporin* and such penicillin derivatives as *nafcillin* and *ampicillin* each known to be effective against a number of strains such as most streptococci while being ineffective against others. He also studied the introduction of members of a family of antibiotics known as *polymoxins* acknowledged to be effective against certain types of yeast and fungi. In addition, Dr. Heggers and staff drew in certain other types of DNA inhibitors known as *quinolones* to combat other pathogens such as *E. coli,* and *Enterobacter* commonly found in tissue adjacent to the wounds undergoing the trauma of healing.

At this point, we realize that the average layperson reading all these fancy descriptions for medicines and diseases with Latin names might find them confusing. But the significance of this study is monumental. So let us simplify.

Simply stated, Dr. Hegger's study underscored a longstanding dilemma facing every health professional engaged in plastic surgery or any surgery involving wound healing of large areas of the skin surface: That is the ability of the body to fight infection in the form of microbes that come from the surgery, the environment, and the toxins on the patient's own skin. Compound that by the fact that, though medications are available to treat all the diseases that might invade, before, during and after surgery, none are entirely effective against all of them. So, certain curative cocktails—both topical and oral—are a possibility.

The challenge lies in finding which of these cocktails, if any, works, and in what combinations they might be used.

What Dr. Heggers and his staff found after extensive laboratory examination of each set of candidates was the confirmation of several of their theories. First was a confirmation that, though many of these drugs were effective against a narrow range of pathogens, they were not, in and of themselves, sufficient to do the job. Second, they found that combinations of these drugs or drug cocktails might often be counterproductive in the extreme. In fact, in some cases it was found that it was better to leave the body's immune system alone to fight the pathogens themselves then to "shotgun" the application of these drugs.

The recommendation at the end of the test was to be very meticulous about the selection of the drugs to be used in tandem. The obvious implications were twofold. In the first place there came into play the danger of overdoing the "broad-spectrum" antibiotics applied against some pathogens that had already begun to mutate to form environmental resistances against many forms of the drugs. The second had to do with the inclination many medications have of anti-doting one another. Not only do many of these medications carry with them a panoply of side-effects that might kick-in if used over too long a period of time, some of them can, if used in combination, create allergic reactions that can be devastating to the patient. Both in terms of tissue reaction on the skin surface and challenges to healthy systemic balance, this bombardment of drug therapies, if not carefully administered, can bring complications as severe as the strains of bacteria, virus and fungi they are put in place to fight.

It is here that we bring in the anticipated subtext of stabilized Aloe Vera as both an adjunct and a companionable therapy. (And we feel reasonably sure it is something that Dr. Heggers knew from the studies of others experiments as well as his own.)

It is here that we bring up a number of tests in the past that point not only to Aloe Vera's profound broad-spectrum bactericidal, fungicidal and virucidal capabilities but also its abilities as an adjunct to a number of other remedies of treatment. A number of tests by Ruth Sims and Eugene Zimmermann as well as those by Dr. Ruth Setterstrom and later by BioSearch Assay rendered solid findings on behalf of Aloe Vera as the broad range destroyer of such cutaneous pathogens as various kinds of staph and strep bacteria as well as such fungi as *T. mentagrophytes, Trichophyton rubrum, Herpes zoster, Tinea pedia, Salmonella and E. coli* just to bring in a few household names among a broad list of skin and systemic pathogens.

And more recently in 1994, as we detailed in our section on "Major Milestones," a bacteriological study was conducted by Dr. Kathleen Shupe-Ricksecker in the late 1980s in which various percentages of Aloe Vera solutions proved highly effective against tissue cultures of four common pathogens—*Streptococcus pyogenes, Staph aureus, Pseudomonas aeruginosa (pseudomonas)* and *E. coli,* all of them noted pathogens toxic both to the human system and very often to the skin surrounding wounds.

Later a separate test, Dr. Shupe studied the germicidal effects of stabilized Aloe vera on *Propionibacterium acnes* (ATCC strain 6919), a test that, on the surface, seems anticlimactic. Upon examination, however, this particular strain of acne is not only persistent, it has also mutated to a point that makes it even more difficult to get rid of than similar strains have been in the past. Since we have used Aloe vera to successfully treat acne vulgaris for decades, the test was less of a surprise to me than it was a warm reassurance that our new formulations of (whole leaf) Aloe were still doing the job against all the nasty microbes to which it was being introduced, including some of the more pernicious mutations.

As is so often the case with Aloe Vera, its broad-spectrum curative potential carries no relative toxicity. As a result, at least in a properly stabilized Aloe Vera, there is also none to be found. This in the issue of wound healing and symbiotic tissue growth is a Godsend.

The Danhof-McAnalley Findings. Nothing perhaps underscores the simple truth better than another series of studies in cell growth conducted in 1993. In the *LSE* (Living Skin Equivalent) in vitro studies reported by William Bowles, Aloe Vera proved yet again that it was a standout at stimulating cell growth activity in promoting epidermal proliferation. and what is referred to as keratinocyte growth. In two LSE tests conducted by our friends Ivan Danhof and Robert McAnalley, stabilized Aloe Vera gel in concentrations of 50% to 100% proved highly effective in epidermal proliferation (surface cell growth). And not surprisingly, the higher the concentrations of the Aloe Vera solids, the larger the increase in "basal keratinocyte regeneration."

LSE or *Living Skin Equivalent* tests have now become standard practice in labs and are highly valued for a number of reasons. First, they require no animal sacrifice. Second, they are found to be 98% as accurate as live tissue studies. Some science professionals think they are even more accurate than active tissue *in vivo* samples due to the unpredicted trauma that might be experienced by the laboratory animals subjected to the tests.

The Pugliese Study. Were it placed on a linear graph, the progress of laboratory research would probably appear in the form of a stepladder—each rung of research forming a base for, and leading the way to, the next.

Well fortified with a great deal of research in skin-cell regeneration and further evidence of Aloe Vera's success against an armada of pathogens, we set about in 1994 to commission Dr. Peter Pugliese, a Pennsylvania dermatologist and skin physiologist, to evaluate the effects of stabilized Aloe Vera gel in context with a 10% glycolic acid exfoliation treatment.

Glycolic acid is a remarkably effective treatment in skin care in that it addresses the issue of dead cells on the surface of the skin (the epidermal layer). Dead skin cells tend to remain on the skin surface and adhere through an almost glue-like bond to the living cells coming up underneath. And by doing so, they refuse to make their exit on cue and sort of hang around on the surface of the skin, leaving it to appear dry, mottled, and lifeless.

Better than most transfer media, glycolic acid is able to get deep down into that bond of tissue, cleanse it and get rid of the dead tissue. It's also anti-inflammatory, antiseptic, fungicidal and quite effective in fighting acne. So, evidently, it has benefits to the skin care that are indeed worth tapping, as well as those that appear (on the surface) to complement those of stabilized Aloe Vera. So, a test of the benefits of glycolic acid when used in tandem with Aloe seemed to us at least to be both self-evident and necessary.

Dr. Pugliese specializes in studies of this sort and was quite happy to conduct this test.

In this case, the test was to be conducted on five female volunteer subjects ranging in ages from 50 to 55, all in good health and free from any dermatological diseases or systemic complications.

The purpose of this preliminary study was "to evaluate the outer canthus of the eye when our own 10% Glycolic Acid Exfoliant was applied to the face. The right volar forearm was also to be applied." (*Translation:* They wanted to determine whether the Aloe Vera and glycolic acid tandem actually worked to get rid of wrinkles.)

From that point, evaluations of the skin were to be made on day one, then at two and four weeks after initial treatment.

From the initial date of the reporting period and on every assigned report day afterward, Dr. Pugliese and his associates made clinical assessments and secured photographic records of the women's progress. In addition to the monitoring, silastic castings were made of the eyes of each woman on the reporting dates and appropriate comparisons were made. As final touches, both ultrasound scans and ballistometric gauges were made of the skin to determine increased skin density and whether or not the elastic properties of the skin were enhanced.

Peter Pugliese's test was exceptional in that it is not often that such high criteria are established at so many levels. Much due to Dr. Pugliese's impeccable sense of detail and his patient's invaluable cooperation, it was a test that provided us with invaluable insights and some irrefutable proof.

The intermediate evaluation (after two weeks) reported that all women in the group showed smoother appearing facial skin, and after four weeks the women reported some improvement in the fine facial lines. Photographic evaluations from that first four-week period revealed that four out of the five women had experienced markedly improved facial tone. And all the women showed improvement in the fine lines of the canthus around the eye after four weeks.

Evaluations of the stabilized Aloe Vera gel on the (volar) forearms of the women showed a marked improvement in primary hydration. What's more, the changes in the epidermis gave evidence of a reparative improvement to that outer layer of the skin as well.

As far as evaluations of skin suppleness were concerned, there was apparently no measurable improvement in the elasticity of the skin after four weeks. (This isn't unusual since it usually takes six to eight weeks for that kind of reformation to take place.) However, upon checking with Dr. Pugliese later, we were delighted to discover that in the subjects still checking in with the doctor, all had measured to have greatly improved skin elasticity.

Due to this test and others similar to it, we are now able to see that Aloe Vera possesses distinct abilities to improve collagen formation and in fact does a better job of helping skin rebuild both in epidermal thickness and elasticity than any other treatment we have experienced. And as reports officially often sound dry and inconclusive, we were happy to note that in a personal report, Dr. Pugliese's evaluations were unqualifiedly laudatory.

In his final report to me, Dr. Pugliese wrote that in addition to this study, his ultimate evaluation came to some other distinct conclusions. In his professional opinion, the Aloe Vera and exfoliant treatment scored a declarative superiority over any other treatment he had tried in the past in at least seven different areas:

1). The skin is brighter and has a greater clarity.
2). The overall tone of the skin shows improvement within 4 weeks with the skin color becoming more uniform.
3). Certain areas of discoloration were noted to fade significantly.
4). There is an overall softening and improvement in skin smoothness that is perceptible within one week of use.
5). The skin appears moister over a longer period of time.
6). There is a significant improvement in elasticity of about 20%.
7). There is an improvement in fine dry lines of about 28%.
8). The surface oil is markedly decreased. (This finding should help prevent breakouts of acne.)[14]

If it had offered greater force of numbers, the Peter Pugliese study would, without question, mark a major milestone in dermatology and skin care, especially as it involves treatments with Aloe Vera.

In our book it still qualifies for that distinction. We mark it here if for no other reason than the fact that it is the perfect fit to punctuate so much of the research done in this area. Once again, it underscores the exceptional and seemingly unlimited capacity Aloe Vera possesses for synergistic combination with other elements. In terms of treatment, cure, and restoration, it seems to have no equal. In instances of usage on its own, it also seems to be one of the best remedies for reparation when someone overdoses on another treatment modality. This is particularly the case in uses on the human skin. And we offer the following example.

Too Much of a Good Thing. Purely in terms of skin care and esthetics, glycolic acid has proved to be an exceptionally effective element as long as you observe the caveats about dosage and don't overdo it.

On the skin's surface there are dead cells on top that are naturally held together by a kind of cellulose glue that bonds them and prevents the live cells just underneath from coming to the surface.

Used in a carefully formulated 5% solution administered every day for six weeks, glycolic acid helps to remove the dead surface cells and the bond that holds them on to the epidermis, which in turn allows live cells to come up from the dermis. Following the six-week period, we suggest that you then use the glycolic acid 5% solution every night for about another month to six weeks.

In two or three months, whoever is going through the treatment should have their skin evaluated by an esthetician, a dermatologist, or other qualified professional.

Additionally, when you apply the 5% glycolic acid solution and Aloe Vera gelly on a dry skin before going to bed, the combination makes for a synergistic anti-inflammatory agent and works overnight as an exceptional means of killing acne and clearing troubled skin.

But unlike Aloe Vera, which may be used with impunity, glycolic acid is a sugar cane based acid and should be used with absolute temperance.

On its own the 5% glycolic acid solution does a remarkable job of maximizing the output of natural collagen and elastin, both necessary for the formation of new cells and the glow of a healthy youthful appearance. On occasion and under the strict supervision of an esthetician, a woman may use a 30% solution of glycolic acid on a dry skin for about two minutes, strictly timed and removed immediately thereafter. Afterward, an Aloe Vera gelly may be applied to enhance both the healing, rejuvenation of the skin, and the stimulation of both collagen and elastin. This very strictly supervised process may be undertaken about once every two weeks; but it is not recommended that it be done more than that.

Unfortunately, too many women in their desire to attain the unattainable look of eternal youth have been known to increase their dosage of glycolic acid to 10% and even 20% solutions and use that on a daily basis. Initially this may produce very positive short-term results by artificially stimulating the system to produce more collagen and elastin. But over the long term, even with the addition of Aloe Vera gelly, the results can be unfortunate and occasionally catastrophic.

In one case, a 35 year-old woman came into the offices of our distributor in Canada in dire straights and somewhat desperate about her appearance. Ignoring all advice to the contrary she had, in order to make herself look even younger, started using a 20% glycolic acid solution. After a time, her body simply rebelled and stopped making sufficient levels of collagen and elastin. And one morning this 35 year-old woman awakened to find a 60 year-old woman looking back at her in the mirror.

When she came to see my Canadian distributor, she put a call in to me. After hearing about the young woman's dilemma, I told her that what I thought might need to be done and referred her to our friend and associate Dr. Pugliese. After meeting with her, he gave the woman a reality check. Rule # 1: *no more overdosing on glycolic acid.* In addition, he ordered her to begin a strict Aloe Vera and vitamin C regimen applied topically to restore the lost nutrients to her face.

"You took some time to get into this condition," he advised her. "So don't expect to turn this around overnight. But in time, if you follow this (Aloe and Vitamin C cream) regimen, you should get back to normal."

This time the woman listened, and eventually she returned to normal—sadder, wiser and finally looking younger again.

Object lesson: Especially when dealing with sensitive areas such as the hair and skin, play inside the lines. There are reasons for disciplines and people to help guide you through them.

Face Time: Some Graphic Examples.

In the previous segments, we have emphasized the significance of Aloe Vera in skin care technology, much of it highlighting its importance as an overall treatment.

When it comes to defining personal appearance, words can never equal the eloquence of pictures. In the following segment we will show three very definitive sets of photographs: one involving a case of acne; another impact of Aloe Vera on a phenol peel; a third involving an esthetician's treatments of a man with burn scars; and a fourth giving illustrations of Aloe Vera's positive impact in treating a case of hyperpigmentation.

Acne: In the following photo, two young women in Oakland, California had for a long time been plagued with Grade IV acne. (Acne is graded from Grade I through Grade V, depending upon degrees of severity.) When the young woman came to an esthetician named Kathryn Leverette from Solutions of Oakland, Kathryn used whole leaf Aloe Vera facial products on both women.

Every night, she would have her clients apply our Aloe Exfoliant Lotion in a 10% glycolic acid tandem with stabilized Aloe Vera gelly as a home treatment one-night and Benzyl Peroxide Solution-sulfur (10%-5%) combination on alternate nights.

Every two weeks, she would have them use our exfoliant lotion solution (30% glycolic acid in Aloe Vera gel) under closely timed supervision.

After just 30 days treatment with the regime we have just described both women's complexions had completely cleared up, as the following photos will reveal:

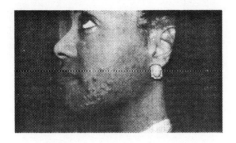

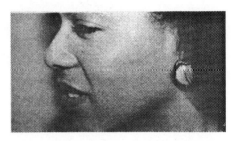

Young woman with Grade IV acne, at the beginning of treatment with the Aloe Vera and glycolic acid regime.

The same young woman 30 days after treatment. The acne has completely cleared up.

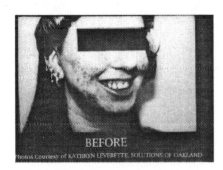

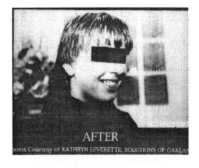

A second young woman with Grades III and V acne, at the beginning of treatment with the Aloe Vera and glycolic acid regime.

The same young woman after just 30 days of the Aloe and glycolic acid treatment. Again, the acne she had been suffering for years has cleared up without apparent trace.

Phenol Peel. Phenol peels are radical but often highly effective treatments for skin that has gone to the north side of 60(or for skin that just looks that way). Since it actually involves the use of carbolic acid to set second degree burns usually on the skin of the face, it has to be conducted under the supervision of a qualified dermatologist. In this case, Dr. Paul O'Neill, a Seattle, Washington dermatologist performed this chemical peel on a 60 year-old woman and followed it by using our Aloe Vera gelly to treat the burn. The reason for using the Aloe Vera gelly was three-fold: to help heal the wound, to dissolve dead revitalized skin, to stimulate rapid cell division and new cell growth, and to prevent bacterial infection and keloid formation (or scarring).

In the following photos, you will see a woman of 60 change before your eyes. (In some ways, it's hard to believe it's the same woman.)

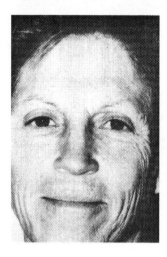 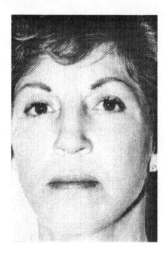

Pre: A woman of 60 before the phenol peel and Aloe Vera treatment.

Post: The same woman the phenol peel and Aloe Vera treatment just 21 days later. Note the loss of lines, the elimination of mottling, and the revitalization of her complexion.

Using Aloe to Heal Burn Scars. Barring plastic surgery and other radical treatments, it is often difficult if not impossible to clear up burn scars. And yet with the right regimen of Aloe Vera in the hands of an astute, caring, and careful skin care professional, these little cutaneous miracles can and do come to pass.

Case in point: a young man caught in a fire, burned all over his face and body and, though healed, severely scarred.

In this case however, the young man was fortunate enough to be treated by Susan Sobel-Guzick. An R.N. and licensed esthetician, Susan is also a specialist in what are called Permanent Pigmentation Procedures.

This is a process that involves gentle but consistent electric scrubs with a soft fan brush and special solutions (in this case Aloe Vera solutions) used in tandem and applied on dry skin like a mask. As a third step in the series, Susan showed the young man how to relax and relieve scarring through gentle massage. And as a fourth step, she used a gentle but potent Aloe Vera mist to treat his entire face.

Treating and eliminating scars that have already formed is not only a delicate process it is also one that requires considerable time and patience. Even with stabilized Aloe Vera as your treatment of modality of choice, the practitioner should be cautiously persistent.

In this particular case, Susan Sobel-Guzek continued with the gentle but persistent treatment for about one year. The results, though gradual in coming were both remarkable and rewarding.

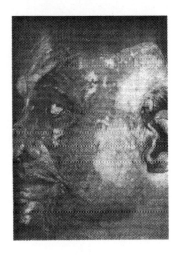
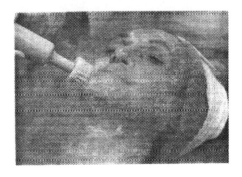

The young burn scar victim at the beginning of treatment.

Stage one of the Treatment.

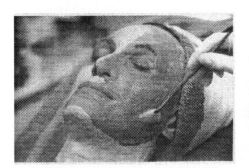
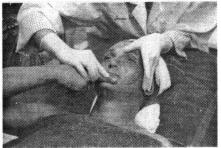

Stage two of the treatment.

Stage three of the regular treatment regimen.

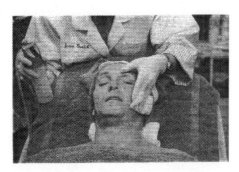

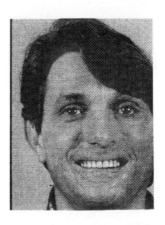

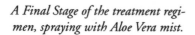

A Final Stage of the treatment regi-
men, spraying with Aloe Vera mist.

The same young man after one year
of treatment. Note that he has healed
virtually without visible scars.

Hyperpigmentation. On occasion we are truly the authors of our own dilemma. Recently in Dallas, Texas, an attractive young nurse was involved in a car crash in which her driver's side airbag opened with such force against her upper body that it left abrasions, scrapes and burns on her face.

In her desire to hasten her recovery and improve her appearance, the young woman went out into the sun too soon, and did so without any sunscreen or protection for her newly forming facial skin and turned them into large brown spots. She went to a plastic surgeon to try and get the spots removed, but the medication he prescribed for her turned her brown spots black instead.

Desperate and distraught, she consulted with four other plastic surgeons all of whom assured her that there was no effective treatment for the black spots; she would just have to get used to them. Determined that she would not have to live with this condition, the young woman went to a fifth dermatologist, Dr. Myles, who in turn recommended an esthetician who was a specialist in replacing pigment lost from burns and vitligo, a post-burn discoloration similar to her own. As synchronicity seems to be the governing law of the universe, this esthetician was Susan Sobel-Guzek who, as we now know, was no stranger to using Aloe Vera for skin pigmentation problems.

Also a registered nurse (RN), Susan set about to put her young associate on a regimen of our Aloe Cleanser, Aloe Mist, Aloe Vera Gelly, and a special cream to put on her face for the removal of the hyperpigmentation.

In 30 days of conscientious application, and to the amazement of some professional skeptics, the young woman experienced a complete recovery. In fact, the plastic surgeon who had recommended that she try the regimen and work with Susan was so impressed with the results that he called me at home to praise what he referred to as our "state-of-the-art" products and find out more about them.

The following four photos chart both the progress and the exceptional result in curing this condition that five specialists had resigned as hopeless.

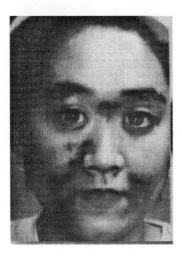

Hyperpigmentation. Stage one: The young nurse when she first came into esthetician for counseling.

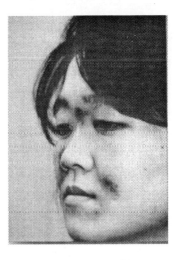

Hyperpigmentation. Stage two: The Aloe Vera regimen already gaining considerable strides.

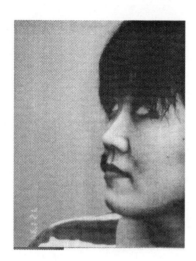

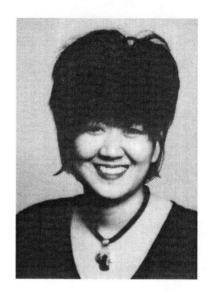

Hyperpigmentation. Stage three: Note a considerable improvement from the Aloe Vera treatment. The discoloration only remains around the critical T-zone areas of the nose and corners of the mouth.

Hyperpigmentation. Stage four: A complete recovery. A young woman's beauty restored.

Dermabrasion: We had earlier mentioned Dr. Robert Fulton's research in the late 1970s that so effectively exposed the comedogenicity of so many popular lines of cosmetics by noting that their key extender ingredient—*isopropyl myristate*—actually contributed toward the causing of acne.

We point again to Dr. Fulton's work, this time in using Aloe Vera to treat patients upon whom he performed strategic *dermabrasion* procedures in his series of acne health care centers.

Dermabrasion is a means of removing scars from acne patients by using high speed brushes to scrape away the scar tissue, usually on both the epidermis and the dermis, and allowing the skin to rebuild. Traditionally, in Dr. Fulton's clinics, patients are treated with the most modern high-speed drills and diamond particles in the brushes. Although far from painless, the process is nonetheless rapid, effective, efficient, and reasonably free of post-operative discomfort. Nevertheless, even under the most ideal conditions, dermabrasion is a serious surgery over a large body of facial skin, and healing is notoriously slow.

In the past, antibiotics were generally looked upon as the drugs of choice for all dermabrasion procedures. Taken both orally and used topically they are believed to cut down the potential for infection and eliminate the possibility of cross-infections to the skin so common to the laying bare of broad areas of skin. Soon, however, Dr. Fulton undertook the use of Aloe Vera—both the liquid and the gelly—to heal the skin postoperatively to prevent infection and as a matter of constant application to promote the rapid cell division for which Aloe is now noted, and accelerate the potentials for healing.

Now having used stabilized Aloe Vera gel and gelly in virtually hundreds of cases, Dr. Fulton has been long convinced that this is the superior way to help his dermabrasion patients move on to a maximum potential range of healing in the shortest time and with the best results. The case we now place before you in graphic study involves photos taken of a young man who underwent one of Dr. Fulton's treatments using stabilized Aloe Vera liquid (gel) and gelly.

Before starting the procedure Dr. Fulton sprayed the Aloe Vera liquid all over the face. Following the dermabrasion, he wrapped the face with gauze (also) soaked in the liquid for a couple of hours. He followed that with Aloe Vera gelly. First he would liberally spray the face with the Aloe liquid and apply the gelly for times daily.

The three photos we include here show the definitive results attained in just seven days of application:

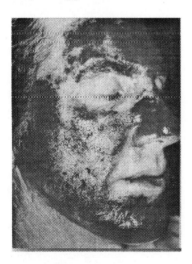

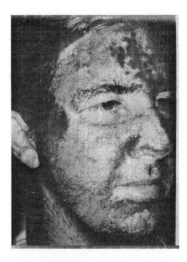

Day 1: A young dermabrasion patient after one day on the Aloe Vera Liquid/ Aloe Vera Gelly tandem treatment.

Day 4: The same young dermabrasion patient after four days on the Aloe Vera Liquid/ Aloe Vera Gelly tandem treatment.

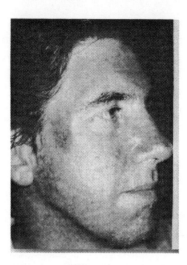

Day 7: The same patient after seven days on the Aloe Vera Liquid/ Aloe Vera Gelly tandem treatment. Normally, this level of healing, repair, and rejuvenation would take two to three weeks to achieve.

The photo study we show here is just one of many examples available to us, all of which illustrate similar dramatic results. This particular perspective however, does nicely summarize the kind of paradigm shift that is now taking place in such significant milestones of cosmetic surgery. What's more, it's one that creates healthy, effective, infection-free alternatives to such a traditional treatment. In our opinion, it is a marked improvement as well.

Just Samples: If we were to try to tell any of these stories without the photos we have included here, we probably would be accused of sensationalizing the accountings. The beauty of these time-lapse photos lies in the fact that they imbed an indelible record of Aloe Vera's effectiveness in the areas of dermatology, plastic surgery and the very underrated science of personal esthetics. What we have shown here, though thorough, is just a sample of the many graphic examples we have that illustrate broad-spectrum uses for treating the human skin, Aloe Vera is without equal.

What about the Hair?

In the last ten to fifteen years, a new area of expertise has arisen in the field of what must be called alternative health practices—the remarkable science of *hair testing* as a primary aspect of what is now being referred to as *tissue mineral analysis, or TMA.*

Rather than being some new brand of high-tech witchcraft, this is based in a centuries old tradition of oriental medicine, inspired by acupuncture pressure points and an understanding of the meridians of the body. In clinics such as the one being administered by Dr. David Nickel in Santa Monica, California men and women are actually able to experience tissue mineral analysis through hair sample testing and have reported reversing many lifetime afflictions such as chronic fatigue syndrome and acute prostatitis through alteration of diet, lifestyle changes and strict regimens of orthomolecular supplementation.

Through chemical analysis and computer readouts of hair fiber samples, acupuncturists, naturopaths and other qualified health professionals such as Dr. Nickel can determine exactly where you are nutrient deficient, where you are perhaps either overvalued or undervalued in the amount and kind of vitamins and minerals you take, whether or not you have a propensity toward certain kinds of systemic heavy metal overload and whether or not you experience a proclivity toward fast or slow oxidation.

If an individual tends to be what is referred to as a "fast oxidizer," he or she will be high in energy, able to make red blood cells more quickly and maintain higher levels of energy. By the same token, that same individual might well be inclined to burn out their vital life candles a little earlier than they should. So, they will require enzymatic balancing to moderate their metabolic burn rate at a certain point in their lives.

According to this kind of naturopathic study, "slow oxidizers" will tend to use their energy less efficiently, tend to age more quickly, and might have problems with digestion, fatigue and autoimmune diseases later in life. By the same token, they're not as likely to experience cardiovascular complications, heart attacks or strokes too early in life as a "type-A" personality fast oxidizer might be. Slow oxidizers are more prone to be calm but at the same time might need to have their metabolism revved up a notch or two by proper diet and blood-building glandular supplementation. Especially as some of these people advance in age, their systems tend to lose their ability to extract live enzymes from their diet. And unless they are able to supplement them properly, they will experience a slow but sure loss of energy and visible breakdowns in both their health and appearance of health; and they may start to do so early in life—in their fifties and even their forties.

So, we are now driven to understand that how we regard the hair on our head is not merely a matter of personal grooming or extensions of our vanity, it might very well be the ultimate window to the triumphs and breakdowns of our systemic selves.

That is absolutely not to say that by improving the health and grooming aids for our hair that we'll be able systemically to improve our lot. It is absolutely to say that our hair may be one of the best weathervanes we have in determining our own personal health horizons.

Example: Through such sciences as (hair testing) tissue mineral analysis, it is now being determined that the turning of one's hair color from its natural brown, black, red or blonde to grey or white is not as much a phenomenon of aging as it is an indication of a deficiency in certain minerals, especially copper. But did you also know that some studies have shown that men who take high doses of most kinds of zinc (presumably to help their prostate gland) are also dramatically increasing their potential for accelerated hair loss?

Did you know that men who start to bald prematurely might not enjoy as high a level of testosterone (as was previously thought) as much as they might simply be chronically constipated? And there is every indication that the lessening of hair strength and content, the loss of hair on the body and the thinning of hair on the head are specific announcements by the body that it is losing its ability to oxygenate and make healthy new red blood cells. It's a phenomenon of aging to be sure. It is also a trend that can be held at bay indefinitely by the introduction of amino acid supplementation, change of diet to low-glycemic natural foods, and some modified increases in the kind and degree of one's regimens of aerobic exercise.

There is still so much to be learned from the complex geography of our own bodies, and yet if anything can be derived from all we have preached on these pages it is that what appears on the outside is so often a reflection of the ongoing struggle for chemical equilibrium that our systems experience on a daily basis.

So, let's *hair* it for those who have learned to strike the balance. And at least part of that balance comes with the understanding that hair, as an extension of skin from the hypodermis and the dermis, goes through its own cycle of cellular death and resurrection. And if we appear to concentrate more on men in this segment, it is because the majority of hair concerns such as alopecia (baldness) and dandruff (seborrhea) are by and large directed at the male of the species Homo sapiens. And, if one were to be honest, hair is to the man as complexion is to the woman—the focus of his vanity and youth.

In truth, women are also well advised to address the health of their hair in terms of systemic analysis because, though they may not be inclined to lose their hair as men do, they often experience a deterioration in body, texture, and resilience that is not nearly as much the result of too much grooming over the years as it is the indication of a body chemistry gone out of balance. The difference with women is that they are more inclined to address their full head of nutrient depleted hair in purely cosmetic terms. They perm it, bake it, tease it, and treat it with finishing sprays, color rinses and straighteners that may work for a week or two but be contributory to long term hair necrosis and gradual thinning that becomes so evident in men and women in their seventies and eighties.

In purely structural terms the hair, in its way, mirrors the complexity of the skin. It consists of two parts, *the root* and *the shaft*. The *hair root* is comprised of *the follicle, the bulb* and *the papilla*. The bulb forms the lower part of the root, the follicle forms the tube enveloping the root and the papilla is a small cone at the bottom of the follicle. The hair shaft is also comprised of three parts, including *the marrow (or medulla)* of the shaft, *the middle layer (or cortex)* which dictates the hair's color and *the cuticle* that gives the hair shaft its strength and elasticity.

Healthy hair grows an average of half an inch per month. Just as the skin does, the hair goes through its own cycle of death and replacement. It is the papilla that brings new hair up through the skin layers to the light of new life. As it does, each strand grows either under or beside the hair it is replacing. And it will usually mimic the hair shaft it is replacing both in its density of structure and its potential for long healthy life. So, healthy hair replaces healthy hair, and conversely: Unhealthy hair is replaced by weak, limp, nutrient depleted hair. And don't look for that lineage to change unless the individual makes conscientious and consistent changes with his or her nutritional intake and hair treatment regimes.

Since real hair growth commences beneath the epidermal layer of the skin, it has to be said that as the scalp goes so goes the hair. Therefore, although a healthy scalp may not necessarily assure the growth of healthy new hair, an unhealthy scalp whose pores are blocked or plagued with conditions such as dandruff are certain to experience erratic growth patterns and unsightly scaling and blemishes.

Essentially, there are two types of dandruff: *seborrhea oleosa* or *oily dandruff*, and *seborrhea sica*, also known as *dry dandruff*.

Oily dandruff not as much of a problem as it used to be back in the 1940s and 1950s when men were taught not to shampoo more than once a week and were subjected to an entire armada of "grooming aids" that actually clogged the sebaceous glands and were largely contributory to premature balding among a large percentage of the male population. Nowadays, education and grooming awareness that parallels those of women have taught men that frequent shampooing and keeping the hair and scalp as clean as possible are both contributory to healthy hair growth

Dry dandruff now occurs more frequently among both men and women and very well might be a reflection of too much grooming, or the use of grooming aids of the wrong kind. Once again, however, we can never discount the toxins in our atmosphere and especially the urban water in some areas of the country.

Whether the dandruff is oily or dry, it reveals itself through the accumulation of white dead cells on the scalp and hair that slough away in unsightly 'flakes."

And whether the causes are internal such as inadequate nutrition and poor circulation or external such as environmental toxins or irregular grooming patterns, they can both lead to premature baldness or what is known as *alopecia* (or *alopecia prematura*). Ordinarily, this is a gradual thinning process that could take years or suddenly come later in life.

No question *alopecia prematura* is often directly tied to the individual's gene bank. But it can also come from all the areas of pathology we have previously noted. Poor diet, high levels of stress, hypertension, anemia, constipation, nutrient deficiency, poor grooming habits, excessive weight, and environmental toxins such as poor quality of tap water—all these factors individually and in combination contribute to the more than 40 million men and women million women in America who have problems with premature balding.

Primarily for reasons of vanity, personal pride and self-confidence, this is a challenge to anyone who experiences, and for that reason there are remedies galore to fix it. Everything from hair plugs (painful and expensive), to minoxydil based hair restoration formulas sold over-the-counter (often replete with side effects) to nutrient packages (usually inadequate and unproven) are being hyped to meet the challenge. But results are mixed and often temporary. Certain enzyme blockers have now emerged that claim near 100% effectiveness, and yet they too fall way short of the mark.

Although certain manufacturers claim to have discovered the magic bullet in this area, none have proven themselves to be a clear-cut winner.

Even now in this age of advanced medical technology, the obsession with keeping one's hair remains a challenge for most men. And though it may seem superficial and vain, what it represents may be more deep-seeded and significant than any of us are willing to acknowledge. Certainly, one can witness, with the passing of the years, the thinness and loss of life in one's own hair. Why then should it be a surprise to anyone that early hair loss and weak hair structure would be anything other than directly related to systemic complications?

Nothing gives more evidence to this fact than a condition called *alopecia aereata,* which is often caused by trauma, injury, disease, or grave systemic imbalances. This aspect of balding can often be temporary and last only as long as the condition that created it. And yet it is indicative of the importance of hair, if nothing else, as the body's weathervane. To be sure, one can be healthy in all other aspects and still have topical challenges presented to the hair and scalp. When those come either as a part of a systemic imbalance or as a part of someone's dispossessed gene bank, one can certainly improve the kind of external care their hair receives in the products they select.

In these cases, we feel that Aloe Vera is the perfect formulation for hair and scalp for a number of reasons:

First, it is bactericidal and fungicidal. This enables it immediately to address and redress the fungi and squalid sebum that accompany some types of dandruff.

Second, its proteolytic enzymatic activity helps slough off dead cells and set the stage for the regeneration of healthy skin tissue around the hair follicles.

Third, the lignin in Aloe Vera helps carry the antiseptic and cleansing power of Aloe deeply into the scalp and forms a healthy basis for new hair growth.

Fourth, the amino acids in Aloe help to build healthy tissue both in the skin and the bulb and shaft of the hair.

Fifth, since Aloe has proven itself to be antipruritic (so it helps stop itching), it helps eliminate the scratching and renewed irritation that accompanies dandruff.

Sixth, the saponins present in Aloe Vera provide a natural sudsing quality of shampoos and soaps that are made with this silent healer.

Seventh, Aloe Vera contains no allergens or side effects to impede its unique abilities to work out infections in the skin and revitalize the epidermal and dermal layers of the scalp, as well as to penetrate even to the hypodermal layers.

These hair and scalp treatments may be accomplished by using properly stabilized Aloe Vera products such as Aloe gel and scrubs specially formulated for the hair and scalp. And they may also be incorporated into Aloe based medicated shampoos and conditioners. Yet even as we proclaim the potential advantages of such products, we add a set of precautions.

Caution 1: Beware of the cheap "aloe vera" imitators. There are unfortunately some marketers of "aloe vera" who cut the Aloe Vera supposedly in their formulations by adding or replacing it either with maltodextrin or calcium and water extenders in ways that mimic the true Aloe. We recommend that you use products that contain at least 50% stabilized Aloe Vera gel accompanied with clinical data that specifically applies to treatment of the hair and skin.

Caution 2: Neither Aloe Vera nor any other exceptional treatment can work effectively if used in tandem with sodium lauryl sulfate, sodium laureth sulfate or any other cosmetic extender that clogs the pores leading to the sebaceous glands. Since this is still the subject of much debate, we cannot issue this caution as a cannon. But we can and will voice our concern that what was once proven about isopropyl myristate for the skin will soon become a truism as regards the negative impact of sodium lauryl sulfate for the hair. If that is the case we want to raise the question: Why use something that is the subject of such controversy when there are viable natural ingredients that can be used in its place? Once again it is the issue of cost of ingredients versus quality of usage horizon.

In the world of health, wellness, and sensible natural alternatives, money cannot be, and should not be, an object.

Summary

Since we believe as Shakespeare once said, "Brevity is the soul of wit," we will clip our inclination to make this chapter about 200 pages long.

In truth there is so much to tell about the strides that have been made in plastic surgery, dermatology, esthetics and skin care that we cannot begin to do them all justice. All we can do in this chronicle is offer samples and signposts; and with them a large neon caution light for the industry that dwells on the edges of this consciousness to continue to monitor itself diligently and with an appropriate measure of pragmatism.

There is in every study of clinical and esthetic breakthroughs involving the skin and hair such enormous potential for establishing new milestones that we are hard-pressed to give adequate attention to them all. Yet even as they occur, there arise in equal number the armies of skeptics and promulgators of doubt. To those, we merely plead the case: Look at the data. Read the reports. And keep an open mind.

We also acknowledge the fact that so much of what has prompted us to probe even further into the nebulous category of personal care has to do with the fact that supervision inside certain organizations is occasionally more defensive than it is proactive. This, as concerns certain bodies governing the personal care industry, is a challenge and a call to honor as well.

If there are still unanswered questions as to standards and practices within certain areas of the CTFA, for example, are they not better served to raise the bar for the entire industry?

Rather than allow marginal standards for acceptable product content to hold sway, would they not be better advised to grade their own products (just as food producers often grade theirs)? Why could there not be a Grade A (pharmaceutical quality) skin treatment, a Grade B (high-end cosmetic) and even a Grade C (general use mass-market) personal care classification for less critical products?

Caveat emptor has often been the theme song of this industry. And yet isn't it time we all change the prevailing ballad to something more like, "Only the Best for You?"

Given our more recent understanding that both the skin and the hair are not only organs but also extensions of organic activity inside the body at large, is it not better to take a more holistic approach to treating the needs of the entire system? We are, after all, not parts but a whole entity. And it is only by addressing that whole being that the world of personal care will ever rise to the level of credibility it should attain, and that frankly should be demanded of it.

Chapter 9

Animal Planet

Sometimes it is difficult for us to grasp that part of our role in the steward-ship of this planet entails the care, feeding and healing of our creature com-panions. In this chapter we give you a look at many of the new innovations that are being employed to treat our creature companions with greater com-passion, insights and understanding. From special Aloe Vera treatments for dogs and cats, we also take a good long look at some treatments for horses, cattle and some of our barnyard friends. Of course, there'll be some dra-matic stories as well as profiles of the courageous professionals who helped make them.

Prophecy is a fool's game, and yet we begin this chapter with a prediction: At some future date in some distant decade centuries from now, every civilization, like those that have gone before it, will be measured by the intelligence, tolerance and compassion with which it has treated its fellow creatures.

Such a mentality cannot be merely dismissed as "new age" or vegetarian as much as it must be understood that this fragile global environment we all share is utterly dependent upon appropriate ecological balance.

That sense of balance comes with an appreciation for the role that our fellow travelers in the animal kingdom have played in the process of scientific discovery, bacteriology, toxicology and healing over the years. Just in the context of estab-lishing credibility for Aloe Vera throughout the world, the impact of endless line-age of dogs, cats, rabbits, rats, monkeys and other designated "lab-test animals" cannot be measured in terms of time, weight, or consideration. Whether they have been the unwitting agents of its respectability or relatively sentient beings aware of their participation in the process is topic for a debate that will no doubt rage for years and, I might add, without probable resolution.

I personally happen to believe that the truth lies somewhere in between—that the awareness of the animal resides in direct proportion to the intelligence of the animal. Don't expect much empathy, for example, from a frog. By the same token, a dog, a cat or a Rhesus monkey might be aware of the procedure and on some occasions (debatably) a cognizant agent in the process of both healing and even experimentation. I come to that belief for a number of reasons. Principal among them was a book I co-authored in 1985 on the holistic treatment of animals and the specific use of Aloe Vera the treatment of choice for literally hundreds of animal pathologies. The book is entitled *Creatures in Our Care.* To our knowledge, it remains the only definitive work ever written on the use of Aloe Vera in the treatment of every kind of creature from tigers to parakeets. And yet its job remains unfinished, because the mural of creature care in the art of healing is constantly subject to new strokes of the brush.

In almost every instance of interaction, there exists a subtext of communication—a permission if you will—that our creature companions and we are partners in the cure. Perhaps because the communication is non-verbal we somehow fine-tune our senses in ways we sometimes forget to use with one another. So we sense their complicity as well as their awareness in our attempts to help them in a way that can only be described as poignant.

By the same token, there is a sense about them that they can make their own contributions to this process, not only in their own treatment but also those of other creatures within their own sphere of influence.

We've all been privy to times where a mother dog will nurse a newborn piglet along with members of her litter and when a mother cat might nurse a puppy. But beyond maternal instincts there are those rare transcendent moments when we witness an extraordinary case of animal rescue, healing or deliverance performed not by the creature Homo sapiens in its dominion but also by one creature to another in the miraculous rhythm of harmony.

When working on the development and research of it with one of my co-authors, Richard Holland (an exceptionally gifted veterinarian), I was privileged to see many animals in his practice that were actively participating in helping to treat, aid, and even heal other animals.

At the time, Richard had a rather homespun, comfortable atmosphere at his clinic in St. Cloud, Minnesota, one in which you could feel a sense of healing and affiliation. It is a field of energy I have since realized, to which our creature companions are most sensitive, and one to which they respond in remarkable ways. In Dr. Holland's rather free-form open-air convalescent center, he introduced us to a dog that as an active blood donor, a cat that acted as a surrogate mother for kittens *and* puppies and a chicken who was a willing suite mate to a recovering bird dog (In fact, they had formed an inseparable bond).

In all these cases there existed a consciousness of participation that could not be ignored any more than it could be denied. And it helped me at least to gain further appreciation of the fact that we share this planet with some very exceptional creatures with whom we are able to learn, share, and mutually contribute.

We bring these instances up as examples of the degrees to which animals can be aware of the process to which they are party. This also serves as the preface to the resolve that no animal experimentation should be undertaken unless it is absolutely necessary. And I personally feel that tortuous and painful lab experiments made on animals just to satisfy someone's intellectual curiosity is cruel, unfortunate, and should be abolished.

Having said that, I am only too aware that there are frequent occasions in which laboratory experiments on animals are often the only ones deemed acceptable by the FDA, the AMA, the AVMA and other national governing health bodies. And if it's the only way open to us to advance the cause of medical science or to gain broad-range acceptance for a treatment, modality or cure, we accept the fact that those are the rules by which we have to play. For that, we ask our fellow creatures' forgiveness and offer our gratitude for their noble participation.

By now, we have already noted that in our past attempts to determine kill ratios or what is known as LD50s on laboratory animals that there is no established LD-50 for Aloe Vera. In other words, it has never been the cause of death to a single laboratory animal. There is simply no measurable toxicity to this plant. Because of it, Aloe possesses a toxicity rating that is lower than anything, including tap water. In fact I often say that the only way you can kill an animal with Aloe Vera is to drown them in a tub of the liquid (not that I recommend it, mind you).

We also underscore the fact that this section will not be dealing with laboratory tests on animals. Those dark necessities of validation are covered extensively in other chapters. Ironically, that is where we first became aware of an animal's need to benefit from this healing plant. But our awareness was long before predated by the ancients. Historically the use of Aloe to treat animals goes deeply into the archives of recorded history.

One of the most enlightening aspects of using Aloe Vera in animal care is and always has been the honesty with which these creatures respond to treatment. When any of our veterinary associates are treating any of the animal species in their care, they are ever aware of the fact that there is little room for debate over the psychological implications of their treatment or whether or not their responses to their disease were psychosomatic.

To this awareness we add another advantage: Because there are fewer restrictions governing the treatment of animals in this country, we have been able to pioneer some major therapeutic breakthroughs not only in veterinary treatment, but also to form the foundation for specific areas of cure and treatment of human maladies.

This is not necessarily the offspring of mere coincidence. We often find that it is through effective long-term veterinary use that a treatment might be submitted for further testing and examination for the human condition. That, under ideal circumstances, is as it should be. Myopia, however, does seem to be a uniquely human affliction. And there are times when potential cures for human diseases have been blocked if for no other reason than the fact that they are viewed as being uniquely applicable to veterinary treatment.

Granted, caution is advised about interspecific applications of certain kinds of medication. There are a number of popular over-the-counter human medications to which cats, dogs, rats, rabbits, monkeys and other animals may be specifically allergic. The lists tend to be extensive and the histories of aversion well documented. In fact, one should always ask a vet or any healing professional for a list of medications that are not to be used on one's dog, cat, hamster, horse or bird. When in doubt about effective non-invasive ways to treat any creature, however, we feel we can recommend one broad-spectrum healant with impunity: stabilized Aloe Vera.

To be sure, Aloe Vera has treated birds and mice as well as elephants and big jungle cats effectively in any number of ways. And it would be easy to expand the landscape of cures to examine some from every species. But for use in the narrow context of this chapter, we'll devote the lion's share of our time on some extensive examinations of treatments for dogs and cats in the small animal category, and horses and cattle in the large. Since treatments for these four species—*equine, bovine, canine,* and *feline*—comprise about 80% of all professional creature care in the USA, we feel these are the areas to which we can do more justice in the limited space allotted us.*

So we proceed with a sense of appreciation and understanding for our fellow creatures that we might not have experienced were there not so many timeless examples of their wise and courageous participation in the healing process.

We also follow with a declaration of admiration for the veterinarians of this world, especially those who treat and care for a wide range of animal species. Where the average M.D., D.O. or N.D. learns all the aspects of the creature

---

*For a detailed examination of all aspects of animal care, we commend the reader to a copy of *Creatures in our Care*—a compendium of holistic animal care for all species, penned by these authors.

Homo sapiens, the D.V.M. has to learn the nature, the physiology and the natural aberrations of a number of species. He has to make intelligent note of their needs for specific response to treatment, to what medications they are averse, and how to create optimum environments to best facilitate their particular needs for repair and recovery. This requires a sensitivity, patience and dedication that can only be defined in all the healing arts as unique.

We acknowledge our reference to healing as an art, simply because science can only take us so far. It can only provide us with the research, the elements and the license to use them with conscientious zeal. It cannot guarantee the pragmatic intelligence, infinite compassion, or scrupulous care that the practitioner will apply in each case. That is the "X" factor that makes the difference in whether or not the patient is healed or not, and often whether that patient lives or dies. That Power comes from a very great Source indeed and humbles the instrument through which it is expressed.

Going to the Dogs.

In a way dogs are the clearest mirrors of our consciousness as a society. No creature with which we interact plays a more varied role—alternately as conscious hero, unwitting villain, constant servant and innocent victim. Whereas there are perhaps 15 breeds of cattle, a dozen breeds of horse, and perhaps 30 breeds of cat, there are more than 450 breeds of dog. Each strain has been specially bred by humankind to serve a specific function, many of which are no longer relevant. This often leaves us on the horns of a dilemma and with a peculiar hybrid creature that may be a total misfit in the world as it has become. Ironically, dogs are the products of what might be considered more advanced societies. (In the developing world, they are too often competition for food and simply too expensive to maintain. So they are often held as close to being feral and not a part of the nuclear family dynamic.)

Historically, dogs have been bred to be everything from hunters to food, from police dogs to smugglers, from palace guard dogs to mountain rescue teams. For millennia, they've herded our cattle, pulled our sleds, helped us hunt our game, guarded our families, been loving comrades to our young, hospice companions for our elderly, and our kind accomplices in medical experiments too numerous to detail. They can be the most pampered animals in all of known creation and yet statistically are the also most abused (due no doubt to their close proximity to the creature homo sapiens). They are the runaway favorites as family pets (whereas cats are more popular with singles). And yet, statistically they rank fourth among creatures considered most dangerous to man.

Every year in the United States alone, there are more than 30,000 reported cases of dog bites resulting in an average of 29 fatalities—more than bites from snakes, scorpions, and spiders combined! The reasons are almost as varied as there are numbers of dogs, but in at least half the cases, the bites come out of some human error of communication, either an improper handling of the dog through a rough or violent motion, attempts to tease, accidental awakenings, startling the creature, or a failure to recognize the dog's training and role in its environment. Dogs that are trained to be herd dogs, guard dogs, police dogs, or work dogs, have a more no nonsense approach to their proximate universe and do not necessarily respond well to intrusions upon their routine. So, suffice it to say, most dog bites come as a result of misunderstandings and improper reactions to what is often a warning bite or reflex bite from the creature itself.***

As far as the rest are concerned, as much as 35% of those could be eliminated entirely by understanding that the dog in question might have what is known in homeopathic terms as a *rabies miasm,* which also means the creature might be successfully treated with infinitesimal doses of an element called *lachesis.* Lachesis lives up to every frontier cliché about "snake oil" in that it is technically just that. It's extracted from the venom of the bushmaster snake, and broken down into infinitesimal potencies. If injected into dogs with certain dark-side tendencies, it has been known to completely turn what are often thought to be rogue dogs into very docile, very good loving citizens. With little exception, *rabies miasms* stem from a biochemical imbalance that is most often genetic in that it is passed down through the gene pools of some breeds of dogs. And yet this phenomenon knows

---

*** Many breeds of dogs come from bloodlines bred to a specific violent purpose, and frankly some of them do not make good pets for that reason. Borzois (Russian Wolfhounds), docile in domestic circumstances, have it genetically encoded into them to run down and kill animals that are fleet of foot and will fly like the wind to any feral movement. Alsatians (German Police Dogs) are part wolf by bloodline and are often trained to be guards, detectives and attack dogs. Staffordshire Bull Terriers (also known as Pit Bulls) have centuries of genetic encoding that bring them instinctively to fight and attack bulls, bears, and others of their own breed. To be sure, these creatures can be trained to some degree to be more obedient, domestic, and perhaps even docile. Still, there is the loaded pistol factor, and there is an often unfounded inclination to favor environment over genetics. So this footnote comes as a caution. Consider your choices of a pet seriously. Do not bring up a dog genetically encoded to do mayhem around small children. Do not coop up a lithe athletic hunting hound in a small city apartment. And do not expect your 200 pound Bull Mastiff, bred to roam the rocky grounds around a castle, ever to feel anything but disoriented in your narrow vertical town house.

no exclusions, and any breed from a diminutive Yorkshire terrier to a Great Pyrenees can exhibit the characteristics. The characteristics are numerous and often present themselves in batches. The most obvious indicator of a rabies miasm is a propensity to bite as a matter of reflex. Whereas it is in the normal dog's nature to bite only as a last resort, it is the nature of the canine rabies miasm to bite as a first line of defense. Dogs with this syndrome also might tend to be incontinent, not easily housebroken, and more susceptible to diseases such as runny eyes, nose, and infections of the mucous membranes.

They might also betray certain rogue behavior such as running away at times, running in packs (often vicious packs), and erupting with sudden unruly outbursts of aggressive behavior without provocation. Rabies miasms do not indicate that the dogs themselves necessarily have rabies, but that they are more likely to contract it. It might well be an indication that this kind of biochemical imbalance would also render them more susceptible to syndromes against which the "normal" dog would have a natural immunity.

We acknowledge that some professionals will view this entire perspective as advancing a daring, if not controversial theory. And yet we make it with a very singular intention. Primarily, it underscores the immense mural facing anyone who is trying to treat 450 different breeds of dogs and an infinite permutation of types of mutts. The challenge is to develop a simpler means of defining their needs and finding the appropriate cure, one that is non-invasive, all encompassing, and broadly effective.

With that in mind, we once again refer you to the healant that has proven universally effective in treating our creature companions time and time again—stabilized Aloe Vera.

If this Silent Healer has proven itself to have a preemptively positive effect on any animal species over the last 20 years it is on the creature *canis familiaris*. In countless tests as well as actual application, dogs have responded with unequivocal recovery to treatments with a number of Aloe Vera compounds.

In the following segment, we will break our treatments for dogs into three categories: 1) the treatment of day-to-day skin conditions; 2) treatment of burns, wounds, trauma and; 3) systemic syndromes, many of which may be dangerous to the dog. It is here that we like to emphasize that dogs often exhibit diseases with topical manifestations that might also have systemic origins. In those instances, we will note the appropriate application of Aloe Vera internally as well as topically.

We also note that dogs in particular seem to respond to Aloe Vera with positive results that are almost spontaneous. As such they are some of our best barometers for the broad-spectrum curative potentials of the healing plant.

Flea Bites, Hot Spots and Allergic Dermatitis.

Fleas are often thought of in comical terms as being a pest. In truth, they are no laughing matter. Fleas are virtually indestructible and in purely historical terms have been the destroyer of worlds. The bubonic plague that killed over 30 million people in the western Europe's sparsely populated nations of the 14th century had its origins in flea infested rats that carried the "buboes" from one host to the next. In modern times, the flea is still the carrier of disease, dirt, and numerous cutaneous allergies that appear on dogs. These include infections and larval parasites that form into such unpleasant intestinal manifestations as tapeworm.

Fleas and dogs are often thought of in synonymous terms in that dogs, especially long-haired breeds, appear to be the perfect host for the nasty little creatures. As is the case with any kind of microbe, fungus, virus, insect or other pathogen born in perverse environments, prevention is the essential proactive step to take. Although our creature companions get tagged as being principal carriers of fleas, the original spawning grounds are often drought, dry hot weather and dry dusty soil. Our pets just get caught with them and carry them into our homes where they love to take up residence in carpeting and furniture.

Especially in hot climates and during summer months, it is important to shampoo rugs, clean fabric furniture and bathe your dogs frequently (every month to six weeks at least). Preventive non-toxic sprays and medications such as Frontline™ have proven quite effective, and there are a number of toxin-free natural repellents such as citronella and penny royal oil that may be sprayed into drapes and carpeting. Once infested with fleas, dogs might need some natural sprays such as those made with pyrethrins. Pyrethrins are flea killing agents made from chrysanthemums and usually do not act as an irritant. Nonetheless, some dogs especially may be allergic to pyrethrins, so it may be necessary to try the spray on a small area of the dog and check for a reaction.

One can also use stabilized Aloe Vera to supersede these treatments, and in fact, a full potency Aloe Vera-jojoba shampoo has proven very effective in driving away fleas. (We have noted before that Aloe Vera is a natural insect repellent. So, although it might not kill fleas, it works very well when it comes to running the pesky little fellows off.)

Invariably there are occasions when every intention of prevention fails. Our canine companions get a plague of fleas, and often do not react well to them. Especially in large covens, fleas left to dance on the skin of dog do a few things that aren't very nice. First, when fleas bite they suck blood and can cause the victim to become anemic. Second, when fleas bite, they release a specific venom into the system of all kinds of mammals, including the creature *Homo sapiens.* Most creatures are immune to that venom and do not react to it. Others, many breeds of dogs included, are not so fortunate.

Dogs, particularly some of the long-haired varieties, are especially easy prey to them. There seems to be an increase in the number of dogs who experience reactions to flea bites that range from moderate skin infections to severe allergies, bleeding and hair loss. Very often it is the result of the owner's mistaken belief that these problems will spontaneously disappear if only the fleas can be killed or driven off.

Eventually, the flea will quit the host either through death or a departure for another victim, but by then the damage is done. And an army of microbes it leaves behind has the virtual power to dig in and cause more serious problems, attracting not only more fleas but other parasites as well.

One veterinary practitioner, now retired, who pioneered much of Aloe Vera's use in the treatment of numerous canine cutaneous conditions, was Dr. Allan Fredrickson. A Washington State vet of some renown, Dr. Fredrickson used Aloe to treat several post-fleabite syndromes such as *hot spots* (also known as allergic dermatitis). Whether the dermatitis is systemic or a externally induced allergy exacerbated by fleas and parasites, Dr. Fredrickson found it very effective to clean the wound either with Aloe Vera liquid or a good disinfectant used exclusively for that purpose. He would then use Aloe Vera gelly and rub it into the sore four times a day. He also found it very effective to mix Aloe Vera liquid with either an Aloe crème or another kind of pure disinfectant cream.

In specific cases of *fleabite dermatitis,* the wound or irritation can be determined as a direct manifestation of a series of fleabites. In such cases, Dr. Fredrickson also found it effective to use 1/2 ounce of Aloe Vera liquid (or gel) and Aloe Vera gelly in a compound to treat any wound that might be caused by a flea-bite allergy. In fact, this proved to be the success rate he got in treating more than 200 cases of fleabite dermatitis and related conditions.

Oftentimes, cases of cutaneous infection such as allergic dermatitis might have a chance of healing were it not for the fact that the dog tries to help it along by licking it. To answer the unasked question: Yes, there are some healing enzymes that flow out of the saliva in a dog's tongue. Unfortunately, there isn't enough to compensate for in an area that the dog is licking constantly for hours on end for several days in a row. This is simply the negative by-product of an overly zealous need to make well, and is defined with a syndrome all its own called *lick granuloma. Lick granuloma* is a common manifestation that causes an already unpleasant skin condition to grow worse—to increase in suppuration, itching, swelling, and infection. Of course, as it does, the dog licks it all the more, and the more the dog licks it the worse it gets. This can easily become a chronic condition if something isn't done to stop the vicious cycle of the overanxious patient trying to heal itself. It is also a phenomenon of lick granuloma that the more irritated the condition becomes, the more often the creature tries to lick it. Part of this is due to the natural process of itching that comes with the rebuilding of tissue.

There are a couple of ways to prevent lick granuloma from becoming even more extreme. One is what is known as an Elizabethan collar. An Elizabethan collar is a high collar, either leather or plastic, that fans out from a dog's neck to prevent it from applying its renowned skills for reaching hard to get to places. Since the collar has to be worn 24 hours a day until the condition improves, it's not a very pleasant experience for our poor companions, and it does nothing to prevent another dog in the same household from licking the wound. Dogs are very sociable creatures and often come one another's aid in times of trouble. So, very often a second dog in a multi-dog family will help the first (especially with hard-to-reach places) by licking the wound to help it. In this case, wrapping or binding the wound is preferable, but it should be done with the right application of healant and a regular changing schedule.

In such cases, and Aloe Vera liquid (gel) and Aloe Vera gelly combination serve as an ideal tandem. The Aloe Vera gel is ideal for cleaning the wound and blocking thromboxane formation (the presence of irregular scabbing). Once the exposed area is cleaned, it has proven most effective to cover the area with Aloe Vera gelly and wrap it. Change the wound every two days and repeat the process until the dog recovers. This process has proved effective in dozens of reported cases from the veterinarians we have worked with over the years, so we feel we can recommend it with great confidence.

Aloe Vera is the ideal healant because it not only fights infection and promotes rapid cell growth, but also because it is antipruritic. So it stops the wound from itching and takes the dog's attention away from the need to lick it, bite it, and constantly tend it.

In the following set of photos, we show something of combination of the syndromes we have just discussed being treated effectively with the Aloe Vera tandem we have just discussed. In this case a Springer Spaniel had contracted a case of allergic dermatitis traceable to fleabite infestation that had turned into a classic "hot spot." Since the reaction was on the back of the dog's head, another dog in the household had attempted to help out by licking the wound, forming a textbook lick granuloma that exacerbated and grew over the next several weeks. The condition reported to our old friend and associate Richard Holland, D.V.M. was treated successfully and turned around within three weeks. The photos tell the rest of the story.

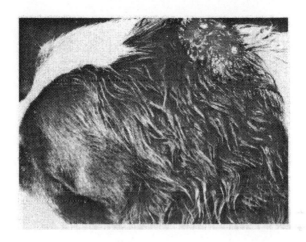

A case of hot spots upon first presentation to the clinic. Upon presentation to the clinic, the wound was cleansed with a mild detergent and Aloe Vera liquid. The scab was removed and the area shaved. Then the lesion was dabbed with Aloe Vera gelly.

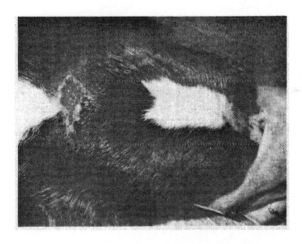

Six days later, healing has advanced markedly. Primary treatment consisted of daily rubbing off scabbing tissue followed by daily applications of Aloe Vera gelly.

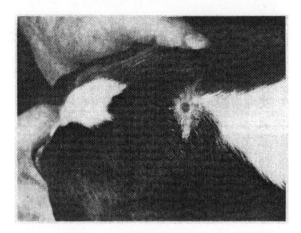

The same hot spot lesion 16 days later. Daily treatment with stabilized Aloe Vera gelly helped reduce the lesion to the size of a match head. and the condition was declared to be in a state of remission. Later, after three weeks, Dr. Holland was informed by the owner that the condition had healed and that normal hair growth was underway.

Wounds and bite wounds.

Of all the wounds dogs receive on a regular basis, bite wounds are by far the most prolific. As they are among the most companionable of all creatures and the most communal, they are also the most dangerous to their own kind and to humankind as well. In fact, second only to auto accidents, bite wounds from dogs are the second most prevalent form of injury to human beings. And bites, dog to dog, are the number one form of pet injury, period.

These statistics are not being quoted to defame "mans best friend." They're just the facts. Dogs' mouths are their primary means of negotiating their universe. They eat with them, health themselves with them, lick and show affection with them and groom themselves with them. Whereas the cat or bird of prey have claws, teeth, beaks and talons, dogs are headstrong (as it were) and so we must understand their need for self-expression. In fact, in terms of self-expression, it's really all they've got.

Other forms of wounds on dogs come of course in various ways. Car accidents, run-ins with feral creatures, and natural traps account for some of the wounds. Human cruelty accounts for the rest. And it must be noted with some degree of disdain for our own kind that the accountings of dog attacks against humans are closely approximated by the instances of human maltreatment of our canine companions. And though they may be reacting to protect themselves, what's our excuse after all?

We must at all times be aware of the redemptive currency of compassion with all the creatures with whom we interact, especially to the one breed of animal who bonds even more closely to us than it does to its own kind.

Invariably when these injuries occur, whatever their source, we would do well to be there with the best available modality for treatment and healing, one that is rapidly becoming the choice of leading veterinarians everywhere: stabilized Aloe Vera.

Once they have occurred, bite wounds particularly should be given the careful scrutiny by both the owner and the vet to whom the dog is taken. Since dogs tend to heal quickly, wounds that may appear to be minor are in fact much more severe and need to be examined thoroughly before appropriate action is taken. If the owner determines incorrectly (and he often does) that the wound has healed more quickly than it has complications can occur. Lick granuloma, advanced infection, cross-contamination and even gangrene can occur. So that's why it is advisable to examine the dog quickly after an accident or an attack. Even though the injury may appear superficial, if the behavior is altered—if the dog appears intemperate, is faltering or is running a fever—chances are the wound is more severe than imagined, and it is definitely time to get it to a vet. That vet, in turn, should take immediate steps.

Initially, a good veterinarian should determine the whereabouts and profile of the attacking dog to determine whether or not the animal was diseased or possibly even rabid. Second, he will give a tetanus injection to eliminate the possibility of further contamination.

All bites from any animal (including and especially the Naked Ape) can be highly infectious. So disinfectants should be promptly administered. If the wound is sufficiently severe and if stitching is necessary, Aloe Vera gelly as an application upon the stitches works very effectively both as a disinfectant and as an agent to accelerate healing, promote rapid cell division and to use under a wrap so that the animal's sensitivity to itching and burning will be minimized.

Many injuries and bite wounds involve torn skin where just the skin is torn. In these cases it is better to trim away the skin flap, which is already dead, and allow new blood to establish itself at the wound site. Skin flaps that are left untended will spread necrotic tissue even to healthy skin areas, creating a greater loss of tissue than is necessary.

Of course there are tears, and there are *tears*. Some are quite severe and require considerable surgical treatment and repair. The following set of photos have been extracted from our earlier work, *Creatures in Our Care*. In it, an injured male poodle had the skin torn completely off part of his left ear, while what remained of his earflap skin was badly bruised and suffering from diminished blood supply. This is typical of so many bite-and-tear wounds in that it is important to be able to determine what is dead tissue and what is not (a decision that should only be made by a qualified health professional). In this case it was necessary to surgically trim the skin and leave a wide gap of injured tissue exposed. The following two photos indicate the severity of the wound and the dramatic degree of recovery.

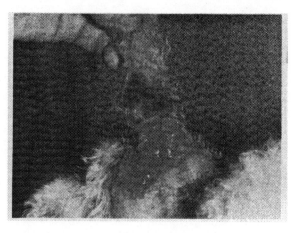

The wound to this poodle was the result of a fight between two dogs in the same household. The skin has been completely torn off the ear and much of the remaining skin is badly bruised. In this case the vet (Richard Holland) surgically trimmed the skin that had lost blood supply and cleansed the tissue with Aloe Vera gel (liquid). After cleaning the wound, he packed the wound with Aloe Vera gelly and followed with numerous applications of Aloe Vera gelly on a daily basis. In this case, Aloe Vera was the sole healing modality used.

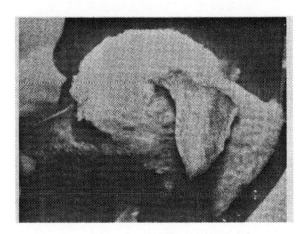

Five weeks later this severe bite wound was completely healed. No scarring was evident, and the skin had grown back over the wound. Hair growth was also normal.

Seemingly the list of topical traumas that dogs might suffer is endless. Such conditions as *ear infections, otitis externa, impetigo, mange, hernias, collie nose, proptosis (distended eyeball), contusions,* and *burns* are many of the conditions not entirely covered here, all of which are treated effectively by various combinations of Aloe Vera in all its presentations. What we have offered here is a sampler, with the understanding that for the true seeker of healing solutions, there are other sources that we also highly recommend.

Systemic infections.

We feel obligated to bring two issues into focus here. First is our awareness that many breeds of dogs have genetic propensities toward certain kinds of systemic illnesses. And we strongly advise that every owner of a pure breed study the needs of that breed and focus in particular upon the miasmic inclinations that creature possesses. Second, we cannot stress strongly enough the issue of diet. Because many dogs show appreciative if not voracious appetites, they are often fed some of the worst junk ever foisted upon any creature in close domestic proximity to civilization as we know it. That requires an understanding that dogs have certain nutritional needs just as people do. And it also prompts us to look into the realization that dogs are carnivores, and need at least 50% of their diets to consist of healthy meat products, at least part of which needs to be in fresh whole foods. Fresh food does not mean canned foods. Canned dog food possesses only trace amounts of live enzymes, is often made of the worst possible "dead" meat products, and might in certain circumstances be harmful to the dog. In feeding the dog live food, it is often good to go to table scraps, especially if those table scraps include healthy meat and dairy products that are fit for human consumption. (Some vets frown on the concept of table scraps for the very specific reason that dogs are very often given desserts and gassy foods that may be unhealthy for the dog. But be conscientious here. If the food involved is your fresh leftovers and they were nutritious for you, they would work well for your companion canine.) In lieu of these there are a number of very good, balanced, vet approved dry foods that would work well for your dog and help keep its teeth sharp. In all cases, it is important to recognize that any dog's individual needs will vary and that they are remarkable mirrors of our care for them. Healthy dogs with healthy coats and buoyant attitudes are visible to the naked senses and a testament to our good care.

There are, however, some occasions in which these creatures in our care may not be getting balance in certain areas. And these need to be looked into in terms of their systemic implications.

It is held as common in many holistic veterinary circles that a majority of ear infections can be systemic in origin and should be treated as such. This particularly applies to cases of *otitis* and *chronic otitis*. In such cases, a Northern California clinic specializing in holistic animal care, Animal Care Services, has come up with an exceptional remedy that accounts for the successful treatment of more than 200 cases of chronic otitis. The modalities used are simultaneous treatment of the ears, skin, and (when needed) the eyes, using an Aloe Vera gel and gelly in a conscientiously applied topical program. Additionally, the clinic recommends a strict change in diet from canned foods to all fresh foods, including a more complete complex of natural grains, vegetables and natural protein, and infusions of stabilized Aloe Vera gel into the drinking water.

Hyperactivity and *hyperkinetic behavior* are systemic conditions that can be specific to certain breeds. Nonetheless they can strike any dog, and when they do some specific treatments are essential. As is now found to be the case with human beings, much can be laid at the table of the junk food diet. With that in mind, Richard Pitcairn, D.V.M. (whose book, *Natural Health for Dogs and Cats,* should be a bible for small pet practitioners) recommends a change of diet from canned and commercial foods to all natural foods, including large measures of natural grains and vegetables, as well as a natural herbal remedy.

In his practice in treating these conditions, Dr. Richard Holland also followed Dr. Pitcairn's routine of diet and herbal remedies, including vervain, valerian, and chamomile to help repair the nervous system and act as calming agents. He also added his own remedy, which included one to three ounces daily of Aloe Vera juice or drinking gel to help calm hysterical behavior and improve the disposition of the dog. Although there is no specificity of data to clinically measure the success in this kind of treatment, Dr. Holland reported over 80 cases in which the overall health and dispositions of the dogs were markedly improved as a result of this kind of treatment regimen.

Canine parvo is a pathology in veterinary circles whose very name is enough to strike terror in any home with dogs in it. Like rabies or distemper, once its gains a hold, there is little that can be done to cure it. There are currently some good vaccines against canine parvo but, unlike rabies and distemper whose immunizations are 98% effective, parvo virus vaccines are only sporadically effective in preventing incidence of the disease and should not be administered to puppies under six weeks of age who are generally targets for the disease.

Since it is a phenomenon of the last couple of decades, theories vary concerning the origins of canine parvo. One of the most prevalent is that it sprang overnight out of a virally contaminated batch of canine distemper vaccinations. Although theories of spontaneous generations are always a bit suspect, there is always the clear and present danger of science gone awry, and it does seem more than a bit bizarre that the disease suddenly just "appeared" in this country a couple of decades ago.

Whatever the etiology (disease origin) of the affliction, it is particularly terrifying in that it tends to strike puppies or young dogs under 12 months old that have even less of a chance of fighting the disease off on their own. Similar in some of its symptomatic manifestations to feline distemper, canine parvo presents itself initially as an intestinal virus, then quickly assumes newer and even more drastic symptoms such as high fever, nausea, chronic diarrhea, intestinal hemorrhaging and severe dehydration. Once these manifestations seize the host body, particularly young puppies will succumb in short order unless something is done quickly. Frankly, that "something" is almost always too little too late. And yet there are several case history studies in which systemic infusions and injections with stabilized Aloe Vera in combination with other modalities did actually turn the condition around.

In one such instance, Dr. Alan Fredrickson was confronted with a litter of eight German shepherd puppies, all of which had canine parvo. Administering large doses of Aloe Vera gel through a rectal injection, along with regular oral doses, Dr. Fredrickson was able to save six of the eight puppies. In applying this treatment regime, he acknowledged that the Aloe, powerful healant though he thought it to be, needed adjunctive therapy in the form of special nutrient fluids and electrolyte solutions to help replenish the dehydrated pups. Dr. Fredrickson also acknowledged the fact that had he kept up the Aloe Vera regimen longer, he might have saved all eight of the puppies.

In its treatment lists, the Holland Veterinary Clinic listed more than 100 cases of canine parvo virus treated successfully, using modalities in which Aloe Vera was the treatment of choice. As had been the occasions of use among other practitioners, Dr. Holland used high enemas with a stabilized Aloe Vera gel in an equal half-half solution with catalyst water. He would then follow that treatment with oral doses of one ounce of Aloe Vera juice or drinking gel—every hour for large dogs, every two hours for smaller dogs—until the situation improved.

Fortunately, some new vaccines have now been introduced that appear to be more effective in the treatment of canine parvo. Nevertheless, in those instances in which the condition does manifest, there are good indications that it can be treated successfully—with stabilized Aloe Vera and compatible therapies.

Toxemia indicates a general poisoning of the body system either through the direct intake of toxins or contaminated tissue. This disease is also often found in goats (and omnivores such as bears) that have broad spectrum eating habits. In fact dogs, even more frequently than goats, get cases of toxemia probably because they are carnivores and because many more toxins can be found in contaminated meat than all other foods combined.

When these conditions do occur, they are usually presented to the veterinarian at a late hour on an emergency basis and when the dog is too far into the syndrome to be saved. In these cases, a number of emergency procedures may be tried. One put into practice by Dr. Richard Holland involved massive doses of Aloe Vera juice or gel taken to detoxify the system. In this case, the recommended dosage is one ounce an hour, every hour, taken orally for two days. This treatment regime was undertaken in nine cases of toxemia, and in all cases the dog survived, and its condition improved dramatically. In six other cases of treatment in which Dr. Holland did not use stabilized Aloe Vera, all the dogs that were treated did not survive either the disease or the treatment. To the best of Dr. Holland's judgment, all the animals in question were presented to his surgery with the same gravity of pathology and opportunity for recovery.

In our interactions with our canine companions, there exists the infinite opportunity for understanding that early care and treatment is the critical issue of caring for dogs. If this kind, loving, loyal species has one thing that favors its soul but punishes its body it is its capacity for enduring injury without complaint. There is a quiet kind of courage about dogs that leads them to accept their condition with a stoic sense of pride. So it becomes even more important for us to be aware of their needs, to tend them early and often, and above all else to treat them with the compassion and proactive care that their noble natures so richly deserve.

The This's and That's of Cats.

No creature on earth has ridden history's rollercoaster of popularity more perennially than cats. Alternately glorified and vilified, they have been perceived as everything from deities to minions of the devil. In ancient Egypt they were worshipped as a creature with godlike attributes. In the fear driven European societies of the middle ages they were held in dread, driven away, hunted down, and often tortured and killed. One thing that favors their longevity and survivability lies in the fact that they've never been considered edible, economically viable or trainable as work animals. As opposed to dogs who have placed their service priorities with humankind, there have never been any herd cats, sled cats, watch cats, police cats, or seeing-eye cats. They do, on the other hand, make unsurpassed rodent-catchers, are actually much better companions for infants and young children and are now viewed as being perhaps the best hospice companions for geriatrics in their final chapters.

As opposed to dogs, who view their bond with us as paramount to their utility as creature companions, cats have remained our nonchalant feral houseguests who allow themselves to be domesticated (but would never admit to it under oath). Dogs, we learn, view themselves as our servants and our children. Cats, we discover, look upon themselves as adults who share space with us. They consider themselves to be our pals, our equals and (in some cases) our superiors.

For the reason of creature dynamics, many experts believe that cats make better pets for families with small children. That's because cats look upon small children and infants as infants. Dogs, on the other hand, too often look upon them as littermates and therefore as possible competition, so there exists the constant pressure valve of territorial imperative. (This of course gives rise to debate until one views the statistics. Instances of dogs biting or attacking children number in legion. Except for the extremely rare mishap when a cat crawls up to cuddle with a newborn and accidentally smothers it, occasions of death by cat are virtually non-existent.)

Generally, cats are viewed as pretty low-maintenance pets. That is at least part of the reason for their popularity in our tightly compacted, career-driven society and no doubt a principal reason that cats have replaced dogs as America's favorite creature companions.

Whereas dogs bond to us, cats bond to territory. Their points of reference are more varied, and so they don't pine away quite as measurably when left alone for long periods of time. They're smarter about what they look upon as acceptable fare, will turn up their very sensitive noses at bad food (and some pretty good food in the bargain) and, as a rule, tend not to overeat. They spend a good deal of their time grooming themselves, so they don't need bathing in the traditional sense as dogs do. Neither do they need to be walked nor long to be taken on trips.

Because of some of these feline traits, there still persists the mythology of "the independent cat." Although they may respond to us on their own timetables, cats can be deeply loving, affectionate, loyal, and emotionally fragile where their measurements of our moods are concerned. So their ability to bond to us should not be underestimated any more than we should dismiss our obligations to them as members of our households. In truth, as any dedicated cat owner will tell you, cats also need their fair share of creature care. Cats, like dogs, need attention, affection, interactive time (play), proper diet, timely health care, and frequent thorough grooming. Despite their apparent sturdy constitutions, they also get fleas, parasites, skin infections, and respiratory infections as often as dogs. Because, they occasionally range about, they are also more likely to contract contagious diseases and so, even more than dogs, need to be vaccinated for a number of potential health hazards.

One issue that needs to be addressed because it affects so many aspects of the creature's health is diet. Contrary to the archaic and inaccurate image of the stock-and-trade alley cat rummaging around in garbage cans, cats, more than most creatures, need a healthy balanced diet, preferably one with at least some fresh foods, and certainly one that contains meat and dairy products that have innate liquid content. The common domestic cat is a direct descendant of desert hunters that lived on the flesh and blood of their prey; that is how they innately absorb most of their liquid nourishment. Cats are not by nature consumers of massive quantities of water. And very often one who is might have nascent symptoms of bladder, kidney or liver malfunctions—or possibly the early stages of diabetes.

Cats certainly have their own sets of wounds, bites, scratches and skin diseases, just as dogs do. And yet many pathologies that manifest themselves topically on the cat have origins in the cat's system. So, we're going to reverse our customary pattern of study and emphasize the systemic ailments that these creatures experience first, as well as the many ways that Aloe Vera can help heal them.

Cats are beset with perhaps as many systemic illnesses as any creature in the animal kingdom. Some of them, we observe, seem to be the direct result of their proximity to the high-tech, high-stress world of human beings, as well as their offerings of synthetic diets, processed foods and environmental toxins. Many of these diseases also come as the result of human misunderstandings of their true needs and nature, and the failure to recognize the differences between dogs, cats and our other creature companions.

As we mentioned, the domestic cat is a direct descendant of wild desert dwellers who had to hunt in order to survive. In every way that instinct resides with them still, and it is a trait they recognize in one another. So it's not at all unusual for wild cats to coexist rather peacefully with common house pets in the same urban neighborhoods; and conversely; many cats when deserted can and do end up surviving on their own…in the hunt, as it were. In fact and in practice, cats are our most feral pet friends, and for that reason are more finely tuned instruments of survival. Like finely tuned instruments, however, they tend to break down more easily under stress in manufactured environments; hence the dilemma.

One of the most common maladies to plague cats is a syndrome called *cystitis*. There is still no general agreement about the causes of cystitis, but one broadly held theory lays blame for its onset at the door of commercially processed dry cat food. Especially if fed as an exclusive diet, especially to tomcats, it seems to hasten the onset of this systemically insidious and often fatal syndrome.

Broadly defined, cystitis is an inflammation of the bladder, but like all broad definitions, this is an oversimplification. More often than not, cystitis is accompanied by dark red or brown and sometimes thick urine, painful or slow urination, and stones, all of which are brought on by the presence of a virus or bacteria. Once a malady believed more common in dogs, cystitis in cats has become a far more frequent occurrence and now carries with it more grave implications as a complete blockage of the urinary tract and uremia, a condition that may become deadly enough on its own to kill the cat outright.

If caught early enough, cystitis can be treated by catheterizing the cat, accompanied by doses of antibiotics, and the use of anti-inflammatory agents. Aloe Vera serves well in fulfilling both of the latter functions and may be used in conjunction with antibiotics or as an anti-bacterial agent on its own.

In his veterinary practice, Dr. Allan Fredrickson found that oral doses of Aloe Vera gel or juice at a level of 5cc three times a day (with a urine acidifier called Curecal) has worked very successfully to help clear out the effects of the disease. Dr. Richard Holland too used oral doses of Aloe in slightly different variations—one to two ounces twice a day until the symptoms cleared up. In both cases, one of the major offshoots of this Aloe Vera therapy was that it seemed to prevent a recurrence of the condition.

Preventing recurrence of or, better still, any occurrence of the syndrome seems now to be a matter of education. In fact, there is a growing contingent of veterinarians who believe that diet is one of the principal culprits and that, especially among tomcats, a large portion of the blame can be directed toward the intake of dry commercial cat food. As we just noted cats are direct descendants of desert hunters who are genetically encoded to still get most of their liquid intake from the blood and juices of animal flesh. Since dry commercial cat food contains no natural fluids and many are laced with preservatives, they can ultimately be hazardous to a cat's health especially if taken over long periods of time. In fact, other than an occasional nibble to keep their teeth sharp, cats should never be subjected to diets primarily comprised of dry cat foods. It has also long since been determined that red meat tuna such as that found in most commercial cat foods is exceptionally high in ash and magnesium. And these are two elements that, in too high a quantity, are hazardous to our feline friends.

As dogs need about 50% animal product in their diets, cats actually require considerably more—at least 70%, preferably in a fresh food formulation. It is true of both species, but particularly cats, that the older they get the more they should be able to enjoy fresh food diets, especially some organ meats. Cats that are often losing body mass and energy as they get older fare quite well when they receive slightly cooked livers, gizzards, hearts and other organ meats from beef and poultry. Cats, like dogs, should never be fed cured pork such as ham and bacon. (The salts, nitrates and nitrites injected in them to treat and preserve them prompt the feline to ignore their other food, have unnatural thirsts, and exhibit subtle but serious toxic reactions over the long term.)

Best bet: Feed them live foods and lots of fresh organ meats, some vegetables (no more than 30%), and go easy on the water. Cats, by nature, have trouble processing the stuff, and any cat that drinks a lot of water might also be providing you with a warning to cut back on the dry food in its diet. One dry-diet bugaboo lies in the fact that some cats start favoring that diet exclusively and will ignore their fresh food entirely. Not a danger over the short term, this can present long-term health challenges.

FRS, feline respiratory syndrome, is a commonly occurring disease suffered by cats under a lot of stress and by litters of kittens where the contagion quickly spreads from one kitten to the other. FRS can also be brought on in part by other stressful situations such as forcing the cat to travel over a long distance in a cooped-up environment, constant shipping from place to place, and frequent changes of environment.

Cats, like some wines, do not travel well. Their central nervous systems and sense of balance are constantly affected by irregular motions they cannot control.

That's the bad news. The good news is that the disease can be treated easily and successfully by long-term doses of antibiotics such as Ampicillin. Holistic vets find that it can also be treated effectively through homeopathic doses of phosphorus.††

---

†† Some holistic practitioners believe that at large number of feline systemic infections are brought on by what is referred to as a leukemia miasm. That is a homeopathic term for a disease base the inclines the feline to be susceptible to certain kinds of diseases. Just as the rabies miasm exists in a considerable percentage of dogs, the leukemia miasm might be found in a significant number of cats. These are the cats that do not like to be petted, are capable of unwarranted and often vicious mood swings, and tend to fight with

Feline Leukemia Virus. (FLV), FAIDS, and FIPS. All related syndromes and somewhat interactive, they in fact spell D-E-A-T-H for the cat in pretty short order if left untreated. Stabilized Aloe Vera gel works well both to treat symptoms such as eye irritations, runny noses and dry itching skin. Nasal infusions of an Aloe Vera gel also work quite effectively to help kill bacteria and eliminate infection in the nasal passages. In these cases, stabilized Aloe Vera liquid (or gel) is inserted into a small plastic syringe with a small curved canula and sprayed into the cat's nostril. Aloe Vera works as an excellent companion therapy to Ampicillin or other penicillin-based derivatives but, significantly, also possesses strong antibiotic properties when used as an exclusive form of treatment. In his treatment of FRS, Dr. Richard Holland also found that following treatment with supplements of Aloe Vera juice either orally or in the cat's diet not only help ameliorate the condition but also help prevent a recurrence of it. If the condition is truly serious, Dr. Holland found that regular daily injections of 2 to 5 cc of Aloe Vera gel intravenously into the cat was not only compatible with other remedies tried but also worked very well on its own to clear up the condition.

FLV is, with improved vaccination techniques, now acknowledged to be highly preventable, and it is certainly recommended that any cat old enough to receive vaccinations get both the booster and the follow-up shots as soon as is physically possible. In the past, there have been instances, before vaccinations were perfected, when some veterinarians actually preferred treating the virus itself. And there were many occasions when stabilized Aloe Vera in large oral and injected doses would do a remarkable job. The challenge with feline leukemia lies in the hydra-headed reality that, like AIDS in humans, there are so many concomitant diseases such as cancer and tumors that can drive the cat down, that it's simply not worth risking discovery, and often that discovery comes too late even for the silent healer to do the job.

What's more, this syndrome, like FIPS or *feline infectious peritonitis* is highly contagious and is often transmitted from male tom to male tom during fights over territory. Since no cat that ventures outside is immune to the occasional wayward claw or fang, the spread of this type of syndrome, if left unchecked, is inevitable.

---

other cats for no apparent reason. Homeopathic vets have determined that the symptomatic pathology that most clearly defines the leukemia miasm is gingivitis. Cats, especially those who contract gingivitis at an early age, are believed in 100% of the cases to be betraying early indications of a leukemia miasm.

On those occasions when there is absolutely no choice, however, we do note one very effective treatment used by Animal Care Services and Ihor Bosko, D.V.M. Addressing that syndrome, Dr. Bosko has treated numerous cases of feline leukemia, FIPS and related syndromes using a "health cocktail" that includes raw liver, stabilized Aloe Vera juice, carrot juice, corn oil, brewer's yeast, corn oil, and a series of special herbs and secret ingredients. Whatever the nature of the cocktail, Dr. Bosko has indicated that the remission rate has been in the range of 90% for what are often badly debilitated cases of the syndrome.

Perhaps the most dramatic and certainly the best documented work involving these rather sinister and challenging syndromes has to have been in the studies of doctors McAnalley and McDaniel in treating FLV and FAIDS stricken cats with the polymannose isolate of Aloe Vera, Acemannan. In dozens of test treatments of both feline leukemia and several cases of *rhino-tracheitis* in cats, the McAnalley/McDaniel research group found that the Acemannan brought the affected cats to dramatic stages of recovery in over 85% of the cases treated.

The "Nine Lives" Legacy? One of the qualities many of our veterinary associates do note, especially in dealing with systemic complications in the cat, is the creature's remarkable ability to recover from hard-to-treat systemic diseases. If given sight of even the smallest window of recovery, our feline friends seem to be able to shoot through it and find the way back to health. In some ways, they are more resilient than some of their cohabitants from the canine world, and yet it may also be true that they are often even more sensitive to their environments.

Very often, feline systemic ailments insidiously creep in from a condition known as "cooped-up cat." No, you won't see this syndrome officially recognized in any veterinary pharmacopoeia, and yet it exists. And just as it exists, it can be prevented by giving more attention, interactive time, and grooming to those tiny friends so ready to adapt themselves (against their nature) to our world.

The operative idea here is to provide them with every physical, emotional, and interactive window possible and to use healthy alternative therapies such as Aloe Vera as leverage to open it.

Crossover Conditions and Typical "Habit" Syndromes. Although the condition may not be as dramatic as some of the syndromes we have just mentioned, *hairballs* are certainly a more common occurrence. Cats, especially long-haired cats, with their rough tongues and their penchant for taking their grooming habits to fastidious extremes, often swallow large quantities of hair which in turn is bound to settle down into their digestive systems. If the cat is lucky, it will be able to absorb these hairs and pass them through its digestive system. If not—and this is often the case—cats can get hairballs that are up to six inches long and three inches in diameter. Traditionally petrolatum based treatments or such oils such as mineral oil have been used to help kitty flush the hairball. But in the last few years a newer player has entered the game that has proven to be even more effective both as a digestive aid and as a dissolving agent—stabilized Aloe Vera gelly. First of all, the gelly tastes pretty good. So cats don't mind taking it. Second, it's effective both as a lubricant and as a natural laxative. Third, certainly in view of the usually quick results it gets, it is cost effective and enjoys a purity of contingent usage that few other remedies can offer.

Skin Diseases, Topical Treatments and Wounds. *Ear Mites* are found more often in cats than dogs and tend to be evident in debilitated or neglected cats. They're microscopic in nature and cannot be easily detected by the naked eye; but they do leave clues. Dirty-looking ears filled with chunks of dark brown wax are good indicators that ear mites are probably setting up housekeeping. Cats innately like to have their ears rubbed. So, when you go to rub your feline friend's ears, if it winces or starts to pull away, that too is a good indication that ear mites are on the rampage.

They're also quite well traveled—that is to say contagious. So if one cat in your family gets them, there's a very good chance that your other cats and possibly your dogs will get them too. So swift proactive treatment is strongly recommended.

Fortunately, there are several good treatments around for mild cases of ear mites. One of them is a safe effective home remedy that includes the combination of 1/2 oz of olive oil and 400 IU of vitamin E squeezed from a gel cap into a dropper bottle. For more severe cases of ear mites, a small 1/2 oz doze of stabilized Aloe Vera liquid, followed by Aloe Vera gelly applied and massaged into the ear have proved to be an exceptionally effective combination. The Aloe liquid (or gel) applied gently with a cotton-tip swab acts as a very good flush and helps clean out irritated areas. Aloe Vera gelly massaged frequently into the ear heals irritations, stops itching, and helps prevent the recurrence of the ear mites later.

For a number of reasons *eye infections* seem to be very common to cats. Its eyes are the cat's primary sensory organs (Yes! They have terrific night vision and can see exceptionally well in dark places.) So, it is imperative that their eye health is kept in balance and that additional attention is given to them to prevent and treat the occurrence of *conjunctivitis.*

The conjunctiva comprises the soft pink inner lining around the eyeball. When it becomes inflamed and swollen for no particular reason it is very often an indication of conjunctivitis. These infections in cats can come from a number of sources. Including, particulate matter in the air, air-borne spores from plants and water, pollens and other creatures such as other cats and dogs. Indeed the condition is both contagious and cross-infectious. It is also controllable, especially if you use stabilized Aloe Vera. When faced with this condition, our old friend and co-author Richard Holland used Aloe Vera as his treatment of choice—one that helps to clear conjunctivitis and accompanying discomfort in about half the time of most preparations traditionally used to address the syndrome either as a primary or an adjunctive therapy.

Customarily antibiotics are used to treat conjunctivitis, but a significant percentage of cats don't respond well to antibiotics and form a systemic resistance to them. In such cases, Aloe Vera serves well as a companion therapy, especially when the vet may be as resistant to the Aloe as the cat is to the antibiotic. And salinated eye drops with Aloe Vera gel work well to treat *conjunctivitis* in the eyes so often concomitant with these conditions.

Abscesses are wounds that have become complicated by their environment of healing. Wounds require oxygen to heal properly, and abscesses are wounds that extend themselves due to a lack of appropriate exposure to healing atmosphere.

Abscesses tend to be a more common occurrence among cats for a few very good reasons: 1) cats tend to get in their fair share of fights (usually with a dog or with another male cat over a female); 2) Cats tend to heal more quickly than dogs or any other creatures for that matter. And since abscesses are wounds that seal over themselves and prevent the flow of oxygen to the affected area, they become impacted, swell up and form a seedbed for bloated infection, pussing, and further unsightly complications; and 3) Cats tend to go away and "lick their wounds," a ritual of self-healing that often creates complications of its own.

By definition, an abscess is any collection of pus surrounded by inflamed tissue. In most cases abscesses occur because the pus has become encapsulated in a wall of connective tissue. It is a natural reaction of the body and in that way is the most negative possible expression of the cat's uncanny facility for rapid healing. In cats, most abscesses form as a result of fighting, but it can also be a blood-borne infection that has apparent systemic origins.

In either case the ground rules for treating abscesses in cats are the same as in other creatures. If an abscess is hot to the touch, it is ready to burst open and should be lanced. (Note: this is a job for a veterinary professional, and should not be tried at home.) Gravity is an ally in this kind of undertaking, so it is important that the wound be lanced at a point low enough to permit appropriate drainage.

Once a wound has been hot packed with gloved hand and a sterile towel soaked in hot water, some vets have found it very helpful to flush out the wound with sterile, stabilized Aloe Vera liquid, using a syringe without a needle or canula. Dr. Richard Holland found that about 20cc of Aloe Vera gel were sufficient to clean out a wound, but also noted that in the case of a smaller wound with thicker pus, placing a pad of gauze soaked with Aloe liquid and leaving it there for about 24 hours is quite effective in helping turn the wound around. Afterward, packing the wound daily with Aloe Vera gelly has proven to reverse all effects of the abscess and to permanently prevent it from recurring.

One of the most unfortunate aspects of treating any creature comes when an owner tries to treat a dog or a cat with a medium to which that species is allergic. It is perhaps the curse of Genesis 5, that we believe what is good for us must therefore be good for our creature companions and decide to forego appropriate historical consideration. This is not merely the error of the lay amateur. It is also a common error committed by scientists in research environments when entire tests are conducted using dogs, cats, rats, or rabbits in a study when their innate susceptibilities are going to be entirely different. In these cases the layperson, though misinformed, may be forgiven. The scientific professional, on the other hand, should be held to a higher standard.

Equus.

It has to be observed, painfully if accurately, that horses have become the gallant ghosts of a world we've left behind. They are rapidly disappearing from our culture without a ripple, and we're scarcely aware of it. It's not that they're an endangered species; it's far more critical than that.

Where they were once the source of our power, the symbols of our opulence and the benchmarks of our military might, they are now merely elegant, noble, and expensive curiosities banished to the racetrack, the rodeo, the ever-diminishing traditional ranch, and the occasional Budweiser commercial.

It's hard to fathom the fact that little more than a century ago, they were the standards against which all our industrial progress was measured. (And do we not today still refer to all of our mobile machinery in terms of *horse power?*) So it is now, with a sense of reverence, a modicum of gratitude, and a fountain of fascination that we still engage our study of horses and their highly complex requirements.

In our studies of veterinary care for horses, we come to realize the essential tenet of creature care: *the larger the creature, the more expensive the care.* Horses underscore this perhaps more than any other "barnyard" animal. In truth, they're much more than that.

As horses can be beautiful and awe-inspiring to watch and ride, they can also be intricate pieces of machinery. While they have traditionally been our draft animals, our battle taxis, and our constant travel companions throughout the dark and perilous passages of history, they are also among the world's finest athletes.

No other animal with which we interact offers the ultimate paradox of both power and fragility. A horse is able to run for short distances at upwards of 50 miles per hour, and yet exerts 100,000 psi (pounds per square inch) on a lower leg bone that is only slighter thicker than the throat on a squash racquet. It is a sturdy animal often able to pull ten times its own weight. Yet it possesses a skin that is as thin as paper and tears open nearly as easily. It is a powerful runner capable of breaching wide distances, and yet it can only breathe through its nose—long, shrill cones of air that are shoved through a passage no thicker in diameter than your little finger.

For these reasons and many others, horses can present treatment challenges that are formidable, unique and costly. So we examine our treatment of them with a canny mixture of awe, caution and daring pragmatism. And since, horses challenge us with a powerful and mysterious perplexity of systemic challenges we will examine those first.

Pathologies of the Equine System. One of the most astute observers and practitioners of the equine condition has been Dr. Allan Fredrickson, a veterinarian from the state of Washington. Dr. Fredrickson is now retired from his active veterinary practice, but he has left a tradition in large and small animal treatment modalities that have formed a role model for others to follow. Dr. Fredrickson had been a veterinarian in mixed practice for a number of years, and later converted extensively to equine medicine during the later years of his practice. As such, he was acknowledged for his innovative uses of Aloe Vera in various modalities of treatment for horses.

Traditionally, one of the more frequently occurring conditions plaguing horses has been *swollen joints*. Although swollen joints are often the result of sprains or work-related strains, they can also come about due to systemic causes or be congenital in the horse's lineage. In all cases of application, Dr. Fredrickson used both topical and oral doses of stabilized commercially processed Aloe Vera compounds first in deep rubs with Aloe liniments (with eucalyptus) or as an alternative by applications of the plain lotion that were wrapped with Saran® wrap followed by Aloe-soaked cotton bandages. These were recommended to be changed daily, and were accompanied by large oral doses of Aloe Vera drinking gel. He found in many cases that the combination of the regular systemic intake of the gel along with the Aloe wrap worked best in treating this condition.†††

Founder or *laminitis* is a pathology common to many breeds of horse, and is quite often the result of too much of a good thing. Frequently a horse, especially

---

††† *Because of the extremely effective counter-irritant qualities in eucalyptus it is not recommended that Aloe liniment be used in a wrap. Otherwise blistering might occur.*

a young one imbued with a voracious appetite will partake of too much pasture grass, drink too much water when overheated, or most often will combine the two excesses and virtually founder, unable to maintain its powerful balance.††††Since founder is the result of toxic build-up in the system, Dr. Allan Fredrickson discovered that it was successfully treated in dozens of instances by flushing the horse's digestive system with massive oral doses of Aloe Vera juice. One of the side-benefits of Aloe is that it increases the appetite, and since appetite loss is often a manifestation of the advanced condition of laminitis, the Aloe Vera works in two ways: as a detox-flush and as a surprisingly effective appetite enhancer.

Horses are noted for being high-strung. And a broad rule of thumb applies in that the finer the breed of horse, the more often the mares are prone to be infertile; so infertility among thoroughbred mares is quite common. It is also not at all unusual for some fillies that arrive at maturity to be unable to come into foal. When this occurs, steps can and must be made to help them.

We call to memory the British Military chronicles of Sir James Watt in which he, while on campaign in India, referred to ancient Vedic texts and folk remedies in which Aloe was credited with helping with infertility in women. Although this is hardly clinical corroboration for use in horses, it does help reinforce our belief in the possibility of it.

In the case of Dr. Fredrickson's treatments for *infertility* in mares, the sole common denominator of change was the introduction of Aloe Vera in large doses as an intrauterine infusion with a saline solution. This infusion was administered once a day for five days, then once a week for twelve weeks. In a number of instances of treatment, mares—who were previously unable to foal—were now able to do so.

We also note with interest that Diamond K Animal Care of Sulphur Springs, Texas recommended the use of stabilized Aloe Vera injections, ranging from 60cc to 100cc per injection, to aid in the artificial insemination of mares, though no specific outcome for this kind of use was indicated.

We propose that serious breeders take careful note here, because it appears that the effectiveness of Aloe Vera has a sperm inducing agent is directly proportionate

††††Founder can also be the result of retained placenta in mares.

to the pH balance set for the gel. At pH levels of 6 and above, it is a profoundly effective sperm enhancer. At levels of 3.4 and below it has proved to be a strong spermicidal agent.

One of the most influential advocates of Aloe Vera for internal uses has been longtime race horse owner Larry Duffy. An owner of a stable of standardbred trotters out of Los Alamitos racetrack in Southern California, Duffy first experimented by using Aloe Vera in nebulizers for his horses. Due to the demands of racing, the stresses of travel, and constant changes of climate, race horses can and do experience more than their share of respiratory complications. Nebulizers are bridle-like hoods that fit over the horse's nose, and are the equine equivalent of oxygen masks for humans, except for the fact that warm medicated vapors are introduced while the horse is breathing. In the case of racehorses, it is used to prevent blockages and to ameliorate occasions of sore and bleeding throats.

Working with a number of veterinarians, including Dr. Ed Hill, one of the California Racing Commission vets, Duffy explained his positive experiences with the healing plant and was able to encourage these professionals to use Aloe Vera for such conditions as *blood in the urine, chronic diarrhea,* and *constipation.* In most instances of treatment, Dr. Hill was able to determine that four to eight ounces a day of Aloe Vera was an effective level of dosage to use until the condition was alleviated entirely.

Dr. Hill went on to use stabilized Aloe Vera compounds in gel, gelly, and lotion form to treat such conditions as uterine infections in mares, dozens of cases of throat infections in trotters (including several chronic cases), and even a few cases of *laryngitic hypoplasia* (a severe infection of the larynx usually accompanied by blisters). In every instance of use, "Doc" Hill found remarkable improvement and de facto cure, and continued to use Aloe Vera as a treatment modality until his passing early in 1995.

Another veterinarian among the Larry Duffy converts, Robert Baker, D.V.M. used Aloe Vera to treat a number of standard-bred and thoroughbred race horses for respiratory infections, including chronic coughs, including a syndrome in horses commonly known as *follicular pharyngitis,* an aggravation of the pharynx (or larynx) accompanied by a pronounced fever. A student of the Aloe applications of Dr. Allan Fredrickson, Robert Baker also found the Aloe Vera treatment to be exceptionally effective in the treating of this complex condition.

In his medical chronicles, however, Allan Fredrickson warns that, "Unfortunately, a good many people wait until the animal is too far gone and then suddenly want the vet to fix it." Nevertheless, Dr. Fredrickson noted that the Aloe Vera treatments did work to ameliorate follicular pharyngitis, even in advanced cases.

Throat infections such as the ones we have just mentioned, along with many similar in nature have become more prevalent in the last three decades. Some racetrack vets including Dr. Ed Hill believe that a significant number of throat infections are man-made. He equates them to the increase in A and B type flu vaccinations that were given to all racing thoroughbreds and standardbreds back in the mid 1960s. At the time, the flu viruses were so severe that horses would fall down coughing onto the tracks. So, many research laboratories came out with a number of vaccines that seemed to help the condition. The challenges with them resided in the fact that the side-effects from the vaccines were often worse than the viruses themselves, giving rise to such conditions as laryngitic hypoplasia, a condition that prompts blisters to form on the larynx of the horse, lesions that appear from no apparent cause.

Whether the cause is apparent or occurs de novo, Dr. Hill always found the condition to be treated with remarkable success by using stabilized Aloe Vera gel as a treatment modality, usually in a nebulizer or as some other form of inhalant.

Cuts, Contusions and Deep Wounds.

Except for the occasional riding stable "pet" horses are still animals that earn their keep, either as athletes (racers and jumpers) or as beasts of burden. If one is going to keep a horse, it is still most often as a work animal. That's why such injuries as *rope burns and wire cuts* are injuries that the working cow pony experiences frequently. If tended quickly, they present problems that are routine and easily remedied. The challenge, however, comes when they are noticed or tended too late. Whenever the cut occurs in the area of the fetlock it can be especially difficult to heal, because the horse's fetlock, situated just above the back of the hoof is the one place that is subjected to constant stretching and extension. In fact, there is so much movement that the horse is often confined to a smaller stall until it starts to heal. This is a situational aid but is neither the short-term nor the long-term answer.

In his extensive photo archives, our veterinary associate Dr. Richard Holland shared with us a classic case of a wire cut on a horse's fetlock that he treated with stabilized Aloe Vera. Using Aloe Vera gelly as the sole medium of treatment, he found that daily applications of the gelly brought the horse to a full level of healing within 2 1/2 weeks;` about a quarter of the time usually required to accomplish the same level of healing for this kind of injury:

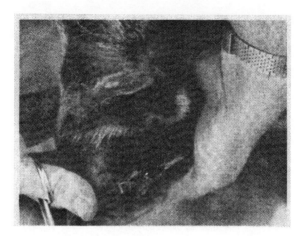

A wire cut on a horse's fetlock shortly after the injury occurred. In this case Aloe Vera gelly was applied to promote enzymatic debridement and rapid healing of the skin.

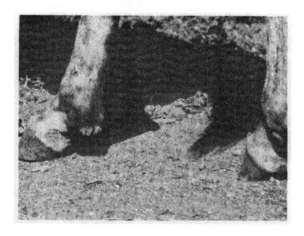

After just 2 1/2 weeks, the area has knit together nicely with no lameness. Ordinarily these cases are treated with antibiotic salves and take anywhere from 6 to 10 weeks to heal. In this case, Aloe Vera gelly was the sole modality used to heal the cut.

Deep Wounds on the body of a horse can be painful, disfiguring and even deadly. Given the horse's surprisingly thin skin, combined with its constant needs for movement, it presents constant challenges to the healing process, both in terms of restraint and methodology. Whereas wounds might be stitched on other creatures, they often tend to tear open on horses. The thin equine skin combined with thickness and swelling around the stitched area is a bad combination. Left unstitched, an area such as the horse's chest can heal rather nicely if the wound is properly cleaned and if serum fluids can be permitted to drain. Aloe Vera liquid is the ideal medium with which to clean a wound, and if the wound is of a sufficient severity, it generally fares quite well if it is packed with Aloe Vera gelly.

The russet mare in the following photos provides a striking before and after point of study of a deep gash wound brought to a remarkably quick heal just two weeks and four days after the original trauma took place. Although Richard Holland was brought in to tend the horse, his was the second treatment rendered. The first had been undertaken by another vet who had tried to use the traditional method of stitching the wound together with large stitches. Unfortunately, these actually tore into the wound, causing it to heal irregularly and appear even more ravaged than it was when the gash was initially sewn together.

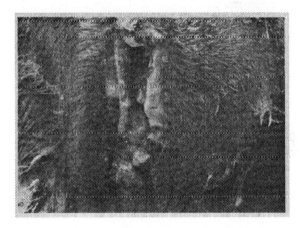

A russet mare with a deep gash in her chest. Four days after the accident, pronounced swelling around the wound has pulled half the stitches loose.

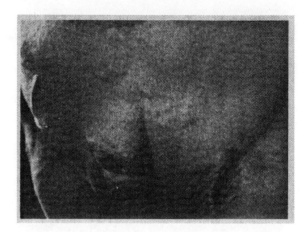

Although this actual photo was taken later, it is entirely depictive of the horse's chest two weeks after the incident of the injury. Even though the stitches tore open, daily applications of Aloe Vera left it healed without a trace of scarring.

Severe hematoma. Even the most superficially educated person knows that horses have very tender feet that need to be shod. For that reason, deep blood borne bruises to the sole of the foot are both commonplace and problematic. The following set of photos reveals the case of a horse that had gotten a sole bruise that had caused a severe hematoma under the sole, causing blood to accumulate underneath and create massive pressure. These cases are very much like abscesses in that the only way to release the pressure is to lance the foot and let the blood and pus run free. In this case, Dr. Holland cleaned the wound with Aloe Vera liquid and then packed it with Aloe Vera gelly, changing the bandage every day for the first two days. With the second change of Aloe Vera gelly dressing, he left the bandage on the wound for a week and then removed it. The wound on the hoof had assumed a pronounced healing within one week, and a complete healing within 10 days, a progressive healing to which the photos give ample evidence.

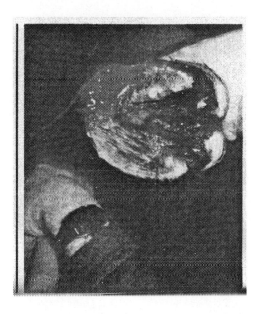

Severe hematoma of a horse's hoof. In this photo, the blood pocket forming under the sole caused the tissue to bleed easily, while the hoof itself remained swollen and spongy to the touch.

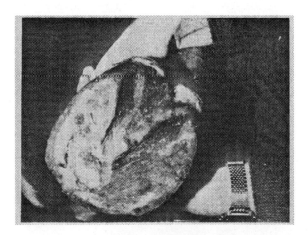

On the second day after applications with Aloe Vera liquid and subsequent packing with Aloe Vera gelly, the hemorrhaging has been controlled and the area surrounding the wound has cleared considerably.

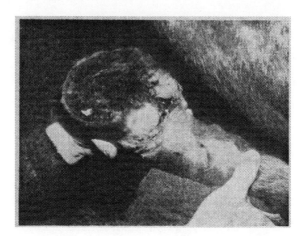

One week after the Aloe liquid and Aloe gelly combination, the hoof is normal in appearance and hardness. This is a remarkable rate of recovery.

What we have learned on these pages only creases the lining of what Aloe Vera has been able to accomplish in the world of equine veterinary treatment. Although many new vistas of holistic care and compatible therapies for horses have been developed, so many more remain to be discovered. The good news is that horse owners are, as a rule, governed by an overriding concern for their creature companions. Especially in the world of trotters, racers, runners and jumpers, horse owners are willing to undergo almost any expense to see to it that their charges are well cared for and given the most up-to-date treatment modality they can receive. This opens wide the gate for new opportunities and even more breakthroughs involving not only the silent healer but also a number of other therapies as well.

There is no doubt that the interaction on several levels between humankind and its equine companions will continue. And often treatments for one species seem to precede treatments for the other. Such remarkable treatments as magnetic blankets for horses are now looked upon as helpful in alleviating many minor injuries and cooling problems that many racehorses experience after a run. Such rehabilitation therapies as water treadmills, first used for horses, are now being used to rehabilitate world-class track athletes and some professional football running backs. One of the key pro-factors for the HRT (Hormone Replacement Therapy) used for women in the 50 plus age group comes from the high estrogen levels found in the urine of pregnant mares.

Granted, some of these treatments are perennial subjects for debate. But progress, however carefully measured, is forever a lightning rod for controversy.

Clearly, such fields of exploration are those of creature care and human care where everyone is willing to be ahead of the curve. And with that kind of approach to healing, we are all the better for it.

Cattle Call.

Although we acknowledge gratefully that all God's creatures were formed and molded by Higher hands, there is no question that where cows are concerned, man had a very strong role in the design.

In truth, cows are viewed as little more than food factories. Even to the most compassionate farmer and rancher, they are a commodity—raw material. For that reason, emotional attachments are seldom if ever an issue, and economic considerations usually come to mean everything. As opposed to dog and cat owners who may spend thousands of dollars to save the lives of their creature companions, cows and steers enjoy no such intimate relationship. As such, they are not members of the family; they are both resource and overhead.

In direct opposition to the horse owner and trainer who may be responsible for a magnificent thoroughbred worth perhaps millions of dollars, the rancher and farmer measures his cattle, sheep, goats or pigs according to whether or not it would be cost effective to save them or give them up for slaughter.

The term "slaughter" is a terribly harsh word. And yet all livestock, even the most pampered registered prize bull, eventually spends its final days camped next to a slaughterhouse. This is not brought up to seem either dispassionate or inconsiderate. It is simply a fact of life that often intentionally goes ignored.

The issue is not whether we cultivate, house, breed, shear, milk and slaughter animals for our purposes, but the energy with which we do it.

Because the business of ranching and farming is based in terms of profit and loss, there has been the universal tendency in the last several decades to press into service all the cost-effective techniques of factory farming. The arguments that always favor the factory farm are those jeremiads you often hear about razor-thin profit margins and the high-cost of doing business. The iron law of economic necessity comes into force, driving the small to medium-sized farmer either into cooperatives or out of business.

Meanwhile, the highly automated, supremely mechanized and deeply impersonal machine of commerce sweeps more and more agri-businesses into the hands of a few large corporations. Somewhere along the way, we lose the human touch, and there are many who believe that this is acceptable, because it keeps our T-bone steaks, mashed potatoes and creamed gravy on the table at a price that, relative to the high cost of living, is still under control.

So, who are we to question the relentless churn of progress, and why should we even think to do so?

We summon you to something called the Law of Manifestation that says "For every action in the universe, there is an equal and opposite reaction."

So, we have cheap chicken and low-cost bacon and some of the worst out-breaks of *E-coli, Salmonella, toxoplasmosis* and *BSE* (bovine spongiform encepha-lapothy) more commonly known as "mad cow disease."

We bring up the last of these because of the flare-up in the year 2001 of this potential pandemic—one that brought the United Kingdom into a near panic, one that spread to the continent of Europe, one that caused tens of thousands of head of cattle to be put down, and one that seemed to interlock almost inevitably to an outbreak of hoof-and-mouth disease that devastated the European beef and dairy industries for nearly two years, beginning early in the year 2000, and put our own North American relative departments of agriculture on full alert.

Even though it was little more than a high interest newsflash for a few days in the United States, it presented a genuine health and food chain nightmare in the EEU, aggravated by the causal subtext of this ruinous chain of events.

As so often occurs in the perilous cycle of food-chain factory farming, process-ing and distribution, it was the expediency of feeding and housing techniques that lay root of the problem.

A series of investigations by British health authorities revealed that the pri-mary cause was "cannibalism." According to investigations provided to the over-sight panels and (almost simultaneously) to the press, dairy and beef cattle growers had been buying cheaply processed, "high-protein" feed from a set of suppliers who had in turn been purchasing dead carcasses of euthanized dogs, cats, various road-kills, cattle that died either of disease or injury, and sheep that had died of a disease known as *scrapie*. Ultimately these euthanized, road-killed, diseased and dead animals were ground up into low-cost high protein bone meal and sold to feed lots all over Europe. Upon closer examination, it was determined that this deadly recipe could ultimately have created no other outcome than the health crises it stirred. And if anyone cares to raise any debate about the source of this, they need look no further than a cheap feed contract by an institutional meat supplier bent on using any means necessary to squeeze food quality on one end in order to reap bottom line profits on the other.

To be sure, appropriate fines, bans, and criminal prosecutions ensued, but not before the real damage had been done. And even though only a handful of people died from the "mad-cow" virus, possibly thousands were made ill from the human form (CSD), and tens of thousands of animals had to be destroyed, including a herd of 1700 elk.

What we fail to realize about the world we now live in is that so many of the fish we eat (including salmon, trout, catfish and some bass) are commercially farmed. So are a number of "game" birds and wild antlered animals such as elk. We bring this up because, the elk who had to be put down were ranch elk fed the same marginal high-protein bone meal that was purveyed to cattle.

The terrifying aspect of this is the marginally indifferent response rendered by a public that has become inured to food-chain scandals of this sort, if for no other reason than the fact that they've come to expect them.

Unfortunately, it may take a major crisis on a global scale to get anyone's attention for any period longer than a weekend tabloid read. And yet we are certain it will come to that unless the beef and dairy industry, the poultry industry, the pork industry and every other industry involved in the slaughter and processing of animal life are willing to amend their approach to the factory farm and institute more humane, more sanitary, and more conscientious applications of their trade.

Even as we sound like prophets of doom, we also acknowledge the many beef herders and dairies in America who maintain the highest possible standards for their herding, housing, growing, and marketing beef and dairy cattle. Such companies as Cactus Feeders, Inc. of Texas and Alta Dena Dairies of Southern California maintain the highest standards, which include banishing all feeds containing subtherapeutic levels of antibiotics and permitting their cattle to lead normal bovine lives with plenty of fresh air, exercise and normal bovine lifestyle experiences. It perhaps sounds patronizing, if not condescending, to make these observations, and yet we find there are Americans in legion who still believe that all cows, especially dairy cows, lead normal diurnal lives filled with pasture grazing and clover, when nothing could be farther from the truth. Many dairy cattle never see the light of the sun, spend most of adult lives either breeding or hooked up to a milking machine, and only live to be a few years old. Whereas the normal life expectancy of a dairy cow could be as much as 25 or 30 years, most factory-farmed milk-cows only live to be five or six.

We're not here to moralize about the pros and cons of factory farming except to note that, even on the most efficiently run factory farms, actual milk production is a long-term challenge. It has already been proven that crop rotation farms with natural plant additives enjoys better crop yields with one seventh of the plowings over a long term than fields that are exposed to commercial fertilizers and pesticides. This illustrates the dramatic erosion that takes place in commercially "driven" crop yields. The same approximate rule of thumb applies to cattle that are organically fed and allowed natural grazing habitats as opposed to those who are forced into the unnatural warehoused environments that prevail in most factory farms.

(Forget the histrionics of the "mad-cow" and hoof-and-mouth pandemonium, although they are highly symptomatic of agricultural dynamic victimized by its own expedient economics, the real drama in the food industry lies in the day-to-day diminished yield of relentless commercial processing, industrial crop cycles, and "strip-mine" farming.)

Anyone who has ever partaken of organic or naturally grown dairy products can tell you that the difference is astounding. There simply is no comparison in the quality, taste and richness of milk, cheese, yogurt, butter or beef that comes from a stress-free naturally fed and housed animal. In addition, the difference in measurable nutrient value in dairy products grown "organically" comes in the form of reports that often boggle the mind to contemplate.

We preach this sermon, because with cows, as with no other creature in our care, there is a direct line in the food chain that goes, uninterrupted, to us. So, we have to be conscientious in our treatment of these animals for reasons that are both humane and selfish.

Not surprisingly, it has been our finding through working with Dr. Richard Holland, Dr. Bob Corbett, Dr. Allan Fredrickson and a number of other highly regarded veterinarians that there are unlimited uses for stabilized Aloe Vera in the beef and dairy industry. Its uses begin at feedlot levels, flourish during the calf and milk cycles, and continue through the life of the cow (or steer).

We have begun by stressing the internal uses of Aloe Vera on cattle, because we believe that is at the crux of what needs most to be addressed in the process of food chain standards and practices.

Since demand drives the market, the need to provide large quantities of viable foodstuffs at a reasonable prices is more than undeniable; it is a matter of survival to the farmer and grower. Livestock need to be fed quantities of food that help them gain weight, maintain healthy weight gain, increase their normal nutrient value and be more resistant to disease, not allowing themselves to become pathogenic growth media.

This opens a door of opportunity through which crawl the marginal player and the unscrupulous processor who sell what they know to be damaged goods to farmers, ranchers and herdsmen, when a food additive like stabilized Aloe Vera offers a viable healthy alternative.

The Perfect Dietary Supplement. The Ideal Systemic Immunizer.

In a significant number of instances with both beef growers and dairy farmers, the introduction of Aloe Vera accomplishes a number of things.

One of the advantages of Aloe Vera over other medications and therapies is that when administered orally, it often acts as an appetite stimulant rather than an appetite suppressant. This bodes well for industries such as ranching where weight gain and healthy stock are not only important but essential to the economic survival of the rancher.

In fact, in one study it was shown that by adding Aloe Vera drinking gel to the drinking water of just fifty dairy cows, one Texas dairyman was able to increase their milk production by as much as three pounds per day. That amounted to an average increase in net income of over $10,000 in one year from fifty cows. Other dairy farmers using the same approximate portions of Aloe Vera experienced similar results, so much so that Aloe Vera has, for years, been the dietary supplement of choice for conscientious Texas dairymen.

This begins an entirely new chapter in the use of Aloe Vera and its potential impact on an industry that brings more than $55 billion in annual revenues directly to the global food chain and untold impact on the general network of usage of animal raw materials.

Still, the very act of being involved in the food production business as it regards "the beasts of the field" tends to rob one of idealism. One thing of which we must be constantly mindful is the fact that, even in the most ideal circumstances, cattle are looked upon purely in terms of utility.

They must be useful in one form or another. So their ability to resist disease and infection is paramount to their very survival. And their survival against numerous diseases and cross-infections often come with the territory. If cattle are food factories, their sheer proximity to waste and cramped conditions causes them to be potential disease factories as well. For that reason, they are the perennial victims of systemic infections that are the direct result of environmental influences.

In his chronicles of holistic animal care, Dr. Richard Holland, was as much a specialist in bovine maladies as any vet in general practice could be. For that reason, some of his treatments of cows and cattle read like an educational primer in the use of Aloe Vera for bovine diseases.

In covering Dr. Holland's work and those of others, we will, again, focus upon internal uses and diseases with internal origins that offer possible topical manifestations.

Abscesses are common afflictions in cattle that may occur for a number of reasons; some of them such as the accumulation of toxins are often systemic. And when they do, the manifestations can be quite dramatic, and some abscesses such as one that Dr. Holland literally uncapped can release much as four gallons of fluid. In all instances of abscess puncture, incision, and cleansing, Richard Holland found that at last 4 ounces of Aloe vera jelly packed into the abscess cavity would bring about rapid healing with virtually no recurrence of infection.

Second only to its role in food production, a cow exists to be a breeder of off-spring.

Particularly in the instance of dairy cows, the heat cycle (in other words, the cycle of mating, reproduction, and resultant lactation) is what keeps the cow a worthwhile investment and the dairy farmer in business. When that cycle is inter-rupted or stopped, cows get to be very expensive pets, and economic conse-quences can get to be disastrous, especially when they experience a condition known as *metritis*.

In fact, metritis occurs so commonly in cattle that all bovine uterine infections are often (erroneously) referred to by that term. Although uterine infections take a number of forms, metritis is most frequently shown to be an inflammation of the uterus accompanied by pus trapped in the uterine cavity. It's almost always a painful infection with nasty complications, the most pronounced of which can lead to the cow's loss of participation in the heat cycle. To complicate the issue further, prior to the introduction of Aloe Vera, there had traditionally been very few ways that are considered reliable treatments for metritis and other uterine infections.

In his veterinary practice, Dr. Holland was able to successfully treat hundreds of cases of metritis, dozens of cases of *prolapsed uteruses* and *everted uteruses* (which occur during calving), and bruised or torn uterine cavities. In most cases he infused infections with 60cc to 100cc of Aloe vera gel and packed the cavity with Aloe Vera gelly to heal the wounded area and prevent the further spread of infection.

Cattle, especially beef cattle, experience their fair share of respiratory compli-cations, though perhaps to a lesser degree than in horses. These usually creep-in during the cold weather winter months, especially affecting herds that may be left out of doors for much of the time. When this occurs, deep coughing, sore throats, and copious nasal discharges may result (just as those that occur with human beings). When such profound respiratory complications do occur, Dr. Holland recommended direct infusions of Aloe vera gel into the windpipe (20 cc for calves and smaller cattle, 30cc to 60cc for full adults). In these instances, the enzymatic activity in the Aloe Vera works to break up phlegm and other block-ages and help control the infection. And vets who have employed this method have enjoyed a remarkable rate of success.

Due to stress, inactivity, and questionable feedlot environments, many cows get diarrhea, a common bovine malady also often referred to as *scours*. Although it is a problem with adult cattle, the situation is seldom fatal. In very young calves, however, it takes on more sinister implications, and can turn into a life and death struggle in a few days time. Usually this takes place because dairy farms, hungry for profit and high milk output, will either take calves off colostrum milk provided by their mothers after just one day or not let them nurse at all. Since colostrum milk that the mother gives, especially in the first days after birthing, contains most of the fortification calves need to build up their immune systems, calves really need three to five days of nursing but, due to the demands of mass market milk production, are often denied even that brief time. So, they lose their ability to fight off disease, and scours result.

In a dozen cases of calf scours treated by Dr. Allan Fredrickson and in over 50 cases of calf scours treated by the Holland Veterinary Clinic, both doctors found that Aloe vera gel or juice administered orally two times a day helped flush the bowel of accumulated toxins, helps combat stress, and helps replace liquid nutrients and electrolytes often missing from the system. Dr. Fredrickson found his treatments were more effective when augmented with 10cc of Aloe Vera juice or gel injected into the muscle for at least three days.

In most cases of the scours treated, both veterinarians found that scours were greatly relieved and recovery was a fact.

Even more sinister than scours are incidences in baby calves of a disease called *coccidiosis*. Common in calves of one to two months of age, it seems to be a more common manifestation of animals confined to small pens. Symptoms of this dread disease are pronounced diarrhea and watery discharges with bloody fluids or clots of blood. The calf becomes depressed, loses its appetite and often dies of the effects. In treating calves for this condition, Diamond K Animal Clinic of Sulphur Springs, Texas found that by adding 2 ounces of Aloe Vera liquid in twice daily doses for about two weeks, the coccidiosis could be turned around and incidences of its reoccurrence could be lessened dramatically. Since it is now often understood that good nutrition, especially the addition of amino acids to the diet, can improve mood and stimulate appetites, Aloe Vera seems to fulfill a dual role with cattle, swine and most livestock in that they add viable nutritional and immunological balance.

Calves, particularly those who are being shipped over long distances, are prone to both weight loss and infections (including diarrhea) seemingly in series. In his veterinary chronicles, Dr. Richard Holland found that calves given Aloe Vera would need only half the antibiotics previously administered and would also show improved weight gain over the same period of time over those calves given antibiotics to the exclusion of Aloe. In fact, it has been anticipated especially in veterinary circles that Aloe vera may soon be the indicative antibody of choice by many veterinary practitioners. It is already enjoying widespread approval for that use, and may soon become a prevalent treatment. Certainly, as we have often illustrated by now, Aloe will not antidote standard antibiotics and, for that reason, serves as the ideal complementary therapy.

Much of what we have discussed thus far has to do with the heat-cycle, milk-cycle and often involves an "overuse' syndrome common to commercial farming practices. Nothing illustrates this challenge more profoundly than a condition of infected teats in cattle known as *mastitis.*

Teat injuries in general are the most common diseases to which dairy cows in particular are susceptible. Many of them such as frostbite and teat fistula are often caused by environmental factors. Others such as mastitis claim diverse causes. And yet it should be noted here that, although mastitis in particular has plagued dairy cows for centuries—and even though it is said to stem from at least 114 known sources—its occurrence since the invention of the commercial milking machine in the 1940s has skyrocketed. So overuse in this case is clearly a smoking gun.

Mastitis is classically defined as *an inflammation of the mammary glands brought about by various strains of bacteria and Candida (yeast), all of which can pollute the cow's milk.* The milk may be lumpy, curd-like and slightly off color, or else very watery. Even worse, there may be no change in physical appearance at all, which may bring about effects that are both deceiving and ultimately infectious. Milk batches are only spot-checked by the USDA. So, common sense and modern ethics dictate that proper self-testing is essential to the survival of any dairy.

When mastitis does occur, its impact can be both devastating and pervasive. In the first place, it is cross-contagious. Since milk machines often feed in chains to a central processor, cows infected with mastitis need to be gotten off the milk chain immediately and isolated for diagnosis and treatment. Most modern dairies have one of many excellent diagnostic kits that determine the degree of infection as well as the level of pus in the milk, and an estimate of how long the cow will be out of production. The most familiar and traditionally accepted is the California Mastitis Test, more popularly known as the CMT.

Traditionally, the treatment of choice for mastitis has been a mixture of broad-spectrum antibiotics, mainly as a quick fix means of reducing the spread of infection. But, even with immediate diagnosis and effective treatment, the cow will have to be left out of the milk cycle for a minimum of two to three weeks. Since at least half that time is required to clear the antibiotic from her system before she can be allowed to continue milk production, this disease and its concomitant treatment can prove very expensive. As of the year 2000, it was estimated that mastitis and related conditions cost the world dairy industry nearly $5 billion a year in lost milk production, primarily because of the extended lapsed time required to get cattle back into the milk cycle.

There are three types of mastitis: *basic mastitis, acute mastitis and gangrenous mastitis.* Acute and gangrenous mastitis are both notable by the hardness of the wound and the degree of density and distention of the teat itself, and either can develop into dangerous and life-threatening syndromes if left untreated, Obviously these latter two stages are less frequent and more severe, and yet any of them can develop into chronic mastitis. And chronic mastitis, if left unremedied, can eventually end the useful life of the cow, and therefore life itself.

Aloe's introduction to the treatment process for mastitis began back in the early 1980s and yet has only recently begun to achieve the attention its positive impact has merited.

A number of vets with whom we have been in contact over the years have used Aloe Vera to treat various types of mastitis, and have done so with surprisingly positive results. Virtually hundreds of cases of mastitis that we know of have been treated successfully with Aloe Vera. The physician's reports have been provided to us and are available upon request.

There are many ways of effectively treating mastitis, and though they may vary slightly from vet to vet, a graphic example of mastitis progressive treatment and cure is included in the following set of photographs:

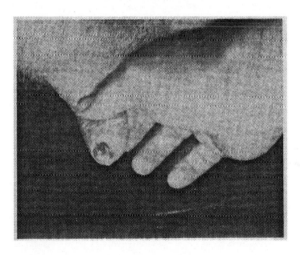

Mastitis may originate from a number of sources—from teat injuries to poor milking practices. When it does, such manifestations as appear in this photo are typical of the infection that occurs.

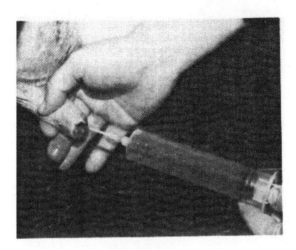

Injections of Aloe Vera gel, or gelly (average dosage 30cc) into each affected quarter is left there for 24 hours, later stripped empty and, in severe cases, repeated.

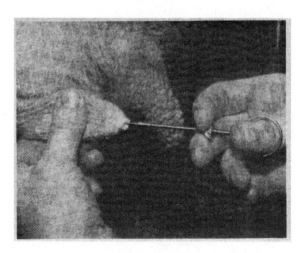

Later, widening of the teat through infusions of Aloe Vera gel or gelly helps to prevent recurrences of the mastitis.

There is a crucial footnote to all of this in the fact that Aloe Vera, when used in place of antibiotics does two things exceedingly well. First, where antibiotics often present challenges in therapeutic compatibility, Aloe doesn't antidote alternative forms of treatment. Second, Aloe Vera dramatically shortens the time required for the cow's recovery and return to the milk cycle. Not only has it proved nearly twice as fast in healing mastitis, it also contains no residual toxicity that would cause it to cling to the physical system. Because broad-spectrum antibiotics leave a presence that often lingers in the cow's milk, dairy cows stricken with mastitis are not allowed to return to that cycle for as much as three weeks, and often longer. With Aloe Vera, most mastitis sufferers are able to be back within a week of discovery and treatment. If properly studied and corroborated, this could amount to billions of dollars in savings to the dairy industry worldwide.

Everything Else.

For a number of reasons, we have focused almost exclusively on Aloe Vera's positive impact on the systemic challenges that face the beef and dairy industry. In truth, Aloe Vera is so universally effective in the treatment of cattle in particular and barnyard animals in general that we have barely creased the immense terrain of its therapeutic potential in other areas. In fact, the following is a brief list of successful treatments by an entire college of forward thinking vets, many of whom have left us with proof positive reports in these areas. We list some of them here: *abscesses, broken jaws, clouded corneas, keratitis, dehorning, embryotomies, everted uteruses, foot rot, prolapsed uteruses, retained placenta, teat fistula, udder swelling (edema), vaginal infections and warts.*

This laundry list of treatments for cutaneous and topical pathologies is incomplete, and yet it underscores just how much Aloe has to offer to the practitioners of bovine medicine, and to all God's barnyard creatures.

It is nevertheless our conviction that it is at the core of compassionate animal care that we should address the thrust of our concentration, especially in the case of livestock. If pigs, goats, sheep and especially cattle can be treated more humanely, be allowed to function in what amounts to a normal "fresh air and free movement" lifestyle, and be fed proper nutrients at the beginning, middle and end of their productive life-cycle, the net return to the farmer in purely economic terms will almost invariably be positive. This requires little more than an "organic" mentality and the willingness to spend a bit more on the care and feeding of our barnyard friends in the beginning. From that, the end result is one that has far-reaching horizons and broad-spectrum implications, ones that will create a more productive and economically sound environment for everyone. For that, health—human and animal—has to become a part of the bottom line.

Certainly Aloe Vera can and should play a significant role in this healthy mix. In fact, in cases where it has been a part of routine, daily use in both beef and dairy industries effective production soars, and loss and downtime from injury and disease are invariably minimized.

Summary

If this chapter on Aloe Vera in use on this "Animal Planet" could have one apt description, it would have to be its emphasis on versatility. No other field underscores its applicability in every imaginable area of use quite as well as this. If for no other reason than its lack of toxicity, it should be termed a staple in every household in the civilized world. It has proven to be nearly infallible in human application. Now, we know "the rest of the story." There is simply no point of reference in which Aloe Vera does not begin to appear as the standard against which all other means of treatment will be judged.

That has so often proved to be the case in the past. And, as we fully ride the crest of this new millennium, it is proving to be the case yet again in the future.

Chapter 10

Aloe's Perfect World

If we were now to paint a portrait of the perfect world of this New Millennium, we would place a great deal of new technology in it. And yet we would also enter it with the understanding that we are not only able to hold onto what is the best of the past, but also to make even more effective use of it. Thus we look upon Aloe Vera's role in the coming decades as an integral part of any triage in the future of medicine and, more importantly, as the perennial helpmate for any preventive wellness lifestyle.

Amid the broad strokes of history new eras are measured distinctly, and somewhat ruthlessly, in terms of progress. And yet as a part of that measurement, we have learned to understand that technology, no matter how advanced, has never been designed to entirely replace what Nature brings to heal us, feed us and otherwise complete our lives. At best, it can enhance it. At worst, it can impede and retard so much of what has been done that we must always be on guard to evaluate it, examine it and, if necessary, check it.

So, let it be with Aloe Vera. We have, in all our research and development of Aloe products, intended to accomplish one thing: to increase the awareness and credible use of Aloe Vera, not only as a viable form of therapy but also as a means of wellness lifestyle enhancement.

We feel that, in this document at least, we have substantiated claims that Aloe Vera can be used reactively as a treatment for scores of pathologies from systemic cancer to AIDS and from athletic injuries to major cosmetic surgery. In many instances, if not a majority, we feel we have also offered profound evidence of its emergence as a "treatment of choice" for a number of pathologies. Especially when confronted by maladies such as autoimmune diseases, that are both difficult to diagnose and to treat, this silent healer has often been sought as the last best hope for cure when in truth many health practitioners would be well served to consider it the element of first resort.

What we find even today is that, although more physicians and osteopaths are familiar with the healing potentials of Aloe Vera, they remain reluctant to put it into practice because there is no manual of common usage that offers guidelines for dosage, combinability and frequency of use.

In our previous works, we have particularized professional usage patterns for Aloe Vera in the fields of athletics, veterinary medicine, general medical usage, and several aspects of cosmetology. And yet we find that we face the same obstacles in each of them: They are read for content and not used as guidelines for application. It was never our intention to use this book as a vehicle for demarcations of usage, and yet one needs to be done.*

What we feel we can emphasize on these pages are the proven quantities about Aloe.

1). It has no established toxicity. So it can be used with impunity and in massive quantities.

2). It is often a case of providing optimum saturation. Oftentimes, the higher and more frequent the dosages, the better.

3). Properly formulated Aloe Vera has no record of antidoting any other known accepted medication. It has proven itself time and again to be the ideal compatible therapy.

4). It offers interspecific benefits. So, it can be used with equal beneficial effect on human beings, their animal companions, every barnyard habitué and all the creatures of the forest.

5). It offers special advantages, with pharmaceutical grade skin care, for the fields of aesthetics and cosmetology.

6). It might well be finding its most eloquent form of expression in the fields of prevention and preventive medicine. In fact, Aloe Vera, taken internally as a part of one's daily regimen, is proving to be the consummate agent of synergy both as a supplement and as a carrying agent for enhancing immune system functions.

---

* In fact, the next work we proposed will be a complete manual for usage of stabilized Aloe Vera in all aspects of professional and personal application.

We offer a set of new findings that illustrate these potentials. To be sure, we recognize that they are not yet fully documented, and therefore deemed inconclusive. And yet for us they are signposts to the future, ones that point the way to a more enhanced quality of life for everyone who chooses to participate in the pathway to total Aloe awareness.

We have already noted the aspirin studies conducted by Dr. Robert Davis that showed how Aloe Vera was able to synergize the pain-killing effects of certain analgesics dramatically by skipping the blood-bond barrier in the stomach and getting straightaway into the blood stream. In the Vinson, Al Kharat studies, we also noted the profound role Aloe exhibited as a carrying agent for Vitamins C and E as well as vitamins in general.

In a recent ongoing calf control group study in 2002 conducted by our friend and associate, Dr. Bob Corbett, a series of 150 dairy calves one to four days after birth were alternately tested for their immune system responses to the addition of Aloe Vera drinking gel in their diet. Since it is commonly acknowledged that 80% of a calf's immune system is built up in the first 96 hours after birth (mostly through the intake of colostrum milk from the mother), this period is of supreme importance in determining the health of the calf later in its development. In Dr. Corbett's study, every other calf (the Aloe test group) is, on the first day of its new life, given eight ounces of Aloe Vera as well as the mother's milk. Meanwhile the control group (every other calf from the same period of birth) is fed exclusively from its mother's colostrum milk. Although the test is not complete and therefore may not be deemed conclusive, the results thus far have led us to some profound conclusions.

In Dr. Corbett's test, all the calves fed the regular daily doses of Aloe Vera as an adjunct to the diet of colostrum milk have shown a number of advantages over the non-Aloe control group. First, they exhibited profoundly improved weight gain. Second, both their appetite and energy levels were far better than those of the control group. Third, they have experienced less difficulty with concomitant diseases, infections and maladies that often befall newborn calves—far less than the control group fed only mother's milk.

Once this study is finished and all the data compiled, we believe this will make a profound impact in a number of areas. If this current set of statistics carry through to completion, this study might not only prove the ultimate panacea for herd stability and healthy alternatives for beef and dairy farmers everywhere, but also serve as a signpost to give direction to other areas of health, wellness and dietary alternatives.

Since we know Aloe Vera offers interspecific benefits that are limitless both in depth and scope of usage, we foresee a number of areas in which Aloe Vera could and should become a part of everyone's daily usage regimen, not just as treatment and cure but more significantly as part of a proactive, preventive wellness plan and as a healthy versatile super-food.

So, we once again find ourselves confronted by the most important challenge facing all true disciples of the healing plant: How do we set the bar higher? How do we get people to understand that this silent healer is a precious gift that must be understood before it can be put to effective use? Once it is, once we have served our purpose both as messengers and educators, we can then share its true potentials as a prime ingredient in the complete wellness lifestyle. In that regard, let us illustrate what a universal blessing Aloe Vera has now proven itself to be and how it can be seamlessly integrated into everything we do.

To accomplish this, we set before you what might be considered A Day of Perfect Health, one that involves an immersion in wellness products replete with Aloe Vera.

Aloe Vera's Day of Perfect Health.

It begins with the moment you get out of bed, use your mouthwash and brush your teeth—both done with Aloe Vera. As a mouthwash, Aloe Vera is remarkably effective both in changing the pH balance of your mouth and in the complete removal of plaque. It is also an exceptional healant in the treatment of aphthous ulcers, canker sores, or other irritations in the oral cavity. Formulated into a toothpaste—and there are some good ones—it is one of the most effective agents known to science in removing plaque (strep mutans) entirely from tooth enamel.

You may continue your Aloe Vera wellness regimen over to the intake of vitamins, minerals, amino acids and any other nutriceuticals you take on a regular basis. If you take your choice of nutritional supplement with four ounces of stabilized Aloe Vera drinking gel you increase the effective assimilation of those nutrients into your system by as much as three to four times the normal rate of absorption. Additionally, you receive the nutritional synergy of Aloe Vera in all its cryptic abilities as its own phytonutrient with profound antioxidant capabilities.

Since the skin needs nutrition of its own, Aloe Vera—when formulated into a properly designed personal care regime—can treat, exfoliate, restore, rebuild and provide constant, impressive nutrition to the human skin. Since Aloe Vera has shown time and again that it senses the subtle shifts in pH skin balances of both men and women, it provides the essential ingredient in the kind of prescriptive skin care that is sure to be the wave of the future in the next 20 years. Not only has Aloe Vera in various preparations proved to be the skin therapy of choice for a number of leading aestheticians in the United States, it has proved to provide some of the most effective, antiallergenic skin care programs available today. The caution here remains constant however: *Caveat Emptor* the Aloe "marquee" products that are diluted beyond any measurable, usable form. Always, in these cases, check out the sources of your Aloe, in what form it is presented to you and what the listed percentages are. Cost, as we have mentioned, is not an infallible indicator of quality and content. (There are, after all, some rather mediocre products that charge a hefty price.) But it is certain that you cannot come by a viable, effective Aloe product on the cheap. Truly efficacious Aloe Vera products require costly means of stabilization, formulation and testing; and all those things bring costs that justifiably must be passed on to the consumer.

As we go through our day, we find that Aloe Vera can be a part of everything we do. In a proper formulation, it can polish our brass and silver. It can coat and preserve our furniture, and even serve as a superb insect repellant.

As we participate in daily exercise or play a sport, our Aloe Vera products can serve us as a lubricant, a rubdown, a counterirritant pre-event massage and most certainly as a healant for any injuries that we might incur.

It's reputation as an anti-burn agent is already legendary. And formulated into a skin-treatment, skin-conditioner, and suntan lotion, it provides the best possible combination of skin conditioning and moisture replacement.

Knowing that Aloe Vera has a GRAS qualification and is, in every sense of the word, a super-food leaves us with the awareness that it can even be used with delicious intelligence in different kinds of juices, smoothies, soups and salads. And yes! There is even a small Aloe Vera cookbook that offers some surprisingly creative recipes.

Of course, we could never overlook its original longstanding purpose as a very effective regulating agent for the digestive system. And we feel it is essential that Aloe Vera be taken in doses of at least four to eight ounces daily to maintain optimum health, body balance, regularity, and anti-oxidant potentials.

Living in today's world is more than stepping through the minefield of life on a very busy planet. It is a place where human traffic, third world health crises, mass production, and wholesale farming of animals leads to environmental challenges that almost go beyond measure. That's why, now more than ever, it's up to us to seize our own destiny where our health is concerned. And that *Carpe Diem* requires of us an intelligent awareness of the potential we have to make healthy choices every time we are challenged to do so.

So very often we are victimized by ignorance of our own surroundings, of the perils that face us as well as the opportunities that surround us. Broadening our health horizons empowers us to do the right thing and step into a realm of life-extension where the longevity of flourishing is more than an option; it is our God-given right.

Summary

It has occasionally been said that in pursuing the truth, one must be both relentless and patient. We have learned that lesson well, and yet we have so much more to learn, teach and pay forward. At the moment we are sponsoring tests in a number areas that are in critical stages of evaluation. So any information we might share about them is both proprietary and incomplete. One of them in the area of bovine medicine could mean billions of dollars of savings to the dairy industry and revolutionize milk production as we know it. Another in the planning stages, could finally bring an end to the global AIDS dilemma and herald an entire new awareness in the preventive treatment of pandemic contagious diseases. There are also ongoing studies, to which we are privy, that provide viable insight into Aloe's treatment and cure of specific autoimmune diseases that have previously been deemed "impossible to treat."

Given the momentous potential for treatment and cure that Aloe Vera offers, it is not only important that we do so, it is our responsibility as well as our life's work. And as long as we are charged to do so, we will continue...

Notes

1. Russell, Richard R. "Letter to Mesquite Independent School District." 1976. *Stabilized Aloe Vera Archives*. Vol. 4—Athletics.

2. Aloe Vera of America, Inc. Archives. "Taped Endorsements." Athletic Product Lines.—"Larry Gardner." *Stabilized Aloe Vera*. Volume IV—Athletics.

3. Aloe Vera of America, Inc. Archives. "Taped Endorsements." Athletic Product Lines.—"Mike O'Shea. *Stabilized Aloe Vera*. Volume IV—Athletics.

4. Coats, Bill C. and Robert Ahola. *The Silent Healer*. Sweet. Austin. 1980 p. 117.

5. Davis, Robert H. "Aspirin and Aloe." *ALOE VERA/ A Scientific Study*. *Vantage Press*. New York. 1997. p. 230.

6. Ibid. p. 232.

7. Vinson, Joe A., Hassan Al Kharrat and Lori Andreoli. "Effect of Aloe Vera preparations on the human bioavailability of Vitamins C and E.' Private Paper. Department of Chemistry. University of Scranton, Scranton, Pennsylvania. June. 1999. p. 10

8. Agarwal, O.P. "Prevention of Atheromatous Heart Disease." *Angiology 36*. Westminster Publications, 1985, p. 490.

9. Ibid. p. 491

10. Engel, Elliot D., DPM, Nelson E. Erlich, DPM, and Robert H. Davis PhD. "Diabetes Mellitus—Impaired Wound Healing from Zinc Deficiency," *Journal of the Podiatric Medical Association*. October 1981, Vol. 71. Number 10. p. 541

11. Ibid, p. 543

12. Pulse, Terry L. M.D. "Nutritional Supplementation Study # 1 and #2. (Clinical Trials)." Based on Walter Reed Clinical Evaluation Scores Compared to the Initial Health Status of the Patient. *Private Paper*. July. 1989.

13. Womble, Debra, and J. Harold Helderman. "Enhancement of Aloe Responsiveness of Human Lymphocytes by Acemannan (Carrisyn™)." *Internal Society for Immunotherapy Journal.* London 1988, Vol. 10. No. 8, pp. 967-974.

14. Pugliese, Peter T., M.D. "Preliminary Evaluation of Coats 10% Glycolic Acid Exfoliant and Coats Aloe Vera Gel." *Private Paper.* Bernville, Pennsylvania. 1994.

References

Chapter 1
The New Face of World Health

Stolberg, Sheryl Gay. "In the AIDS War: New Weapons and New Victims." *The New York Times. New York.* June 3, 2001.

Gergen, David. "Breaking a Solemn Promise." *U.S. News and World Report.* New York. April 1, 2002.

Mallaby, Sebastian. "The Arthur Andersons of Medicine." *The Washington Post.* Washington, D.C. April 28, 2002.

"A Majority of Americans Seek Alternative Treatments." *USA Today.* New York. April 1998.

Pilzer, Paul Zane. *THE NEXT TRILLION. Why the wellness industry will exceed the $1 trillion health care (sickness) industry in the next ten years.* (Abridged Version). Video Plus Publications. Lake Dallas, Texas. 2001.

Hatch, Orin. Harkin, Thomas. "Freedom of Health Information Act. U.S. Statistical Abstract. Washington, D.C. 1995.

"Stem-Cell Research." *Newsweek.* New York. February 23. 2001.

Wade, Nicholas. "Teaching the Body to Heal Itself..." *The New York Times.* New York. November 7. 2000.

Nickel, David, PhD., N.D. "Organotherapy." Primezyme International. Santa Monica, California. 2002.

"High Technology meets Ancient Medicine," *Alternative Medicine.* Tiburon, California. March 2002.

Grady, Denise. "A User's Guide for Those Who Choose Hormone Replacements." *The New York Times.* June 23, 2002.

Pulse, Terry L. M.D. "Nutritional Supplementation Study # 1 and #2. (Clinical Trials)." Based on Walter Reed Clinical Evaluation Scores Compared to the Initial Health Status of the Patient. *Private Paper.* July. 1989.

McDaniel, H.R., M.D., B.H. McAnalley, Ph.D. and R.H. Carpenter, D.V.M. "The Basic Science and Principals for the Use of Acemannan in Clinical Medicine." *Fisher Institute for Medical Research at Dallas-Fort Worth Medical Center.* Carrington Laboratories Research Division. Irving, Texas. 1991.

Plaskett, G. Lawrence, PhD. "Aloe Vera and the Human Immune System." *The Aloe Vera Information Service.* Three Quoins House. Trevalett, UK.

Chapter 2
Aloe Vera Q&A

De Werth, A.F., H.T. Blackhurst, and B.A. Perry. "Aloes," *Texas Agricultural Progress.* 1970. Vol. 6. pp. 13-17.

Bovik, Ellis. G. "Aloe Vera/ Panacea, or Old Wives' Tale?" *Texas Dental Journal.* 1966. p. 14

Harrison, R.K. "Healing Herbs of the Bible." *Janus,* 1961. Vol. 50, p. 16.

Heyne, KJ. *Useful Seed Plants of Indonesia,* Vol. 1, 3rd Edition. 1950.

Kent, Carol Miller. *Aloe Vera.* Arlington, Virginia. 1979. pp. 5; 8; 28-29; 40-41.

Plinius, Gaius Segundus. *Natural History.* (John H. Bostock and H.T. Riley Translators. 1856. Volume 5. Book 27. pp. 222.

Watt, Sir George. *A Dictionary of the Economic Products of India.* Superintendent of Government Printing. Delhi, 1908. (reissuance 1972). Volume 1, p. 179.

Morton, Julia. "Folk Uses and Commercial Exploitation of Aloe Leaf Pulp." *Economic Botany.* 1963. Vol. 15. pp. 314-315.

Coats, Bill. R.Ph. and Robert Ahola. "Chapter 6. A Matter of Chemistry." *The Silent Healer.* Sweet Publishing. Austin, Texas. 1984, pp. 46-59.

Rowe, Tom D., and Lloyd M. Parks. "A phytochemical Study of Aloe Vera Leaf," *Journal of American Pharmaceutical Association.* 1939, Vol. 39. pp. 262-265.

Begnini, Renzo. *Chemical Abstracts.* 1950, Vol. 44. p. 10036A.

Lorenzetti, Lorna J., Rupert Salisbury, Jack Beal, and Jack N. Baldwin. "Bacteriostatic Property of Aloe Vera," *Journal of Pharmaceutical Sciences."* 1964, Vol. 53. p. 1287.

Ikawa, Myoshi, and Carl Niemann, "Further Observations on the Behavior of Carbohydrates in Seventy Nine Percent Sulfuric Acid." *Archives of Biochemistry and Prophysics.* 1951. Vol. 3161. pp. 70-71.

Professional Service Industries, Inc. "Effect of Aloe Vera MPS Formula 38/100% Against Four Microorganisms. Sample 1000-A," *Special Report.* BioSearch Laboratories. Arlington, Texas. 1988.

Danhof, Ivan E., Ph.D. M.D. "PurAloe Test Samples." *Private Paper.* North Texas. Research Laboratory. 1987.

Dorn, Gordon L., Ph.D., "A Summary SWINS Analysis of the Aloe Samples," *Sponsored Report.* Dorn Microbiological Consultants, Inc. Dallas, Texas. 1988.

McDaniel, H.R., M.D., B.H. McAnalley, Ph.D. and R.H. Carpenter, D.V.M. "The Basic Science and Principals for the Use of Acemannan in Clinical Medicine." *Fisher Institute for Medical Research at Dallas-Fort Worth Medical Center.* Carrington Laboratories Research Division. Irving, Texas. 1991.

Coats, Bill C. and Spanky Stephens. *Healing Winners. Sweet.* Austin, Texas. 1983.

Passwater, Dr. Richard and Dr. Neil Solomon. "Science Behind Aloe Vera." *Optimal Health Journal.* Apprise Publishing. Canada. 1997.

Chapter 3
Aloe Super Stars

Dallas, Cowboy's Trainers' Reports, *Stabilized Aloe Vera Volume VI,* 1993. Dallas, Texas.

Sheehan, George. *Running and Being.* Simon & Schuster. New York. 1978. p. 136.

Gray, Henry, F.R.S. *Gray's Anatomy.* Bounty Books. New York. 1977.

Coats, Bill. Coats Aloe Archives. "Major Professional Sports Account List." Vol. II. Garland Texas 2002.

Man's Body. An Owners Manual. Bantam Books. New York. 1977.

Coats, Bill C. and Robert Ahola. *The Silent Healer.* Sweet. Austin. 1980

Flagg. J. "Aloe Vera Gel in Dermatological preparations." American Perfumer. 1959. Vol. 74. p. 27

Russell, Richard R. "Letter to Mesquite Independent School District." 1976. *Stabilized Aloe Vera Archives.* Vol. 4—Athletics.

Aloe Vera of America, Inc. Archives. "Taped Endorsements. Athletic Product Lines.—'Larry Gardner.' "*Stabilized Aloe Vera.* Volume IV—Athletics. 1983.

Coats. Bill C. and Spanky Stephens, A.T.C. *Healing Winners.* Sweet. Austin. 1982.

Aloe Vera of America, Inc. Archives. "Taped Endorsements. Athletic Product Lines.—'Mike O'Shea.'" *Stabilized Aloe Vera.* Volume IV—Athletics. 1983

Chapter 4
Major Milestones

Grossman, Mervin H. and Henry Cobble. "Final Report—Acute Oral Dose Range (Dogs). Acute Dermal Application. (Rabbits)." Lakeland Laboratories. 1966. *Aloe Vera of America Archives.* Vol. 1. pp. 124-134.

Busey, William M. Marcelina B. Powers and Richard Voelker. "Final Report. Acute Oral (rats), Acute Dermal Application (rabbits)." Hazelton Laboratories, Falls Church Virginia, 1968. *Aloe Vera of America Archives.* Vol. 1. pp. 137-184..

Brasher, James. Eugene Zimmermann, and C.K. Collings. "Effects of Prednisolone, Indomethacin and Aloe Vera on Tissue Culture Cells," *Federal Dental Services.* 1969. pp. 122-125.

Coleman, Martin E. "Single Level Acute Oral Toxicity Study of Aloe Aqueous Extract #10209 in Rats," Dawson Research Corporation. Orlando, Florida. 1977. 1981.

Chopia, R.N. and N.N. Gosh. Arch Pharmacy. 1938. Vol. 276. p. 246.

Davis, Robert H. "Aspirin and Aloe." *ALOE VERA/ A Scientific Study.* Vantage Press. New York. 1997. pp. 226-263.

Vinson, Joe A., Hassan Al Kharrat and Lori Andreoli. "Effect of Aloe Vera preparations on the human bioavailability of Vitamins C and E.' Private Paper. Department of Chemistry. University of Scranton, Scranton, Pennsylvania. June. 1999.

Coats, Bill. R.Ph. and Robert Ahola. "Chapter 6. A Matter of Chemistry." *The Silent Healer.* Sweet Publishing. Austin, Texas. 1984, pp. 58-59.

Rowe, Tom D., and Lloyd M. Parks. "A phytochemical Study of Aloe Vera Leaf," *Journal of American Pharmaceutical Association.* 1939, Vol. 39. pp. 262-265.

Begnini, Renzo. *Chemical Abstracts.* 1950, Vol. 44. p. 10036A.

Ikawa, Myoshi, and Carl Niemann, "Further Observations on the Behavior of Carbohydrates in Seventy Nine Percent Sulfuric Acid." *Archives of Biochemistry and Prophysics.* 1951. Vol. 3161. pp. 70-71.

Professional Service Industries, Inc. "Effect of Aloe Vera MPS Formula 38/100% Against Four Microorganisms. Sample 1000-A," *Special Report.* BioSearch Laboratories. Arlington, Texas. 1988.

Danhof, Ivan E., Ph.D. M.D. "Aloe Vera/ The Whole Leaf Advantage." *Private Paper.* North Texas. Research Laboratory. July. 1992.

Agarwal, O.P. "Prevention of Atheromatous Heart Disease," *Angiology.* Vol. 36. Westminister Publications. 1985, pp. 485-492.

Dixit, V.P. and Suresh Joshi, "Effect of Aloe Barbadensis and Clofibrate on Serum Lipids in Triton-induced hyperlipedemia in Presbytis Monkeys." *Indian Journal of Medical Research, Volume 78,* September, 1983, pp. 417-421.

Joshi, Sureshi, and V.P. Dixit. "Hypolipidemia effect of Aloe barbadensis (Aloe Fraction I) in cholesterol-fed rats in Lipid and Lipoprotein metabolism." *The Process of National Academy of Sciences of India,* 1986. Sect. B. 56, pp. 339-342.

Coats, Bill C. and Robert Ahola. *Physicians and Trainers Reports. The Silent Healer.* Sweet. Austin, Texas. pp 152-238.

Heggers, John P., Ph.D., and Martin C. Robson. "Chapter 11. Eicosanoids in Wound-healing." *Prostaglandins in Clinical Practice.* Edited by W. David Watkins et al. Raven Press, Ltd. New York. 1989. pp. 183—194.

Heggers, John P. "Wound-healing Potential of Aloe & Other Chemotherapeutic Agents." *Private Paper.* Presented at the 6th International Congress on Traditional and Folk Medicine, December 1992.

Heggers, John P., Wendell. D. Winters, *et al.* "Beneficial Effect of Aloe Vera on Wound Healing in an Excisional Wound Model." *The Journal of Alternative and Complementary Medicine. Volume 2. No. 2.* pp. 271-277

Sims, Ruth M., and Eugene R. Zimmermann. "Report on Aloe Vera on Certain Microorganisms," (Baylor College of Dentistry). Aloe Vera of America Archives—Bacteriology. *Stabilized Aloe Vera.* Vol. I. pp. 230-234.

Coats, Bill C. "Telephone Report from Jean Setterstrom, Ph.D. Bacteriology. Research Institute/ Walter Reed Hospital." Aloe Vera of America Archives. Stabilized Aloe Vera. Vol. III. June 1978.

Sims, Ruth M., and E.R. Zimmermann. "Report—the Effect of Aloe Vera on Mycotic Organisms (Fungi)." Aloe Vera of America Archives. *Stabilized Aloe Vera.* Volume I. pp. 237-238.

Sims, Ruth M., and E.R. Zimmermann. "Effect of Aloe Vera on Herpes Simplex and Herpesvirus (Strain Zoster)." Aloe Vera of America Archives. *Stabilized Aloe Vera.* Volume I. pp. 239-240.

Sims, Ruth M., "Effectiveness of undiluted Aloe 99 Gel against Trichomonas vaginalis," Dallas Microb—Assay Service, 1971." Aloe Vera of America Archives. *Stabilized Aloe Vera.* Volume I. pp. 241-242.

Shupe-Ricksecker, Kathleen, PhD. "Germicidal Properties of Coats Whole Leaf Aloe Vera Gel." *Private Paper.* University of Dallas. Dallas, Texas. 1994.

Shupe-Ricksecker, Kathleen, Ph.D. "Germicidal Properties of Aloe Vera Gel on a Strain of Propionibacterium Acnes." *Private Paper.* University of Dallas. Dallas, Texas. 1994.

Burns, Frank S. (Substance Abuse Counselor). "Substance Abuse and the Use of Aloe Vera Products During the Early Stages of the Recovery Process." *Private Paper.* Spokane, Washington. 1982.

Chapter 5
Autoimmune Disease Meet the Aloe Vera "Orchestra"

Lemonick, Michael D., J. Madeleine Nash, Alice Park, Mia Schmiedeskamp and Andrew Purvis. "Revenge of the Microbes," *TIME.* New York. September 12,1994, pp. 62-69.

Mitchison, Avrion. "Will We Survive?" *Scientific American.* September, 1993. pp. 136-144.

Marrack, Phippa and John W. Kappler. "How the Immune System Recognizes the Body." *Scientific American.* September, 1993, pp. 82-89.

Nagourney, Eric. "The Kinder Side of a Scorpion Sting—Health and Fitness." *The New York Times*. New York. July 11, 2000.

Robinson, James W. *et al.* "Toxic and Hazardous Substances Control (Part A) and Environmental Carcinogenesis Reviews (Part C)." *Journal of Environmental Science and Health*. 1992, pp. 54-71.

Steinman, Lawrence. "Autoimmune Disease." Scientific American. New York. September, 1993.

Huang, Huei-Chen, Jin-Hsia Chang, Shiu-Fend Tung *et al.* "Immunosuppressive effect of emodin, a free-radical generator." Department of Pharmacology. College of Medicine. National Taiwan University. Taipei, Taiwan. Elsevier Science Publishers. BV. 1992.

Paul, William E. "Infectious Diseases and the Immune System," *Scientific American*. New York. September 1994.

Chapman, M. Lynne, Dan Dimitrijevich, Julia C. Hevelone, Dudley Goetz, Jack Cohen, Gary E. Wise, and Robert W. Gracy. "Inhibition of Psoriatic Cell Proliferation in In-Vitro Skin Models by Amprilose Hydrochloride." *In Vitro Cell. Dev. Biol.* Tissue Culture Association October, 1990. pp. 991-996.

Janeway, Charles A. Jr., "How the Immune System Recognizes Invaders." *Scientific American*. New York. September 1993, pp. 73-79.

Davis, Robert H. "The Conductor-Orchestra Concept of Aloe Vera." *ALOE VERA/ A Scientific Study*. Vantage Press. New York. 1997. pp. 290-310.

Nagourney, Eric. "Promising Progress in Lupus Research—Health and Fitness." *The New York Times*. New York. Sept. 7. 1999.

Coats, Bill C. and Robert Ahola. "The Rita Thompson Story." *The Silent Healer*. Sweet. Austin, Texas. 1984. pp. 104-106.

Engel, Elliot D., DPM, Nelson E. Erlich, DPM, and Robert H. Davis PhD. "Diabetes Mellitus—Impaired Wound Healing from Zinc Deficiency," *Journal of the Podiatric Medical Association*. October 1981, Vol. 71. Number 10. pp. 536-544

Davis, Robert H., Mark G. Leitner, and Joseph Russo. "Aloe Vera—A Natural Approach for Treating Wounds, Edema, and Pain in Diabetes." *Journal of the Podiatric Medical Association.* February 1988, Volume 78. Number 2. pp. 60-68.

Davis, Robert H. and Nicholas P. March. "Aloe vera and Gibberellin. Anti-inflammatory Activity in Diabetes." *Journal of the Podiatric Medical Association.* Volume 79. Number 1. January 1989. pp. 24-26.

Coats, Bill C. and Robert Ahola. "Brenda's Story." *Aloe Vera/ The Inside Story.* Dager Press. Dallas. pp. 205-208.

Chapter 6
Memories and Miracles

Coats, Bill C. and Robert Ahola. *The Silent Healer.* Sweet. Austin. 1980

Aloe Vera of America, Inc. Archives, "Asian Files." *Stabilized Aloe Vera.* Volume VI—Private Records Since 1996.

Coats, Bill C. and Robert Ahola. "Brenda's Story." *Aloe Vera/ The Inside Story.* Dager Press. Dallas, 1995. pp. 101-107.

Chapter 7
AIDS, Cancer and the Aloe Answer

Winters, W.D., R. Benavides and W.J. Clouse. "Effects of Aloe Extracts on Human Normal and Tumor Cells in Vitro." Economic Botany. Volume 35. New York. 1981. pp. 89-95.

Danhof, Ivan E. "Are Aloe Anthraquinones Genotoxic and/or Carcinogenic?" North Texas Research Laboratory. Omnimedicus Press. Grand Prairie, Texas. 2000.

Danhof, Ivan E. "The Antitumor Effects of Aloe Vera?" North Texas Research Laboratory. Omnimedicus Press. Grand Prairie, Texas. 2000.

Plaskett. G. Lawrence. "Aloe Vera and Cancer." *Biomedical Information Services.* Camelford, Cornwall, U.K. 1996.

Stolberg, Sheryl Gay. "In AIDS War, New Weapons and New Victims." *The New York Times.* New York. June 3, 2001.

Greene, Warner C. "AIDS and the Immune System." *Scientific American.* September 1993, pp. 100-105.

Kahlon, Jashir B., Dr. PH, Maurice C. Kemp Ph.D., Robert H. Carpenter DVM, Bill H McAnalley, Ph.D. H.R. McDaniel, M.D., "Inhibition of AIDS Virus replication by Acemannan *in vitro."Molecular Biotherapy,* 1991. Volume 3. September, pp. 127-135.

Pulse, Terry L. M.D. "Nutritional Supplementation Study # 1 and #2. (Clinical Trials)." Based on Walter Reed Clinical Evaluation Scores Compared to the Initial Health Status of the Patient. *Private Paper.* July. 1989.

McDaniel, H.R., M.D., B.H. McAnalley, Ph.D. and R.H. Carpenter, D.V.M. "The Basic Science and Principals for the Use of Acemannan in Clinical Medicine." *Fisher Institute for Medical Research at Dallas-Fort Worth Medical Center.* Carrington Laboratories Research Division. Irving, Texas. 1991.

H. Reg McDaniel, M.D. Sue Perkins, and B.H. McAnalley Ph.D. "A Clinical Pilot Study Using Carrisyn™ in the Treatment of Acquired Immunodeficiency Syndrome (AIDS). *Abstracts of Papers. AJCP.* October, 1987.

Womble, Debra, and J. Harold Helderman. "Enhancement of Aloe Responsiveness of Human Lymphocytes by Acemannan (Carrisyn™)." *Internal Society for Immunotherapy Journal.* London 1988, Vol. 10. No. 8, pp. 967-974.

Davis, Robert H. "Does Aloe Vera Have a Place in AIDS Therapy?" *ALOE VERA/ A Scientific Approach.* Vantage Press. New York. 1997.

Chapter 8
More Than Skin Deep.

Fulton, James E. "Let's Talk Cosmetics." Acne Research Institute, Inc. Miami, Florida. 1973.

BioSearch Laboratories. "Summary Report—Independent Analysis of Various Aloe Vera Products." Stabilized Aloe Vera. Vol. III. 1979.

Milloy, Stephen. "AMA, Disinfect Thyself." JunkScience.com. FoxNews.com. July 7, 2000.

Coats, Bill C. and Robert Ahola. "Chapter 6. "The Care and Feeing of the Human Skin." *The Silent Healer.* Sweet Publishing. Austin, Texas. 1984, pp. 129-137.

Heggers, John P., Wendell. D. Winters, *et al.* "Beneficial Effect of Aloe Vera on Wound Healing in an Excisional Wound Model." *The Journal of Alternative and Complementary Medicine.* Volume 2. No. 2. pp. 271-277

Skovan, Stephen J. and Robert H. Davis. "Principles of wound Healing and Growth Factor Considerations." *Journal of the American Podiatric Medical Association.* Volume 83. No. 4. April 1993.

Kaufman, Teddy, A.R. Newman *et al.* "Aloe Vera and Burn Wound Healing." *Plastic and Reconstructive Surgery.* June 1989.

Heggers, John. P. PhD. "Antimicrobial Therapy for the Plastic Surgeon." *Advances in Reconstructive Plastic Surgery.* Volume 9. *Mosby Year Book.* 1993.

Bowles, William. B. " MTTEC50 "Determination in TestSkin™ Living Dermal Equivalent Rapid Assay. " In Vitro Alternatives, Inc. Project Number. 0-0084. 1990.

Bowles, William. B. "Aloe Vera Gel and Its Effect on Cell Growth." (Cell Growth Study). Aloe Vera In Vitro Studies, Inc. 1994

Heggers John P. "Wound-healing Potential of Aloe & Other Chemotherapeutic Agents." *Private Paper.* Presented at the 6th International Congress on Traditional and Folk Medicine, December 1992.

Shupe-Ricksecker, Kathleen, PhD. "Germicidal Properties of Coats Whole Leaf Aloe Vera Gel." *Private Paper.* University of Dallas. Dallas, Texas. 1994.

Shupe-Ricksecker, Kathleen, "Germicidal Properties of Aloe Vera Gel on a Strain of Propionibacterium Acnes." *Private Paper.* University of Dallas. Dallas, Texas. 1994.

Pugliese, Peter T., "Preliminary Evaluation of Coats 10% Glycolic Acid Exfoliant and Coats Aloe Vera Gel." *Private Paper.* Bernville, Pennsylvania. 1994..

Coats, Bill. C. "Human Case Studies/ Skin Care Case Studies—Utilizing Whole Leaf Aloe Vera Gel and Glycolic Acid. *Coats Aesthetics.* Volume II. Garland Texas. 2000-2002.

Nickel, David, PhD., N.D. "TMA/Tissue Mineral Analysis." Primezyme International. Santa Monica, California. 2002.

Chapter 9
Animal Planet

Brumbagh, Robert S. "Of Man, Animals, and Morals." *On the Fifth Day.* Acropolis. 1978.

Fogle, Bruce. *Pets and their People.* Viking. New York. 1984.

Fox, Michael. *Massage Program for Dogs and Cats.* New Market Press. 1981.

Coats, Bill. C., R.Ph., Richard Holland, D.V.M. and Robert Ahola. *Creatures in Our Care.* Hurst. Dallas, 1985.

Fox, Michael. *Understanding Your Cat.* Bantam Books. New York. 1975.

Pitcairn, Richard, and Susan Hubble Pitcairn. *Dr. Pitcairn's Complete Guide to NATURAL HEALTH FOR DOGS AND CATS.* Rodale Press. Emmaus, Pa, 1982.

Coats, Bill. C., R.Ph., Richard Holland, D.V.M. and Robert Ahola. *Creatures in Our Care.* Hurst. Dallas, 1985.

McDaniel, H.R., M.D., B.H. McAnalley Ph.D., and R.H. Carpenter, D.V.M. "Use of Acemannan (Carrisyn™) in FLV and FAIDS stricken Cats." *Fisher*

Institute for Medical Research at Dallas-Fort Worth Medical Center. Carrington Laboratories Research Division. Irving, Texas, 1991.

Schwabe, Calvin H. *Cattle, Priests and Progress in Medicine.* The University of Minnesota Press. Minneapolis. 1978, p. 153-166.
Prion Disease Center. "BSE and Mad Cow Disease Compendium Reports." *Mad Cow Home Page. www.mad-cow.org.* pages 1-24. Dec. 2002.

Burros, Marian. "Eating Well: The Greening of the Herd." *The New York Times.* New York. July 1, 2002.

Smithcors, J.F. *The Veterinarian in America. 1825-1975.* American Veterinary Publications, Inc. Santa Barbara. 1975. pp. 89-92.

Fredrickson, Allan, *Animal Treatment Compendium.* Mt. Vernon, Washington. 1982.

Coats, Bill. C., R.Ph., Richard Holland, D.V.M. and Robert Ahola. "Chapter 7. Horse Sense." *Creatures in Our Care.* Hurst Publishing. Dallas, 1985. pp. 67-96.

Coats, Bill. C., R.Ph., Richard Holland, D.V.M. and Robert Ahola. "Chapter 8. Barnyard Bravos." *Creatures in Our Care.* Hurst. Dallas, 1985. pp. 97-135.

Corbett, Bob, D.V.M. "Report on Mastitis." *Private Paper.* El Paso, 1999.

Diamond K Animal Care. *Animal Care and Aloe Vera.* Big Spring, Texas, 1981. pp. 11-13.

Coats, Bill C. "Suggested Treatments and Dosage for Animals." *Coats Whole Leaf Aloe Vera. Archives.* Animal Case Studies. Volume. III. Garland, Texas. 2002.

Chapter 10
Aloe's Perfect World.

Davis, Robert H. "Aspirin and Aloe." *ALOE VERA/ A Scientific Study.* Vantage Press. New York. 1997. pp. 226-263.

Vinson, Joe A., Hassan Al Kharrat and Lori Andreoli. "Effect of Aloe Vera preparations on the human bioavailability of Vitamins C and E." Private Paper.

Department of Chemistry. University of Scranton, Scranton, Pennsylvania. June. 1999.

Corbett, Bob. "Aloe Vera Control Group Calf Study." *Coats Whole Leaf Aloe Vera Archives.* Animal Case Studies. Volume. III. Garland, Texas. 2002-2003.

Index

A

AMA, 189-190, 227, 290

Acne vulgaris, 85, 194-195

acne

    Grade I, 210

    Grade IV, 210

    Grade V, 210

Addiction, 86, 97, 107

Addison's disease, 100

Agarwal, O.P., 279, 286

AIDS, 2, 10-11, 13, 85, 97, 106, 152, 159, 161-162, 164-166, 170-172, 174-178, 180-184, 199-200, 220-221, 247, 273, 278, 281, 289-290

AIDS related dementia, 166

Aloe Action for Athletes, 36

Aloe Barbadensis, Miller, 18

Aloe Chinensis, 16, 155

Aloe emodin, 27, 67, 156-157

Aloe polysaccharides, 19, 25, 27-29, 61, 64, 67-68, 104-105, 198

Aloe saponaria, 155

"Aloe Vera and Aspirin", 62-63, 121

Aloe Vera

    history, 19, 52, 55, 58, 61, 67, 71, 75, 81, 123, 156, 162, 187, 203, 227, 241, 243, 251, 273, 282

    "Orchestra", 99, 105-106, 155, 167, 287

    stabilization, 21-22, 56, 64-67, 69, 82, 277

ALOE VERA/A Scientific Approach, 103-107

Aloe Vera's Day of Perfect Health, 276

alopecia, 31, 189, 220, 222

    aereata, 31, 222

    prematura, 222

Alta Dena Dairies, 263

American Society of Cosmetic Chemists, 34

amino acids

Ampicillin, 204, 246-247
Amyozocolictryptomiacin, 164
analgesic effects
Anger, 31, 87, 94-95
Anthraquinones, 18, 24, 26-27, 30, 57, 67, 105, 156-157, 289
antibiotics, 12, 70, 80, 97, 103, 123, 142-143, 156, 160, 183, 190, 204-205, 217, 245-
    246, 250, 263, 267-268, 270-271
    broad spectrum, 80, 86, 98, 120, 181, 242
antigens, 11, 100-101, 103, 177, 179
anti-inflammatory activity, 42, 62-63, 66, 121, 288
"Antimicrobial Therapy for the Plastic Surgeon", 203, 291
antipruritic, 28, 58-59, 75, 190, 223, 234
antiseptic, 42, 46, 66, 75, 182, 190, 198, 206, 223
"Antitumor Effects of Aloe Vera", 158, 289
Anxiety, 31, 86-87, 89
Appetite, 87, 91, 93, 118, 253, 265, 267, 275
Arginine, 170
Arizona Cardinals, 40, 47
aspirin, 23, 62-63, 77, 97, 121, 134, 275, 279, 285, 293
    and Aloe Vera-1, 63, 66, 146-147, 158, 181, 209, 212, 221, 233-235, 271, 285, 293
autoimmune diseases, 10-13, 19, 31-32, 85, 99-101, 103-104, 106-107, 110-112, 115-
    117, 125, 157, 167, 170, 183, 219, 278
AVMA, 227
AZT, 57, 164-166, 171, 174, 179-181, 184

B

B-Cells, 100, 155, 163
Baby Boomers, 2, 13, 186, 192
Baker, Robert, 254
Baltimore Colts, 47
Barefoot, W.R., 148-151
bee pollen, 87-97
bee propolis, 135
Bell Curve, 166
Bijon Frises, 144
blisters, 31, 40, 83, 127, 134, 168, 254-255
Botox™, 158
Boyer, John, 172

Brasher, James K., 58-59
Brenda's Story, 121-122, 124, 289
Buffalo Bills, 35, 40
Burns, Frank S.
burns, 20, 30-31, 40, 42, 46, 48, 51, 75, 86-87, 97, 102, 121, 123, 136-137, 190, 203, 211, 214, 231, 239, 255, 287
    sunburn, 30-31, 136-137
    radiation, 31, 147, 160, 190
    turf, 31, 40, 42, 46, 48, 51-52, 168, 190

C

Campbell, Earl, 41, 44, 131-132
Campbell, Tim, 44
Cancer
    colon, 81, 157
    skin, 11-12, 14, 28, 31, 33-34, 37, 46, 58, 61, 74-75, 81-82, 85, 100, 102-103, 107-108, 110-111, 113, 122-124, 130-131, 133, 145, 153-154, 158, 162, 177, 185-212, 214, 216-218, 220-221, 223-224, 231, 233-234, 237-240, 244, 247, 249, 251, 256-257, 274, 276-277, 288, 290-292
Candida albicans, 11, 81-82, 187
Caveat emptor, 33, 224, 277
Cactus Feeders, Inc., 263
carcinoma, 153-154, 156, 202
cardiovascular disease, 63
cats
    bites, 20, 31, 158, 162, 230, 232-233, 236-237, 244
    conjunctivitis, 31, 249-250
    cystitis, 245
    FAIDS(feline anti-immune deficiency syndrome), 247-248, 292
    FIPS (feline infectious peritonitis), 247-248
    FLV (feline leukemia virus), 10, 29, 176, 247-248, 292
    FRS (feline respiratory syndrome), 246-247
    rhino-tracheitis, 178, 248
    scratches, 244
    topical treatments, 124, 249
    wounds, 16, 30, 74-76, 78, 81-82, 100, 119-121, 155, 168, 202-205, 231, 236-238, 244, 249-250, 255-256, 288
cattle

    abscesses, 31, 250, 258, 265, 271
    calves and calving, 267-270
    colostrum milk, 266, 275
    broken jaws, 271
    BSE (bovine spongiform encephalapothy), 262
    CSD, 262
    Coccidiosis, 267
    clouded corneas, 271
    dehorning, 271
    edema (udder swelling)
    embryotomies, 271
    everted uterus, 271
    factory farming, 2, 261-263
    immune system, 7, 11-12, 19, 29, 76, 100-104, 111, 116, 154-155, 159, 161-170, 174, 176, 179-180, 182-183, 194-195, 197, 201, 204, 275, 282, 287-289
    mad cow disease, 2, 262, 292
    mastitis, 267-271, 293
    metritis, 266
    Prolapsed uterus, 271
    scrapie, 262
    vaginal infections, 271
    warts, 31, 154, 271
cephalosporin, 204
cell division, 28, 61, 69, 74-75, 212, 217, 237
Clofibrate, 73, 286
cholesterol
    HDL, 72-73
    LDL, 70, 73, 108
    VLDL, 73
chemotherapy, 147-148, 159-161, 164
Chow, Danny, 138
Chronic fatigue syndrome, 5, 8, 31, 82, 187, 219
CMT (California Mastitis Test), 268
Coats, Kimberly, 128-129
Coats, Shannon, 129-130
Coenzyme Q 10, 197
Cobble, Henry, 58, 66, 284
collagen formation, 120, 208
Collings, C.K., 58, 285
cloning, 1, 7

colitis, 29, 100, 178-179
control group studies, 22, 118, 120, 164
contusions, 31, 40, 46, 75, 239, 255
Corynebacterium xerosis, 81-82
Corbett, Bob, 293
Cosmetic Toiletries and Fragrance Association, 189
Creatures in Our Care, 32, 226, 228, 240, 292-293, 313
CTFA, 189-190, 199, 224
    "crocodile's tongue", 16
Crohn's disease, 12, 29, 100, 178-179
Curecal, 245
cuts, 20, 31, 40, 42, 46, 75, 192, 255

D

DNA, 102, 112, 118, 204
Dallas Center for Immunology, 112
Dallas Cowboys, 32, 40, 45-47
Dallas Mavericks, 40, 46
Dallas, Texas, 58, 81, 156, 214, 281, 283, 287, 291
Dawson Research Corporation, 60, 285
Danhof, Ivan, 61, 69-70
Davis, Robert H., 279, 285, 288, 290, 293
Dead Sea, 108
Decadron, 127
Denver, Colorado, 149-150
Depression, 31, 86-88
dermabrasion, 34, 186, 195, 216-217
dermis, 12, 193, 200, 209, 216, 220
Desire
    to drink, 87, 96, 130, 140, 196
    to return to drugs, 96
Detroit Lions, 40
De Materia Medica, 16, 131
detached leaf, 69
diabetes, 5, 12, 30-31, 71, 99-100, 102, 104, 116-122, 168, 244, 279, 288
    type 1, 12, 71, 99-100, 102, 104, 116-118, 121-122, 144, 168
    type 2, 71, 102, 116-117, 203
Diamond K Animal Clinic, 267

Dioscordes, 16
"Disease with No Name", 148
Dixit, V.P., 286
dogs
  bite wounds, 236-237
  Borzoi
  Burns, 20, 30-31, 40, 42, 46, 48, 51, 75, 86-87, 97, 102, 121, 123, 136-137, 190, 203, 211, 214, 231, 239, 255, 287
  Canine parvo, 241-242
  Great Pyrenees
  otitis, 239-240
  poodle, 144, 238
  rabies miasm, 230-231, 246
  skin conditions, 75, 82, 194, 231
  Yorkshire terrier, 231
  wounds, 16, 30, 74-76, 78, 81-82, 100, 119-121, 155, 168, 202-205, 231, 236-238, 244, 249-250, 255-256, 288
Duffy, Larry, 254

E

Ebola, 2, 31
ECG (electrocardiogram), 71-72
E-coli, 2, 262
eicosanoids, 76-77, 286
Eicosanoids in Wound Healing, 76
Electrodermal Screening (EDS), 9
endocrine, 11, 19, 100-103
  glands, 7-8, 11, 100-102, 154, 158, 169, 189, 193-195, 221, 223, 268
  system, 3, 7, 9, 11-12, 19, 24-25, 29-30, 38, 62, 73, 76-77, 81, 100-105, 111, 114, 116-119, 121, 129, 135, 145, 149, 154-155, 158-170, 173-174, 176-177, 179-180, 182-184, 186-187, 192-199, 201, 204-205, 209, 224, 233, 240, 242, 244, 248, 252-253, 267-268, 271, 275-277, 282, 287-289
Engel, Elliot, 279, 288
Enzymatic debridement, 42, 75, 121, 190, 256
Energy level, 87, 92
enzymes
  hydrolyzing, 25
  protein bonding, 25

proteolytic, 25, 28, 30, 105, 198, 223
Environmental Protection Agency, 169, 171, 196
EPA, 169, 171, 196
epidermis, 192-193, 198, 209, 216
Erlick, Nelson, 118
Essential fatty acids
    cis-linoleic, 169
    eicosopentanoic, 169
    gamma-linolenic, 169
eucalyptus, 18, 20, 186, 252
Evans, Pat, 45

F

factory farming, 2, 261-263
fatty acids
    Omega 1, 6, 169-174
    Omega 3, 6, 169-174
    Omega 6, 169
FDA, 4, 6, 19, 21, 24, 46, 58, 65, 110, 125, 164-165, 171, 177-178, 181, 189, 198, 227
Feline Leukemia Virus, 10, 29, 176, 178, 247
Fibromyalgia, 31, 82
fish
    oil, 158, 169, 171, 193-195, 208, 230, 232, 248-249
    tropical, 130-131, 141-142
flesh eating bacteria, 2-3
four factors
    age-2, 8, 13, 70-71, 85, 115-117, 130, 134, 144, 159, 168, 183, 185, 188, 194, 196, 201-202, 219, 222, 225, 241, 247, 260, 267
    environment, 1, 60, 80, 108, 111, 131, 162, 190, 192-193, 195-196, 199-200, 202-204, 225, 230, 246, 250, 271
    heredity
    nutrition, 5, 7, 61, 91, 110, 117-118, 131, 160, 166, 169, 182-184, 188, 191, 194, 196, 198, 222, 267, 276
Fredrickson, Allan, 293
Freedom of Health Information Act, 6, 281
Frostbite, 126, 142, 268
Fulton, Robert, 188, 216

G

GABA, 170, 197

GLA, 169, 171

Gardner, Larry, 45-46, 279, 284

Genomics, 1, 7

Georgia Tech, 40

glucose, 27, 105, 116

glucosamine sulfate, 170

glutathione, 170, 197

glycolic acid

    exfoliation, 202, 206

    solution, 26, 28, 51, 62-63, 79, 82-83, 101, 113, 119, 123, 133-134, 142, 182, 190, 209-210, 242, 253

    treatment, 2, 4, 7-8, 10, 12-13, 16, 18-19, 23, 30, 33-34, 36, 40-43, 46-48, 50, 52-54, 56, 70, 73, 75, 79, 85-87, 97, 99, 102-103, 106, 108-110, 112, 119-120, 122-125, 127-130, 137-138, 143, 147, 153, 159-162, 164, 166, 169-170, 173-178, 180-181, 190, 194, 197, 202-203, 205-214, 216-218, 221, 223-224, 226-229, 231, 233, 235-237, 240-242, 247-249, 252-255, 257, 260, 264, 267-273, 276, 278, 290, 293

Glycolic Acid Exfoliant, 207, 280, 291

Gergen, David, 281

GRAS, 6, 9, 24, 33, 60, 171, 182, 277

Grossman, Mervin, 284

H

HLA molecules, 103

hair, 113, 118, 147, 159-160, 187, 189, 191-194, 197-198, 210, 218-224, 233, 236, 239, 248

    analysis, 69, 116, 219-220, 283, 290, 292

    bulb

    testing, 15, 21, 23-24, 26, 47, 58, 60, 64, 68-69, 71, 73, 82, 84-85, 156, 158, 160, 164, 171, 174-176, 178, 182, 184, 219-220, 228, 277

    follicle, 221

    papilla, 221

    root, 108, 158, 221, 262

    shaft, 221, 223

Hazelton Laboratories, 59, 285

Headaches, 41, 158, 167
healing, 8-10, 13, 15-19, 22, 25-28, 30-36, 42, 46, 50-52, 55-58, 60-62, 64, 66-70, 74-81, 85-86, 97-99, 103-107, 113, 116-122, 124-127, 129-132, 134-135, 137, 139, 142, 144-145, 151-153, 155, 166, 173, 176, 178, 181, 203-204, 206, 209, 216-218, 225-229, 232-233, 235, 237-239, 250, 254-256, 258, 261, 265, 271, 274, 276, 279, 282-284, 286, 288, 291, 313
    acceleration, 42, 75
    impaired, 116-119, 279, 288
    rapid, 49, 74, 77, 79, 120, 166, 212, 216-217, 234, 237, 250, 256, 265, 291
Healing the Heart, 70
Healing Winners, 51, 283-284
Heggers, John, 286, 291
hematoma, 30, 41-42, 44, 74, 258-259
hemp, 18
Herpes II, 31, 83
Herpes simplex, 10, 31, 83, 134-135, 176, 178, 180, 183, 286-287
Herpes zoster, 31, 83, 187, 205
HGHs, 2, 170
Hill, Ed, 254-255
histamine, 77
histidine, 77
HIV, 2, 10-11, 29-31, 85, 155, 161-168, 170-180, 183-184
HMOs, 3
hogs, 133
Holland, Richard, 226, 235, 238, 240, 242, 245, 247, 249-251, 255, 257, 264-265, 267, 292-293
Holland Veterinary Clinic, 242, 267
Hormone Replacement Therapy (HRT), 8, 260
horses
    cuts, 20, 31, 40, 42, 46, 75, 192, 255
    contusions, 31, 40, 46, 75, 239, 255
    deep wounds, 255-256
    founder, 252-253, 313
    hematoma
    laminitis, 252-253
    magnetic blankets, 260
    swollen joints, 252
    standardbreds, 255
    thoroughbreds, 255
Human Growth Hormones, 2, 170, 184

Human Immunodeficiency Virus, 2, 162
Hunt, H.L., 65, 145-146
hyperpigmentation, 210, 214-216
hypodermis, 193, 220

I

Ikawa, Myoshi, 283, 285
immune system, 7, 11-12, 19, 29, 76, 100-104, 111, 116, 154-155, 159, 161-170, 174,
    176, 179-180, 182-183, 194-195, 197, 201, 204, 275, 282, 287-289
immunotherapy, 11, 280, 290
"Impaired Wound Healing from Zinc Deficiency", 118, 279, 288
Indomethacin (Indocin), 58-59
inflammation, 4, 37, 62-63, 76-77, 120-121, 182, 245, 266, 268
Isabgol, 71-73
isopropyl myristate, 188-190, 216, 223

J

Japanese Health Ministry, 156
Jennings, J.R., 81
Joshi, Suresh, 73, 286

K

Karnofsky Quality of Life Scale, 172

L

Lakeland Laboratories, 58, 284
Lane, Eddie, 47, 54
LD50, 47, 58, 227
L-Glutamine, 111, 170, 197
lesions, 31, 40, 100, 102, 107-108, 112-114, 128, 149, 167-168, 190, 195, 255
lignin, 18, 24, 26, 30, 61, 105, 120, 198, 223
Locker, Ken, 48-49, 54
Lorenzetti, Lorna, 283

leukocytes, 76, 100
LSE (Living Skin Equivalents), 206
Lupus erythematosus
     discoid, 111
          systemic, 5, 8-9, 11-12, 16, 20, 31-32, 82, 100, 102-103, 106-108, 110-113, 115,
          125, 135, 147, 154, 160, 165, 170, 190, 197, 203-205, 207, 219-220, 222, 231,
          233, 239-241, 244, 246, 248, 250, 252, 264-265, 271, 273
lymphocytes, 100, 155, 178-179, 280, 290
lysine, 197

M

McAnalley, T.H, 29, 174-179, 290-292
Macaw, 140-141, 143
     Golden, 70, 140, 143
McDaniels, H.R., 174-179, 282-283, 290, 292
McDaniels/McAnalley Studies, 174-179, 282-283, 290, 292
McClung, Coy, 127-128
macrophage, 11, 101, 111, 168, 177, 179-180
Malaysia, 17, 136, 138, 313
mannose, 10, 27, 29, 105, 176, 182
mannose 6-PO4, 105
melatonin, 170
Medicare, 3-4
Medina, Frank, 43-46, 51, 54, 132
Melanosis coli, 157
"Memories and Miracles", 126, 160, 289
miasm, 230-231, 246-247
     leukemia, 10, 18, 29, 155, 176, 178, 246-248
     rabies, 158, 230-231, 241, 246
microbotics, 1, 7-8
monocyte, 179
Multiple sclerosis, 31, 100, 102-104, 125
Myasthenia gravis, 100, 104

N

NBA, 40, 53-54

NCAA, 35, 39-40, 43, 132
NFL, 35, 40-41, 47, 49, 53
Nanocytes, 7
National Taiwan University, 156, 288
Natural Health for Dogs and Cats, 240, 292
"Nature's Pharmacy", 55
neutrophils, 11-12, 100-101
Niemann, Carl, 27, 283, 285
Nickel, David, 281, 292
Nugget, 140-143

O

Olympics, 45
Olympic, Montreal, 45
Olympic Committee, 45
O'Neill, Kevin, 36, 54
O'Neill, Paul, 211
Oral Toxicity Studies, Acute, 60
Organotherapy, 1, 8, 169, 281
O'Shea, Mike, 49-50, 54, 279, 284

P

pain
    relief, 30, 42, 46, 75, 122, 133, 135-136, 150
    symptoms, 9, 72, 93, 97, 100, 102-103, 106-108, 111-113, 117, 148, 150, 167, 171, 181, 241, 244-245, 247, 267
Parks, Lloyd, 27
parrot, 140, 142
Pearson, M.A., 128
Pemphigus vulgaris, 111
penicillin, 80, 204
pernicious anemia, 100, 125
Pierce, Charlie, 129-130, 161
Pierce, Dot, 129-130, 161
Pitcairn, Richard, 240-241
Plaskett, Lawrence, 11

Pliny, the Elder, 16
polymoxins, 204
Post, Troy, 65
Prednisolone (Prednisone), 58
Presbytis monkeys, 73, 286
Prescriptive Skin Care
    cleansing, 197-198, 200, 202, 223, 265
    moisturizing, 133, 200, 202
    protection, 166, 180, 202, 214
    pure aloe vera liquid, 200
    stimulation, 7, 12, 200, 209
    sunscreen, 200-202, 214
    toning, 200, 202
Propionibacterium acnes, 85, 205, 287, 291
Providone-iodine, 204
Prostaglandins
    PGE-1, 102, 167-169
    PGE-2, 29, 63, 102, 167-168
    PGE-3, 102, 167-169
Pseudomonas aeruginosa, 84, 205
Pulse, Terry, 279, 282, 290
penetration, 25, 30, 42, 46, 56, 61-62, 66, 98
pH balance
    acid, 27, 31, 44, 64, 73, 77, 107, 120, 169, 184, 196-197, 201, 206-211, 220, 280, 283, 285, 291-292
    alkaline, 197
phagocytes, 76
Pseudomonas aeruginosa, 84, 205
Psoriasis, 12, 31, 104, 107-111, 125, 193
pyrethrins, 232
pyridoxine, 184

Q

quinolones, 204

R

Radiation, 31, 147, 160, 190
Rays
    UVL, 201
    UVB, 201
reduction of swelling, 69, 75
Reeves, Dan, 48
rehabilitation, 39, 41, 46, 87, 260
relief of pain, 42, 75
Rheumatoid arthritis, 30-31, 100, 104, 106, 111-112, 148, 197
Robson, Martin C., 76, 286
Rowe, Tom D., 283, 285
Russell, Richard, 279, 284

S

SDA, 189
Salmonella, 2, 158, 183, 205, 262
saponins, 18, 24, 26, 30, 105, 120, 223
sarcoma, 154
scleroderma, 31, 100, 104, 111, 115-116, 125
seborrhoea
    oleosa, 221
    sica, 221
Self-esteem, 86-87
Setterstrom, Jean, 82, 134, 286
Shupe-Ricksecker, Kathleen, 287, 291
silver sulfadiazine, 78, 204
Sims, Ruth, 286-287
Sims-Zimmermann, 28, 134
Smith, Emmitt, 35-36, 132
SLE, 111-112
Sleep disturbances, 87, 90
snakebite, 66, 144-145
Sobel-Guzek, Susan, 213-214
sodium hypochlorite, 79, 204
sodium lauryl sulfate, 189-190, 223
sodium laureth sulfate, 189, 223

Southwestern Medical Center, 112, 179
sprains, 31, 40, 42, 46, 48, 51, 252
Stabilization, 21-22, 56, 64-67, 69, 82, 277
Staphylococcus aureus, 12, 81
Streptococcus mutans, 82
Streptococcus pyogenes, 84, 205
stem cell research, 7-8
Stephens, Spanky, 50
Strains, 2, 10, 12, 31, 34, 39-40, 42, 46, 48, 51, 80-85, 104-105, 190, 204-205, 252, 268
Streptococcus viridans, 81
Skin
    combination, 9, 20, 26-27, 34, 43, 61-63, 67, 73, 78, 100, 107-108, 116, 121, 151, 158, 160, 171, 177, 180-181, 183, 193, 195, 200, 204-205, 208-210, 222, 234, 241, 249, 252, 257, 260, 277
    dry, 16, 31, 46, 82, 107, 192, 194-195, 206, 208-209, 212, 221, 232, 240, 245-247
    oily, 195, 221
    problem, 6, 99, 110, 119, 122, 134, 142, 146, 161, 189, 195, 221, 262, 266
    sensitive, 58, 69, 195, 200, 210, 226, 243, 248
Sydney
    Australia, 135, 313
    Opera House, 135

T

T-Cells, 100, 155, 162-163, 165, 168, 177, 179
TMA (tissue mineral analysis), 219, 292
T. mentagrophytes, 205
tendonitis, 31, 41-42, 45-46, 48
tendons, 41, 51
Tenny, Lynne, 133
Terry Pulse Studies, 170
Thompson, Rita, 112-114, 116, 140, 288
Tinea pedia, 205
tomatoes
    hydroponic, 146
    Aloe growth medium, 146
toxicology, 19, 24, 46, 56-58, 60, 198, 225
triglycerides, 70-73

tubercule bacilli, 81
Trichophyton rubrum, 205

U

University of Florida, 40
University of Iowa, 40
University of Louisville, 40, 50
University of Miami, 36, 40
University of Texas
    Galveston, 76, 203
U.S. News & World Report, 3, 281
USA Today, 281
USDA, 6, 268

V

vitamins
    A, 77, 108
    B
    C, 63, 111, 275, 279, 285, 293

W

Wakeland, Edward K., 112
Waters, Charlie, 36, 48-49
Washington, Redskins, 40
wound healing
    athletics, 10, 32, 34-35, 37, 41-43, 45, 47, 51, 274, 279, 284
    cats, 29, 181, 225, 228, 230, 240, 243-251, 262, 292
    cattle, 8, 33, 140, 169, 190, 225, 228-229, 261-268, 271, 292
    dogs, 58-59, 143-144, 181, 225, 228-234, 236-246, 249-251, 262, 284, 292
    horses, 31, 41, 225, 228, 251-255, 257-258, 260, 266
    laboratory studies, 47, 84, 188

X

x-factor, 121, 157, 186
x-rays, 129

Y

Young, Marty, 140-141, 143

Z

Zimmermann, Eugene, 28, 58, 181, 205, 285
zinc, 118-120, 184, 220, 279, 288

About the Authors

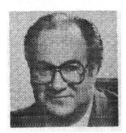

Bill C. Coats, R.Ph. C.C.N is one of the world's foremost experts on Aloe Vera and is the founder and CEO of Coats Aloe International. In his capacity as lecturer, teacher and world authority on the healing plant, he often tours and lec tures annually in several countries, including Taiwan, Hong Kong, Australia, Indonesia, Malaysia, Japan, Spain, Portugal, Mexico and Canada. Nominated by the Society of Cosmetic Chemists three times for its prestigious Merit Award, he has also co-authored five books on Aloe Vera, including, *Aloe Vera/ The Inside Story, Creatures in Our Care* and *the Silent Healer. ALOE VERA/ The New Millennium* marks another milestone in Mr. Coats career as a pioneer in the wellness movement.

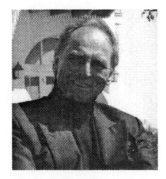

Robert Ahola is a writer, producer and director who lives in Malibu, California. As CEO of Galahad Films he has written and produced over 300 films, videos and documentaries for television, satellite, and independent theatrical release. He is the author of five plays, including *The Year of the Tiger* and *Judas Agonistes,* and he has authored or coauthored 11 published books including *Delusion is Good,* the *GODWIN/ The Boy Magician* series and *The Return of the Hummingbird Wizard. ALOE VERA/ The New Millennium* is his fifth collaboration with Bill Coats.